D1810634

History and Theory
of Human Experimentation

GESCHICHTE UND PHILOSOPHIE DER MEDIZIN

HISTORY AND PHILOSOPHY OF MEDICINE

Herausgegeben von
Andreas Frewer

Band 2

Ulf Schmidt / Andreas Frewer (Eds.)

History and Theory
of Human Experimentation

The Declaration of Helsinki and
Modern Medical Ethics

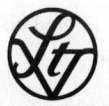 Franz Steiner Verlag Stuttgart 2007

With the kind support of / Mit freundlicher Unterstützung von
Medizinische Hochschule Hannover, Germany
Wellcome Trust, United Kingdom

Cover
The representatives of the Finnish Medical Association present the Declaration of Helsinki (1964) to the President of the Republic of Finland, Urho Kekkonen.

Editors:

Prof. Dr. Ulf Schmidt
Professor of Modern History
University of Kent
Rutherford College
Canterbury, United Kingdom
CT2 7NX

Prof. Dr. med. Andreas Frewer, M.A.
Geschichte, Ethik und Philosophie der Medizin
Medizinische Hochschule Hannover
Carl-Neuberg-Str. 1, D – 30625 Hannover

Institut für Geschichte und Ethik der Medizin
Professur für Ethik in der Medizin
Friedrich-Alexander-Universität Erlangen-Nürnberg
Glückstraße 10, D – 91054 Erlangen

Bibliografische Information der Deutschen Nationalbibliothek
Die Deutsche Nationalbibliothek verzeichnet diese Publikation in der Deutschen Nationalbibliografie; detaillierte bibliografische Daten sind im Internet über <http://dnb.d-nb.de> abrufbar.

ISBN 978-3-515-08862-6

ISO 9706

Jede Verwertung des Werkes außerhalb der Grenzen des Urheberrechtsgesetzes ist unzulässig und strafbar. Dies gilt insbesondere für Übersetzung, Nachdruck, Mikroverfilmung oder vergleichbare Verfahren sowie für die Speicherung in Datenverarbeitungsanlagen.
© 2007 Franz Steiner Verlag, Stuttgart.
Gedruckt auf säurefreiem, alterungsbeständigem Papier.
Druck: Printservice Decker & Bokor, München
Printed in Germany

Table of Contents

Ulf Schmidt, Andreas Frewer

History and Ethics of Human Experimentation: The Twisted Road to Helsinki
An Introduction 7

I. History and Theory of Medical Research Ethics

Ulrich Tröhler

The Long Road of Moral Concern:
Doctors' Ethos and Statute Law Relating to Human Research in Europe 27

Dietrich von Engelhardt

The Historical and Philosophical Background of Ethics in Clinical Research 55

Ulf Schmidt

The Nuremberg Doctors' Trial and the Nuremberg Code 71

Till Bärnighausen

Communicating "Tainted Science":
The Japanese Biological Warfare Experiments on Human Subjects in China .. 117

II. The Helsinki Declaration in an International Context

Susan E. Lederer

Research Without Borders:
The Origins of the Declaration of Helsinki 145

Povl Riis

Forty Years of the Declaration of Helsinki:
Progress in Medical Ethics? 165

Kati Myllymäki

Revising the Declaration of Helsinki:
An Insiders' View 173

Robert Carlson, Kenneth Boyd, David Webb

The Interpretation of Codes of Medical Ethics:
Some Lessons from the Fifth Revision of the Declaration of Helsinki 187

David Willcox

Medical Ethics and Public Perception:
The Declaration of Helsinki and its Revisions in 2000 203

Dominique Sprumont, Sara Girardin, Trudo Lemmens

The Helsinki Declaration and the Law:
An International and Comparative Analysis 223

III. History and Ethics of Research – International Perspectives

Andreas Frewer

History of Medicine and Ethics in Conflict:
Research on National Socialism as a Moral Problem 255

Ulf Schmidt

Medical Ethics and Human Experiments at Porton Down: Informed
Consent in Britain's Biological and Chemical Warfare Experiments 283

John Williams

The Declaration of Helsinki
The Importance of Context 315

Jonathan D. Moreno

Helsinki into the Future
An Epilogue 327

IV. Key Documents on the History of Research Ethics

Circular of the Reich Minister of the Interior Concerning Guidelines
for New Therapy and Human Experimentation (Berlin, 1931) 333

The Nuremberg Code (1947) 337

World Medical Association: Declaration of Helsinki I (1964) 339

World Medical Association: Declaration of Helsinki II (Tokyo, 1975) 341

Council of Europe: Convention on Human Rights and
Biomedicine (Oviedo, 1997) 345

World Medical Association: Declaration of Helsinki (2004) 357

List of Contributors 363

Acknowledgements 365

Illustrations 367

Ulf Schmidt, Andreas Frewer

History and Ethics of Human Experimentation: The Twisted Road to Helsinki

Introduction

In March 2006, eight healthy male volunteers, aged nineteen to thirty-four, took part in a clinical trial at the Pharmacological Research Unit, Northwick Park Hospital in London. The trial went badly wrong.[1] The men were the first group of thirty-two subjects who were meant to be subjected to a new drug, called "TGN1412", a monoclonal antibody, in a phase I, single-centre, double-blind, randomised, placebo-controlled, single escalating-dose study.[2] Shortly after having been injected with the drug, six of the volunteers suffered from headaches, rigours, high temperature, nausea, vomiting and a drop in blood pressure. One of the two men who had received a placebo later recalled: "The men went down like dominoes. They began tearing their shirts off complaining of fever, then some screamed that their heads were going to explode. After that they started fainting, vomiting and writhing around in their beds".[3] Eye-witnesses also recalled that one of the men became bloated like an "Elephant Man".[4] Twelve hours after the start of the trial, the conditions of the men had deteriorated to such an extent that they were transferred to the hospitals' Critical Care Unit. Almost all of them were by now suffering from multiple organ failures. The management of the hospital was so shocked by events that they called in the Metropolitan police to see whether a crime had been committed. The UK Medicines and Healthcare products Regulatory Agency (MHRA), which had approved the experiments, as well as other investigative bodies, later concluded that there was no evidence of a crime or technical error, and that the agent had probably triggered a toxic "cytokine release syndrome" which had left the men in a critically ill condition.[5] Although all of the men have since been released from hospital, it is far too early for any predictions about their long term health and there is some evidence that they might develop autoimmune diseases or lymphatic cancers.[6]

---

1   See also the film *Dispatches: A Drug Trial that Went Wrong*, screened on Channel 4, 28 October 2006.
2   MHRA, Investigations into Adverse Incidents During Clinical Trials of TGN1412, May 2006.
3   Ho/Cummins (2006).
4   Ibid.
5   Expert Scientific Group on Phase One Clinical Trials, Interim Report, 20 July 2006.
6   Leigh Day & Co (2006); see also Suntharalingam et al. (2006).

The drug had been developed by the German company TeGenero, a small biotechnology firm based in Würzburg, to combat inflammatory conditions such as leukaemia or rheumatoid arthritis.[7] Parexel, a US-based company commissioned by TeGenero to carry out the trial, had originally been refused to perform the trial in Germany. The German regulatory authority, the Paul Ehrlich Institute in Langen, had returned the application with a long list of "deficiencies" which needed to be addressed before testing would be granted. After the problems had been resolved, the German authority granted Parexel permission to carry out the tests, but by then the company had already approached the MHRA, the British regulatory authority, to conduct the experiments in the United Kingdom. A subsequent investigation by the MHRA found a number of shortcomings in the conduct of the trial. Parexel "failed to complete the full medical background" of one of the subjects and one principal investigator "did not update the medical history file in writing" after a verbal consultation with one of the participants.[8] Not only was there no contract in existence for the "bank screening physician" but Parexel's principal investigator "failed to authorise" the "full work remit for the bank physician" before the tests commenced.[9] Following an interview with the bank physician, the UK inspectors concluded that they were "not satisfied that the individual had adequate training and experience for their role".[10] Parexel failed to review TeGenero's insurance policy in case some of the subjects developed serious adverse reactions. The two subjects, who had been given the placebo, "were permitted to leave the trial before appropriate checks were undertaken to confirm that they were the two subjects that had received the placebo".[11] Finally, there was no contract in place between TeGenero and Parexel at the start of the experiments, although one was subsequently issued.[12] Parexel is one of the world's largest pharmaceutical outsourcing companies which conducts operations in 36 countries, with a revenue of 169.5 million dollars in the quarter which ended on 30 June 2006. It is likely that the company will weather the storm, perhaps because a discussion or reference to the events is conspicuously absent from its website, except on one occasion.[13] TeGenero, on the other hand, filed for

---

7   Bhogal/Combes (2006), p. 89.
8   MHRA, Investigations into Adverse Incidents During Clinical Trials of TGN1412, May 2006; see also Day (2006), Maley (2006), Rawbone (2006).
9   Ibid.
10   Ibid.
11   Ibid.
12   Ibid.
13   See www.parexel.com. Following the report by the MHRA, the head of Parexel International Clinical Pharmacology, Herman Scholtz, commented: "Although there were certain discrepancies identified in the MHRA report, there were no issues that contributed to the adverse reactions experienced by the volunteers, despite the fact that this was a highly challenging situation. It is inevitable that following a highly detailed examination of systems and documentation, there would be areas cited for improvement. We are committed to continuous improvement, and are reviewing, as we always do, ways to enhance our processes and systems".

insolvency in July 2006 after it became clear that it could no longer attract sufficient investment to continue with its business.[14]

The case has not only sent profound shock waves through the pharmaceutical industry, but has raised serious questions about the safety and ethics of human experiments among patient organisation and the global research community. Given the extensive media coverage of the case, questions are being asked whether the existing control and regulative mechanisms for clinical trials in Europe, the United States and the world are adequate in assessing the risks of new biomedical agents and in protecting the safety of experimental subjects.[15] Three days after the incident, the United States Food and Drug Administration (FDA) and The Critical Path Institute (C-Path) announced the creation of a "Predictive Safety Testing Consortium" to reassure investors and the public alike. According to the interim-findings of an independent Expert Scientific Group (ESG), set up by the UK Department of Health, the case has "highlighted an urgent need to review the safety of first-in-man trials of novel agents, and to examine how risks in medicine development are currently assessed and minimised by sponsors, investigators and regulators".[16] Experts have all been astonished, to say the least, about the outsourcing of clinical trials to lucrative contract research organisations (CROs) such as Parexel, an industry which is worth 14 billion dollars in the United States alone. Others have highlighted the methods of assessment of preclinical data, the ethical and regulatory review process, the management of risk, the excessive provision of incentives to the trial subjects, the training of researchers, the lack of informed consent and insurance cover of trial subjects or problems in the sharing of information of positive and negative results of clinical trials. In other words, the pharmaceutical industry and international research organisations are currently undergoing one of the most comprehensive review processes since the end of the Second World War, when news of German medical atrocities led to the formulation of new guidelines for the protection of human subjects in clinical trials, first in 1947 in the Nuremberg Code[17], and in 1964 in the Declaration of Helsinki, the focus of this book.[18]

---

14 See www.tegenero.de; see also Hall (2006).
15 For some of the media coverage and comments in the academic press see Day (2006), Laurence/Paterson (2006), Maley (2006), Mayor (2006), Randerson (2006), Rosenthal (2006a), Rosenthal (2006b), Sample/Maley (2006), Waldman (2006).
16 Expert Scientific Group on Phase One Clinical Trials, Interim Report, 20 July 2006.
17 For the history of the Nuremberg Doctors' Trial and the legacy of the Nuremberg Code see Schmidt (2004); see also Frewer/Wiesemann (1999) and the contribution by Ulf Schmidt in this volume.
18 In July 2006, the Expert Scientific Group reviewing the Northwick Park Hospital trial put forward three recommendation for future clinical trials: First, that "doctors should consider using ill patients as test subjects rather than healthy volunteers; subjects should be given the experimental drug sequentially, rather than all at once; and doctors should be more conservative about the dose given to the first human subjects", Randerson (2006), see also Goodyear (2006). In a parallel development, the pharmaceutical industry has recently been accused of "endangering public health through wide-scale marketing malpractice, ranging from covertly attempting to persuade consumers that they are ill to bribing doctors and

Although opinions differ whether the problems experienced with the drug were "foreseeable", experts agree that the case may have a lasting impact on the industry and the enforcement of ethics standards more generally. Under the headline "London's disastrous drug trial has serious side effects for research", the science journal *Nature* predicted that the case could "change restrictions on clinical research and closer scrutiny of the private companies that carry out the majority of clinical trials".[19] Arthur Caplan, a leading bioethicist from the University of Pennsylvania, remarked: "Was informed consent adequate? Were the right subjects selected? Were the right doses given? This better have [has] been done right, or some tough questions are going to come up for the private, commercialised research sector".[20] Indeed, there is evidence that the consent of the subjects, one of the most basic and most important requirements in non-therapeutic human experiments, may not have been fully informed. One commentator questioned whether the "standards of science and ethics" had "collapsed in the new ethos of the 'knowledge economy' that promoted wealth creation above all else".[21] The Northwick Park trial has thrown into sharp relief the complex problems with which national regulators and ethics committees are confronted in today's global research community in which the profit margins of newly developed drugs and therapeutic methods can take precedence over the safety and integrity of the research subjects. The problems and issues raised in the current debate are all but new. Indeed, experimental scientists, general practitioners, state officials, legislators, drug companies and patient organisations have been concerned with them for over half-a-century.

Following the Second World War, the international medical community was forced to reflect about its conduct. The Nuremberg Doctors' Trial heralded a period of great uncertainty for health professionals and national medical organisations, not just financially, but more with regard to the role that the medical profession was supposed to play in a post-war society. Nazi medical experiments had seriously undermined the reputation of medical practice and had damaged doctor patient relationships. Doctors in Great Britain and elsewhere feared that a sweeping condemnation of the Nazi physicians could negatively effect the profession as a whole. Large-scale funding for experimental research or the foundation of research institutes was potentially at risk. Medical lobbying for the autonomy of medical scientists therefore reached new heights. Any government scheme that advocated a greater degree of central or state planning of medical research was denounced as totalitarian by organisations such as the Society for Freedom in Science. The *British Medical Journal* declared that the individual conscience of the researcher would surrender to the "mass mind of the totalitarian state".[22]

---

misrepresenting the results of safety and efficacy tests on their products"; Boseley (2006), p. 1, p. 9.

19   Waldman (2006), pp. 388-389.
20   Ibid., p. 388.
21   Ho/Cummins (2006).
22   Weindling (1996), p. 1469.

Critics of the National Health Service alleged that a greater state direction of science would apparently lead to a Nazi or Soviet system of government. Overall, it was an attempt by British and American medical lobbyists to shift the responsibility for medical war crimes away from individual scientists onto an authoritarian state, a strategy that the Nuremberg defendants had themselves tried.

The foundation of the World Medical Association (WMA) happened largely in response to the revelations in the Doctors' Trial.[23] At the end of 1946, 100 delegates representing thirty-two national medical associations gathered together in London to form an international medical organisation in the world. The WMA was also established to function as the successor organisation of the *Association Professionelle Internationale des Médecins*, which had been founded in 1926, but which had ceased to operate after the outbreak of the Second World War.[24] The objectives of the WMA were to maintain the honour of the medical profession, the promotion of world peace and the helping of all peoples to attain the highest possible level of health.[25] Behind these laudable aims stood a calculated policy, namely to protect the interests of the medical profession in the forthcoming power struggle with national governments. On 17 September 1947, only weeks after the Nuremberg judgement had been pronounced, the French Minister of Public Health opened the first annual meeting of the WMA in Paris.[26] Costa Rica's suggestion that the organisation should call itself *World Medical Confederation* was dismissed, as was the proposal by Czechoslovakia to exclude the German medical profession from membership for a period of 25 years.[27] The organisation was nonetheless unambiguous in its moral condemnation of Nazi crimes. Not only was the "widespread criminal conduct of the German medical profession since 1933" acknowledged, but the delegates also expressed their "astonishment" that "no sign whatever had come from Germany that the doctors were ashamed of their share in the crimes, or even that they fully realised the enormity of their conduct".[28] German medical associations were invited to make a formal declaration that would help to rehabilitate German medicine in the eyes of the world.

There were other, more material, yet less publicised, issues at stake which set the tone for the following years. For example, the WMA discussed what it called the "principles of social security". This meant that all doctors were to be free to choose their location and type of practice. All medical services were to be controlled by physicians. The WMA delegates announced that it would "not be in the public's interest that doctors be full-time salaried servants of government or social-security bodies" and that the "remuneration of medical services" should not depend directly on the financial conditions of the insurance. Finally, doctors were

---

23 See also the contribution by Susan Lederer in this volume.
24 Schaupp (1994), p. 171.
25 Bundesarchiv Koblenz (BAK), ZSg 154, box 70.
26 World Medical Association (1947), p. 4. We are grateful to Sev Fluss, policy advisor to the WMA, for supplying this material to us.
27 Ibid., p. 11.
28 BAK, ZSg 154, box 70.

to be given the freedom to choose their patients except in cases of emergencies or other humanitarian considerations.[29]

The stated model of medical practice stood in contrast to what almost all industrialised nations were favouring in Europe at the time: a universal, egalitarian, health care system based on social welfare, irrespective of class, gender, race or economic considerations. Issues of medical ethics now became a propaganda weapon in the increasingly hostile battles between the WMA and the respective national governments. In 1949 the WMA declared in its "International Code of Medical Ethics" that it was "unethical" to take part in "any plan of medical care in which the doctor does not have complete professional independence".[30] This had little to do with the welfare of patients or with the social and moral responsibilities of physicians. The WMA at this point was largely influenced by, and showed allegiance to market interests. During the first meeting in 1947 the organisation accepted a "gift" of $ 50,000 US dollars a year for five years from "a group of American industrialists" for the "development" of the organisation. It was an attempt by North American pharmaceuticals and other business interests to exercise considerable influence over the WMA from the moment it was established.

The Nuremberg Code, a set of medical ethics principles designed to protect experimental research subjects, hardly figured in the discussions of the WMA. Only the medical associations from Denmark and the Netherlands proposed to "devise measures" which would prevent the participation of physicians in unethical medical conduct in future.[31] It took another six years, until 1953, that a position paper on human experimentation was tabled and another year until the "Resolution on Human Experimentation: Principles for those in Research and Experimentation" was adopted by the WMA in Rome in 1954.[32] These principles were less comprehensive and far-reaching than those of the Code and excluded a number of key provisions, for example that the subject can withdraw from the experiment at any time.[33] The "informed, free consent" principle, which was "absolutely essential" to the Code, was now listed almost at the end of the document. Above all, the principle indicated a shift away from the rights of patient-citizens to the duties of physicians, a shift which ten years later, in 1964, was formalised in the first Declaration of Helsinki.[34] The process of watering down the Nuremberg Code had begun.

What becomes apparent in this brief historical overview is that the political climate of the time is central not only to the efficiency with which medical ethics regulations are being introduced and disseminated, but, more importantly, to the extent to which the rules are being followed by medical professionals, funding

29   Annas/Grodin (1992), pp. 303-304.
30   Beecher (1970), Appendix A, p. 236.
31   World Medical Association (1947), p. 10.
32   Fluss (1999), pp. 19-20.
33   Ibid.
34   For the history and role of the Declaration of Helsinki see Schaupp (1994); Fluss (1999); Hohnel (2005); see also the chapter by Susan Lederer in this volume.

and state agencies. But the history of post-war medical ethics also tells another story, namely that the public perception of government and private sponsored research, and of the medical profession more generally, increasingly began to play a central role in shaping Western medicine. The first indication that criticism against the prevailing medical ethics standards might be mounted from within the medical profession came during the 1950s, when a few experts started to question the existing research culture. A crisis of trust in the social relations of doctors and patients which was a part of a long history of estrangement was further amplified by growing tensions between hospitals and communities, and by the arrival of new and costly biomedical technologies. Controversies over the allocation of resources for, and beneficiaries of medical research propelled the issue of morals into the public and academic domain.

Medical professionals, lawyers, philosophers and sociologists increasingly incorporated the issue of morals, however vaguely and randomly defined, in their professional debate. Quite often a debate on morals was motivated by deeper political and ideological objectives. In 1954, Joseph F. Fletcher contested the traditional doctor patient relationship in his book on *Morals and Medicine. The Moral Problem of the Patient's Right to Know the Truth.*[35] The image of the paternalistic doctor who was acting in the best interests of the patient, whether as a healer or as a researcher, was increasingly challenged by minority and other interest groups. By the late 1950s the call for greater transparency and accountability in medicine and experimental research grew significantly louder. This resulted in a situation where the medical profession was nervously following sensitive disclosures about its practices, most notoriously in the Thalidomide scandal from 1962.[36]

What today's bioethics community, in the attempt to construct its own, often greatly biased historical narrative, likes to see as a number of courageous whistleblowers like Henry Beecher and Maurice Pappworth was in fact a largely opportunistic and measured response by some of the leaders of the profession to a significant change in the political, social and cultural climate that challenged the status quo and power of medical science.[37] The 1964 Declaration of Helsinki must likewise be seen in the context of a largely successful project by the international medical community to supplant the Nuremberg Code with research regulations that were in line with the "realities of medical research", and which reaffirmed and protected the position of the researcher. To see the early 1960s as a time of medical whistleblowers who, intentionally or not, gave "birth" to modern bioethics would retrospectively turn professionals under pressure into heroes. These men were surely not heroes as such but experts who knew how to secure their professional status and, above all, their financial interests. Change, if at all, was gradual and slow.

---

35   Fletcher (1954).
36   See, for example, Kirk (1999) and Stephens (2001).
37   See Katz (1993), pp. 31-39; also Moreno (1997), pp. 347-360.

The response by the medical establishment deserves nonetheless attention as an indicator for new pressures in the profession in all areas related to research involving human participants. Changes in both research culture and medical ethics regulations were driven by the realisation among scientists that further resistance against human and civil rights issues in experimental medicine could only be counter-productive. The best strategy in order to remain in control over the issues was to take the lead. This insight was not the result of an acceptance or even admiration for the Nuremberg Code. On the contrary, since the late 1950s, American medical scientists tried to water down the Code's "rigid rules" which, it was argued, would stifle medical progress. Ironically, those resisting the effective implementation of the Code in the late 1950s were, in many cases, the same people who in the mid-1960s became known as the "whistleblowers". Foremost among them was Beecher himself. In an act of moral transformation, those attacking the Codes' impracticability changed tack to become the most outspoken advocates for the inviolability of patient-citizens. Looking at it retrospectively, it was not just a master stroke in image management, but in the calculated preservation of professional power.[38]

In 1961 the Medical Ethics Committee of the WMA, chaired by Hugh Clegg, editor of the *British Medical Journal*, produced a draft "Code on Ethics on Human Experimentation" which, after some discussion, was published in the fall of 1962.[39] Two years later, the WMA officially adopted parts of the draft Code during its General Assembly in June 1964. The document became known as the Helsinki Declaration. Important provisions of the draft Code, however, such as the prohibition to use prisoners of war, whether military or civilian, or persons confined to prisons and mental institutions in human experiments, were deleted from the text.[40] In the Helsinki Declaration the doctor "should, if at all possible, consistent with the patient's psychology" obtain the patient's consent. At the same time the personal, non-transferable, legal responsibility of the physician for his research subjects was deleted from the Declaration, as was the right of the subject to terminate the experiment at any time.

Compared to the Nuremberg Code, the Helsinki Declaration is a researchers' paradise, full of legal loopholes. Words like "should" or "if at all possible" or "consistent with the patients psychology" meant that the medical community had gained substantial leverage in shaping experimental research practice. From its early conception, the Helsinki Declaration was trying to adapt to the current research culture. But it thereby undermined the central importance of the informed consent principle of the Nuremberg Code and re-introduced it with a paternalistic value system of the traditional doctor patient relationship. In 1964 a crucial shift was initiated in the Declaration of Helsinki about the quality of international medical ethics codes, from the rights of patients and the protection of human

---

38   United States Advisory Committee on Human Radiation Experiments (1996), pp. 88-92; Moreno (1997), pp. 357-358; Beecher (1970), Appendix A, pp. 214-244.
39   Fluss (1999), p. 19; also Medical Ethics Committee (1962), p. 1119.
40   Katz (1992), p. 233.

subjects in experimental research to the protection of patient welfare through physician's responsibility. It was a move away from the essential requirement of informed consent as stated in the Code, beginning a watering down process of the Code that continues to this day.

This book is the result of a collaborative effort between Hanover Medical School, Germany, and the School of History at the University of Kent, United Kingdom, to study the history of research ethics and mark the 40th anniversary of the Declaration of Helsinki in 2004.[41] Most of the chapters in this volume are a continuation as well as an original contribution to scholarly work which has recently been conducted on the history and ethics of human experimentation, and which primarily focused on the achievements and aberrations of modern medical science in the 20th century.[42] The discourse highlighted the age-old tension between the desire for medical progress in the service of society, on the one hand, and the need to protect vulnerable groups and individual human subjects, on the other. As Wolfgang Eckart has recently pointed out in *Man, Medicine and the State*, the debate not only looked at the institutional and organisational structures which facilitated experimental research on human beings in prisons, prisoner-of-war camps and the military, but raised the central issue of onwership of human bodies: "… who is actually the owner of a human body at what point in time, who may use and misuse it to what purposes, and, finally, who is in a position to make demands on it and to realise these demands, and with what right".[43] The recent surge in studies about the history of human experiments has thrown into sharp relief the issues of human rights and professional regulations when it comes to the protection of individual human subjects. Here the Declaration of Helsinki has undoubtedly secured its rightful place among the key ethics documents which provided researchers with a landmark to guide their research over the last forty years.

Despite having been revised and criticised over the years, the Declaration of Helsinki remains one of the most important and internationally known ethics codes in the world. Yet we know relatively little about its historical origins or about the prolonged revision process which accompanied this "living document" to this day.[44] As early as 1969, Jay Katz not only highlighted the general problems of medical ethics codes in effectively protecting experimental subjects but also pointed out that we know little about them:

---

41   In October 2004, Andreas Frewer and Ulf Schmidt organised the conference on 'The Standards for Research. 40 Years of the Declaration of Helsinki. Progress in Medical Ethics?' at the International Expert Conference Center, Leibnizhaus, Hanover, Germany.

42   See, for example, Annas/Grodin (1992), Lederer (1995), Elkeles (1996), Frewer (2000), Goodman et al. (2003), Goliszek (2003), Roelcke/Maio (2004), Schmidt (2004), Eckart (2006).

43   Eckart (2006), p. 9.

44   For some of the historical and analytical work which has so far been conducted on the Declaration of Helsinki see, for example, Winton (1978), Osterwald (1990), Toellner (1990), Schaupp (1994), Fluss (1999), Human/Fluss (2001), Lederer (2004).

"Taking as a point of departure the ten 'basic principles' set forth by the Nuremberg judges, numerous attempts have been made to propose 'improved' codes of ethics to guide medical research. The proliferation of such codes testifies to the difficulty of promulgating a set of rules that does not immediately raise more questions than it answers. At this stage of our confusion, it is unlikely that codes will resolve many of the problems, though they may serve a useful function later. Even the much endorsed Declaration of Helsinki – praised, perhaps, because it is the newest and therefore the least examined – will create problems for those who wish to implement it."[45]

The aim of the book is to reconstruct the "twisted road" to "Helsinki" and current research ethics, with its many pitfalls, professional and financial interests as well as national and cultural differences. It examines how the Declaration evolved and changed over the last forty years, partly as a result of innovative developments in biomedical technologies, partly as a result of external pressures from drug companies and researchers. The book also looks at the legacy of the Declaration by examining the impact which the Declaration had on European and international laws and regulations, on state-sponsored military experiments, or as part of the ongoing discourse on the ethics of human experiments in the public domain. Many of the authors in this volume ask whether measurable progress has been achieved in medical ethics since the days of Helsinki. The book not only wants to question whether researchers pay sufficient attention to the Declaration and if not, why not, but it also explores the difficulties for scientists in making sense of an enormous body of ethics standards and legal regulations. There is a sense among experts that we need to redouble our efforts so that research subjects enjoy greater protection in the future, and not less. At the same time, there is a need, perhaps greater than ever before, to develop and institutionalise new mechanisms to hold global research and drug companies to account. "There's going to be a lot of soul searching", one bioethicist remarked after the recent Northwick Park Hospital incident.[46]

The chapters presented in this volume look at the history and theory of human experimentation, assess the role of the Helsinki Declaration in an international context, and illustrate specific issues about the history and practice of research ethics through a number of case studies in the United States, Asia and Europe. In Part I, *Ulrich Tröhler* examines the range of ethical arguments that related to human experiments in the past, establishes why, when and where these arguments were formulated, and where ethics standards were introduced. His primary focus is on international codes of ethics but he also draws attention to the moral dilemmas of experimental scientists who were caught between patient care, on the one hand, and the advancement of scientific knowledge, on the other. In a fitting reminder of the current debate, he looks at an unregulated, expanding pharmaceutical industry which needed to come to terms with a greater public awareness that drugs could have devastating effects, for example in relation to the Thalidomide scandal; he also draws attention to the more recent attempt by the American

---

45   Katz (1970), p. 295; see also the contribution by Dominique Sprumont, Sara Girardin and Trudo Lemmens in this volume.
46   Waldman (2006), p. 388.

Medical Association (AMA), under the chairmanship of Robert Levine, to deregulate the pharmaceutical industry in view of commercial interests in new biomedical technologies. His paper provides an overview of some of the contentious historical and theoretical issues which are further explored by *Dietrich von Engelhardt*, who examines the philosophical and historical roots of biomedical research ethics and places them in the context of the philosophy of medicine and history of ideas. Von Engelhardt argues that despite a chequered history of medicine and the relative nature of ethics codes, certain fundamental principles such as dignity, autonomy, beneficence, non-maleficence, justice, virtue, freedom and responsibility have manifested themselves in the canon of medical ethics, principles which were severely violated by German physicians during the Second World War. *Ulf Schmidt* examines the origins of the Nuremberg Doctors' Trial in 1946/47 which charged twenty-three defendants with war crimes and crimes against humanity. He explores the political and legal environment in which the Doctors' Trial took place and reconstructs the authorship of the Nuremberg Code, a catalogue of ten principles which were meant to protect the rights of experimental subjects and other vulnerable groups in the future. Although the Code was largely ignored by the medical community in the immediate aftermath of the trial, Schmidt argues that the Code has nonetheless significant symbolic and in many ways an influential role in the contemporary field of medical politics, ethics and law. The part concludes with a chapter by *Till Bärnighausen* on "tainted science". He examines the channels of communication by which scientific information from unethical Japanese wartime experiments entered publicly accessible medical knowledge, while the nature and conduct of the experiments largely remained secret. His chapter raises the question about the extent to which society should permit scientific data to be published, if it has been procured by unethical means, but if there is the possibility that society might benefit from the results. Bärnighausen's contribution challenges the widely held assumption that scientists present their methods and research findings correctly and in good faith. On the contrary, his is a story of scientists misrepresenting and manipulating the evidence to ensure the publication and "cleansing" of ethically problematic research data to advance their professional careers.

In Part II, *Susan Lederer* shows that the "road to Helsinki" was neither straight nor smooth; she provides a contextualised historical analysis of the decade-long discourse among WMA delegates before the Declaration was finally adopted by the WMA General Assembly in 1964. Lederer not only analyses the WMA's departure from the principles of the Nuremberg Code, but demonstrates that American interests and influence was instrumental in shaping the final form of the "weakened" Declaration of Helsinki. Two of the authors in this volume have been directly involved in the revision process of the Declaration. *Povl Riis*, one of the three authors of the second version of the Declaration of Helsinki, the Tokyo version, adopted in 1975, provides insight into some of the contentious issues and ethical dilemmas which WMA delegates attempted to resolve at the time, for example in relation to randomised controlled trials, the establishment of ethics committees and new biomedical technologies in a globalised medical market place. *Kati Myllymäki*, former president of the Finish Medical Association, was part of the group of "three wise women", who revised the Declaration of Helsinki in Edinburgh in 2000; her contribution provides an original insight into some of the internal discussions and consultations which accompanied the most recent revision of the Declaration. By offering a detailed textual analysis of the recent revisions of the Declaration, *Robert Carlson, Kenneth Boyd and David Webb* come to a better understanding of how medical ethics codes are formulated within the Byzantine organisational and voting structures of the WMA. Their contribution shows the extent to which experts struggle over the precise wording of one of the most important ethics codes in the world, thus shaping its character as a prescriptive as well as aspirational medical ethics code. *David Willcox* looks at the public and professional debate surrounding the 2000 revisions of the Declaration and examines some of the issues which related to the exploitation of research subjects, the use of placebos, the profiteering of drug companies, the role of informed consent and the future function of medical ethics standards. He argues that the public perception of medical ethics issues altered little despite the academic debate about the Declaration. The part concludes with a chapter by *Dominique Sprumont, Sara Girardin and Trudo Lemmens*, who provide, for the first time, an international and comparative law analysis of the Declaration. The authors show that explicit references to the Declaration in national and international laws and regulations for biomedical research are far and few between. Their chapter provides valuable insight into the legislative context of human experimentation in countries such as Switzerland, Germany, France, the United Kingdom and Canada. By examining the extent to which the Declaration is embodied in the laws of these countries, they are able to assess the legal force of the Declaration in different national, cultural and legislative environments. *Sprumont, Giradin and Lemmens* conclude that the most recent references to the Declaration are to the 1996 version rather than to the revisions which were passed in Edinburgh in 2000 and thereafter. As a result, researchers are faced with a "conflict of norms"; on the one hand, they are legally bound to follow the 1996 version whereas, on the other, they may feel obliged from a moral and professional perspective to adhere to the most recent version of the Declaration. This dilemma can only be overcome by going back to the underlying principles of the Declaration which largely remain unchanged.

In Part III, the authors look at a number of case studies which highlight issues of historical research and medical ethics from an international perspective and which raise important questions for human subject protection in the future. *Andreas Frewer* provides a reassessment about the historiography of medicine under National Socialism, as well as the culture and politics of memoralisation in post-war Germany, addressing moral issues which have shaped and plagued research and open debate on this complex subject over the last fifty years. Whilst being aware that much has been achieved, he poignantly examines a number of case studies which have hampered transparent research and critical discourse in the past, and which have, in some instances, tarnished the reputation not only of the representatives of the post-war German medical profession but challenged the ethics of medical history as well. The chapter provides a narrative from the early beginnings and aims of the WMA to the pitfalls of current research and practice. In his chapter on the history of medical ethics at Porton Down, *Ulf Schmidt* examines the ethical, political and legal dimensions of Britain's biochemical warfare programme in the early stages of the Cold War. Porton's scientists appear to have carried out a series of dangerous experiments on the Leading Aircraftsman Ronald Maddison in 1953, and on other subjects, which demanded, given the nature of the experiments, that the highest degree of safety and the most rigorous standards of research ethics known at the time should have applied. He concludes that Maddison's death from exposure to the nerve gas Sarin was an accident waiting to happen which resulted from an inadequate level of disclosure and an understatement of risks, despite the fact that there was widespread consensus in the UK that the principles of the Nuremberg Code should govern these types of experiments. The material presented also shows that the principle of informed consent was in place in UK legal doctrine and medical practice from at least 1933 onwards, long before the promulgation of the Nuremberg Code. *John R. Williams'* important synthesis on the Declaration of Helsinki focuses on the issue of context in discussing research ethics and medical research; by examining a range of scientific, political, commercial, professional, socio-cultural and ethical dimensions, *Williams* demonstrates that the overall research environment in which the Declaration of Helsinki was first conceived has fundamentally changed and that, as a corollary, research ethics had to evolve as well without compromising the general ethos and principles of the Declaration. In the final contribution, *Jonathan Moreno* looks at the global state of affairs of research ethics where, on the one hand, "much has been clarified and much international consensus has been reached", but where, on the other, certain subjects, notably those concerned with national security issues and military studies, remain under-researched. Human experiments which were conducted in a secretive military environment during the Cold War and after, whether with biological, chemical or radiological agents, continue to pose challenging questions for contemporary biomedical ethics and biodefence politics. *Moreno's* paper looks at the role and ability of the Declaration of Helsinki in regulating cutting-edge civilian and military research in a post-9/11 context, and identifies a number of critical areas where research ethics and ethics codes may have to evolve if they want to play a part in protecting human research subjects in the 21st century.

To this day, the Declaration is one of the most important landmarks in human subject research which is aimed at protecting experimental subjects in society. The current volume hopes to offer a better and historically-informed understanding of the Declaration to ensure that the existing safeguards for human experimentation are not only preserved but developed and improved in the future.

References

Annas, G. J./Grodin M. A. (eds.) (1992): The Nazi Doctors and the Nuremberg Code. Human Rights in Human Experimentation. New York, Oxford: Oxford University Press.

Baker, R./McCullough, L.B. (eds.) (2007): A History of Medical Ethics. Cambridge, New York: Cambridge University Press (in press).

Beecher, H.K. (1970): Research and the Individual. Human Studies. Boston: Little, Brown.

Bhogal, N./Combes, R. (2006): TGN1412: Time to Change the Paradigm for the Testing of New Pharmaceuticals, ATLA 34 (2006), pp. 225-239.

Boseley, S. (2006): Drug Firms a Danger to Health – Report. International Research Exposes Flaws in £33bn Marketing Budget. The Guardian. 26 June 2006, p. 1 and p. 9.

Day, M. (2006): Agency Criticises Drug Trial, British Medical Journal. 3 June 2006.

Dispatches (2006): A Drug Trial that Went Wrong. Channel 4. 28 October 2006.

Eckart, W. U. (ed.) (2006): Man, Medicine, and the State. The Human Body as an Object of Government Sponsored Medical Research in the 20th Century. Stuttgart: Franz Steiner Verlag.

Elkeles, B. (1996): Der moralische Diskurs über das medizinische Menschenexperiment im 19. Jahrhundert. Stuttgart, Jena, New York: Gustav Fischer.

Expert Scientific Group on Phase One Clinical Trials, Interim Report. 20 July 2006.

Fletcher, J. F. (1954): Morals and Medicine. The Moral Problem of the Patient's Right to Know the Truth. Contraception, Artificial Insemination, Sterilisation, Euthanasia. Boston: Beacon Press.

Fluss, S. (1999): How the Declaration of Helsinki developed, Good Clinical Practice Journal 6 (1999), pp. 18-22.

Freund, P.A. (ed.) (1970): Experimentation with Human Subjects. New York: The Deadalus Library

Frewer, A. (2000): Medizin und Moral in Weimarer Republik und Nationalsozialismus. Die Zeitschrift „Ethik" unter Emil Abderhalden. Frankfurt am Main, New York: Campus Verlag.

Frewer, A. et al. (eds.) (1999): Medizinverbrechen vor Gericht. Das Urteil im Nürnberger Ärzteprozeß gegen Karl Brandt und andere sowie aus dem Prozeß gegen Generalfeldmarschall Erhard Milch. Bearbeitet und kommentiert von U.-D. Oppitz. Erlangen, Jena: Palm & Enke.

Goliszek, A. (2003): In the Name of Sciences: A History of Secret Programs, Medical Research, and Human Experimentation. New York: St. Martins Press.

Goodman, J./McElligotz, A./Marks, L. (eds.) (2003): Useful Bodies: Humans in the Service of Medical Science in the Twentieth Century. Baltimore: The John Hopkins University Press.

Goodyear, M. (2006): Learning from the TGN1412 Trial, British Medical Journal. 22 March 2006.

Hall, S. (2006): Drug Trial Company Files for Insolvency, The Guardian. 5 July 2006.

Ho, M-W./Cummins, J. (2006): London Drug Trial Catastrophe – Collapse of Science and Ethics. Institute of Science in Society. 7 April 2006.

Hohnel, B. (2005): Die rechtliche Einordnung der Deklaration von Helsinki: eine Untersuchung zur rechtlichen Grundlage humanmedizinischer Forschung. Frankfurt am Main: Lang.

Howard-Jones, N. (1982): Human Experimentation in Historical and Ethical Perspectives, Social Science and Medicine 16 (1982), pp. 1429-1448.

Human, S./Fluss S. (2001): The World Medical Association's Declaration of Helsinki: Historical and Contemporary Perspectives. Unpublished manuscript.

Katz, J. (1970): The Education of the Physician-Investigator, in: Freund (1970), p. 295.

Katz, J. (1992): 'The Consent Principle of the Nuremberg Code: Its Significance Then and Now', in: Annas/Grodin (1992), pp. 227-239.

Katz, J. (1993): 'Ethics and Clinical Research Revisited – A Tribute to Henry K. Beecher', Hastings Center Report 23 (1993), pp. 31-39.

Kirk, B. (1999): Der Contergan-Fall. Eine unvermeidbare Arnzeimittelkatastrophe? Zur Geschichte des Arzneistoffs. Stuttgart: Wissenschaftliche Verlagsgesellschaft.

LaFleur, W. R./Boehme, G./Shimazono, S. (eds.) (2007): Dark Medicine. Rationalizing Unethical Medical Research in Germany, Japan, and the United States. Bloomington: Indiana University Press (in press).

Laurence, D. (2006): Ethics Committees and Drug Trials, The Guardian. 2 May 2006.

Laurance, J./Paterson, T. (2006): Drug Firm 'had not Tested on Humans before', The Independent. 17 March 2006.

Lederer, S. (1995): Subjected to Science. Human Experimentation before the Second World War. Baltimore and London: Johns Hopkins University Press.

Lederer, S.E. (2004): Research without Borders: The Origins of the Declaration of Helsinki, in: Roelcke/Maio (2004), pp. 199-217.

Leigh Day & Co (2006): Devastating News for Northwick Park Drug Trial Victims. 31 July 2006.

Maley, J. (2006): Watchdog Criticises Firm Behind 'Elephant Man' Drug Trials, The Guardian. 26 May 2006.

Mayor, S. (2006): Severe Adverse Reactions Prompt Call for Trial Design Changes, British Medical Journal. 25 March 2006.

Medical Ethics Committee (1962): Draft Code of Ethics on Human Experimentation, British Medical Journal 2 (1962), p. 1119.

MHRA (2006): Investigations into Adverse Incidents During Clinical Trials of TGN1412. May 2006.

Moreno, J. D. (1997): Reassessing the Influence of the Nuremberg Code on American Medical Ethics, Journal of Contemporary Health Law and Policy 13 (1997), 2, pp. 347-360.

Moreno, J. D. (1999): Undue Risk. Secret State Experiments on Humans. New York: Freeman.

Moreno, J.D. (2006): Mind Wars. Brain Research and National Defense. New York, Washington, D.C.: Dana Press.

Osterwald, G. (1990): Die Deklaration des Weltärztebundes von Helsinki in den revidierten Fassungen von Tokio und Venedig, in: Toellner (1990), pp. 31-35.

Pappworth, M. H. 1967): Human Guinea Pigs. Experimentation on Man. London: Routledge.

Randerson, J. (2006): Rethink on Human Drug Trials, The Guardian. 26 July 2006.

Rawbone, R. (2006): Editorial. Research Ethics Review 2 (2006), 2, pp. 37-39.

Roelcke, V./Maio, G. (eds.) (2004): Twentieth Century Ethics of Human Subject Research – Historical Perspectives on Values, Practices, and Regulations. Stuttgart: Steiner.

Rosenthal, E. (2006a): When Drug Trials go Horribly Wrong, Herald Tribune Europe. 9 April 2006.

Rosenthal, E. (2006b): Ill-Fated U.K. Drug Trial Bares Testing Loopholes, Herald Tribune Europe. 30 July 2006.

Rothman, D. J. (2003): Strangers at the Bedside. A History of How Law and Bioethics Transformed Medical Decision Making. 2. ed. Hawthorne, NY: De Gruyter.

Sample, I./Maley, J. (2006): Interest Surges in Trials Despite Patients' Plight, The Guardian. 18 March 2006.

Schaupp, W. (1994): Der ethische Gehalt der Helsinki Deklaration. Eine historisch-systematische Untersuchung der Richtlinien des Weltärztebundes über biomedizinische Forschung am Menschen. Frankfurt am Main: Peter Lang.

Schmidt, U. (2004): Justice at Nuremberg. Leo Alexander and the Nazi Doctors' Trial. Basingstoke: Palgrave.

Steiner, T. J. (2006): Guinea Pig Duties: 6. Non-Consensual Clinical Research, Research Ethics Review 2 (2006), 2, pp. 51-58.

Stephens, T.D. (2001): Dark Remedy: The Impact of Thalidomide and its Revival as a Vital Medicine. Cambridge, Mass.: Perseus Publishers.

Suntharalingam, G./Perry, M.R./Ward, S./Brett, S.J./Castello-Cortes, A./Brunner, M.D./Panoskaltsis, N. (2006): Cytokine Storm in a Phase 1 Trial of the Anti-CD28 Monoclonal Antibody TGN1412, The New England Journal of Medicine 355 (2006), 10, pp. 1018-1028.

Toellner, R. (ed.) (1990): Die Ethik-Kommission in der Medizin. Problemgeschichte, Aufgabenstellung, Arbeitsweise, Rechtsstellung und Organisationsformen medizinischer Ethik-Kommissionen. Stuttgart, New York: Fischer.

Tröhler, U./Reiter-Theil, S (eds.) (1998): Ethics Codes in Medicine: Foundations and Achievements of Codification since 1947, Aldershot (UK), Brookfield (USA), Singapore, Syndney (AUS): Ashgate.

Tröhler, U. (2002): Human Research: From Ethos to Law, from National to International Regulations, in: Maehle/Geyer-Kordesch (2002), pp. 95-117.

United States Advisory Committee on Human Radiation Experiments (1996): Advisory Committee on Human Radiation Experiments Final Report. New York, NY; Oxford: Oxford University Press

Waldman, M. (2006): London's Disastrous Drug Trial has Serious Side Effects for Research, Nature 440 (2006), pp. 388-389.

Weindling., P.J. (1996): Human Guinea Pigs and Experimental Ethics: the BMJ's Foreign Correspondent at the Nuremberg Medical Trial, British Medical Journal 313 (1996), pp. 1467-1470.

Welsome, E. (1999): The Plutonium Files: America's Secret Medical Experiments in the Cold War. New York: Delacorte Press.

Winton, R.R. (1978): The Significance of the Declaration of Helsinki. An Interpretative Commentary, World Medical Journal 25 (1978), pp. 58-59.

Weyers, W. (2003): The Abuse of Man. An Illustrated History of Dubious Medical Experimentation. New York: Ardor Scribendi.

World Medical Association (1947): Minutes of the First Annual Meeting of the General Assembly, Paris, 17-20 September 1947.

I.
History and Theory
of Medical Research Ethics

Ulrich Tröhler

The Long Road of Moral Concern: Doctors' Ethos and Statute Law Relating to Human Research in Europe[1]

I. Introduction

Not unfamiliar to Antiquity, human experimentation emerged again in the 17th century only to become ever more prevalent after the middle of the 18th century.[2] The reasons for this were manifold, rooted in medicine, culture and science. To stay with medicine, the discovery of the circulation of the blood in the first half of the 17th century led to further physiological investigation and to attempts at an intravenous application of traditional drugs. Unwanted effects of new drugs were also tested in various ways in the 18th century.[3] New surgical procedures, too, were evaluated comparatively.[4] Finally, there was the inoculation of smallpox – constituting in fact a series of experiments in preventive medicine carried out throughout Europe. However, in this period, testing (new) therapeutic or preventive interventions was not differentiated specifically from evaluating (patho-) physiological experiments that aimed at understanding bodily functions in health and disease.

This chapter examines ethical arguments related to human research, looking at why, when and where they were formulated and where regulating practices emerged. It also briefly considers the question of researchers' compliance with such regulations. The emphasis will be on international codes of ethics.

II. "For the Good of Mankind":
Little Need for Formal Regulations Prior to World War II

Under the ancien régime doctors had little difficulty finding participants for various kinds of human experimentation, provided one was in a position simply to order patients or, alternatively, to pay them to undergo such procedures, even if they did not understand them. Thus, in the 1660s, the effect of a transfusion of the "good" blood of a lamb (whose "bad blood" was evacuated by copious venae-sec-

---

1   This is an expanded, revised and updated version of a previously published chapter, see Tröhler (2002), with permission by the editors and the publisher.
2   Howard-Jones (1982), Bynum (1988).
3   Maehle (1999a).
4   Tröhler (2000a).

tion) was tested on an insane patient in Paris who was also paid for volunteering. This test caused moral concerns, due partly to its unexpected effects, which proved to be life-threatening. Such experimentation was subsequently forbidden by the Paris parliament.[5] In the second half of the 18th century new ways of amputating limbs, of treating wounds, and of operating on cataracts were tried on military pensioners and on the battlefield. The effectiveness of various antiscorbutics and drugs against different types of fevers were tested on sailors by comparing them with the traditional treatments (see below).

These 18th century clinical trials raised the same moral concerns subsequently associated with controlled human experimentation. Often enough this did not apply to haphazard trial-and-error actions, frequent enough in daily practice (see below). Some army surgeons discerned no problem in allocating soldiers to groups during a battle, for instance, to find out whether the mortality of amputation was lower immediately after the injury or if the intervention was delayed for a few days. Rational arguments existed for both methods. Others hesitated.

When it came to carrying out a study on the benefits of delayed versus immediate amputation during the Napoleonic Wars, the British Army Surgeon, George James Guthrie, had scruples about surgery after the "success" he deemed to have seen with immediate intervention. He felt himself not "authorised to commit murder for the sake of experiment".[6] He preferred to rely on a retrospective analysis of his casebooks instead, despite a theoretical insight into the necessity of conducting prospective comparative trials and the unique opportunities a commanding military surgeon had to enforce them. Another author, Charles McLean, however, realised in 1818 the ethical double standard involved in this pretended "reluctance to try experiments with the lives of men [...] as if the practice of medicine, in its conjectural state, were anything else, than a continued series of experiments, upon the lives of our fellow creatures".[7] This reflection on the morality of acting in the light of evidence gathered in traditional ways remained an isolated one, however, while Guthrie's argument represented the widespread opinion that those participating in research themselves "should benefit from the trials to which they were subjected and that they must not be put in danger for the sake of scientific curiosity".[8]

Indeed, fifty years earlier, James Lind had reacted in exactly that way, but the case ended quite differently. When starting a trial of the "malt-wort" ordered by the Admiralty, Lind acknowledged the "murmur and disgust" after withholding vegetables from scurvy patients at Haslar (because of the belief that this would improve their condition) and stopped it. But the Admiralty ordered it to be taken up at sea "where it was expected that patients would cheerfully submit".[9] Although there was a climate of "ethical awareness", in that some research-

5   Starr (1998), Tröhler (2000a).
6   Guthrie (1815), p. 39.
7   McLean (1817-18), vol. 2, pp. 500-504.
8   Maehle (1999a), pp. 268-269.
9   Macbride (1764), pp. 174-175.

minded doctors felt the dilemma between patient care and the advancement of knowledge, giving relevant information and obtaining consent were obviously not a major issue. Hierarchical power was central in this and other trials, particularly in the Navy, but also in the Army and probably in civilian institutions.

There was another way to circumvent the harm potentially present in the use of any new method. Because he felt "it would be unjustifiable to neglect for the sake of experiment any means of safety", James Currie in 1804 "superadded" his cold water bathing to the traditional fever treatment – in other words, he used today's "add-on design".[10] This implied, of course, that he considered traditional bleeding safe (on what evidence we do not know). These discussions about risk, even sacrifice "for the sake of experiment", and of safety, illustrate the ambiguity of the notion of experiment. Many 18th century doctors understood its everyday meaning, that is, a straightforward test with unknown (yet sometimes hoped for) beneficial results. For some this meant a planned intervention under well-controlled conditions and circumstances with respect to the selection of patients, the treatment(s) given and the particular care with which the patients were attended. Finally, Charles McLean held routine clinical practice based on "conjectural", in other words, inferior, evidence as nothing other than an uncontrolled experiment, an important statement which has often enough not been understood by doctors and the public alike.[11]

These issues, arguments and possible solutions continued to be advanced throughout the 19th century when the ethos of increasing scientific knowledge as a basis for progress also prevailed in medicine. But there were still others. Further safeguards against the apprehensions of inflicting damage to humans "for the sake of experiment" were formulated, such as the quest for previous animal studies and/or self-experimentation by doctors, and there is evidence that these principles were actually followed.[12] The first had been observed since the 17th century, although the transferability of results to humans was sometimes questioned.[13] 19th century surgery again offered many examples of this strategy, such as trying new techniques of ovarectomy and nephrectomy as well as thyroidectomy on animals and observing their consequences before operating on patients.[14] Auto-experimentation played a role in the history of inhalation anaesthesia. Because of the prevailing ethos and/or doctor and patient insistence on surgery as a "last hope", however, other "first operations" were directly done on patients. A case in point was the first successful heart suture performed in 1896 by Ludwig Rehn of Frankfurt in an emergency situation.[15] After the success of vaccination against smallpox and with the rise of microbiology, preventive and therapeutic measures against other infectious diseases, too, were tried throughout the 19th century, some directly

10   Currie (1804), p. 408.
11   Tröhler (2000a), pp. 56-57.
12   Tröhler/Maehle (1990).
13   Maehle/Tröhler (1990).
14   Tröhler (1993).
15   Tröhler (1998).

on patients in order to advance more quickly. This was the case for both Louis Pasteur's anti-rabies serum and his German competitor Robert Koch's tuberculosis treatment with Tuberkulin.[16] Pasteur's treatment ultimately proved a success, Koch's rapidly became a failure.

Clearly, there were no acknowledged rules for the type of evidence seen as sufficient for an innovation to be considered safe enough for general practice. This held true for modern surgery as well as for new drugs, chemical and others, produced by an expanding pharmaceutical industry. No licensing body existed. There was also no set of rules on the ethics of generating scientific evidence.[17] While the need for planned, well-controlled interventions was stressed as indispensable for the advance of medicine in the many editions and translations of Claude Bernard's *Introduction à la médecine expérimentale* (1865), this and texts of the same kind had no explicit headings on the ethics of (human) research. Instead, Bernard reaffirmed the traditional caution of "never performing on man an experiment which might be harmful to him to any extent, even though the result might be highly advantageous to science, i.e. to the health of others".[18] He held that "many physicians attack experimentation believing that medicine should be a science of observation". But, he pointed out, as McLean had done fifty years before him, that "physicians make therapeutic experiments daily on their patients, so this inconsistency cannot stand careful thought. Medicine by nature is an experimental science, but it must apply the experimental method systematically".[19] On the other hand, the 18th century British advocates of professional medical ethics, John Gregory and Thomas Percival, had in fact dealt with ethical issues inherent in therapeutic tests as a form of human experimentation, the former quite extensively,[20] the latter simply insisting on their usefulness "for the public good", provided they were scrupulously and conscientiously carried out and passed a process of prior peer review.[21] It was left to the responsibility and the individual doctor's conscience to judge what that meant. The idea and meaning of giving information and obtaining consent were not heeded[22] and the whole subject became conspicuously absent from the subsequent British and German deontological literature up to 1930 – with one exception. Nor was hardly any misdemeanour in this area dealt with by the professional courts of honour of these two countries, although cases of what we would today call "severe abuse" had occurred.[23]

The exception concerned Albert Moll of Berlin. As a practising neurologist he was interested in medicine related to sexual diseases and sexual reform. He was certainly not representative of mainstream medicine. In his 650-page *Ärztliche*

16   Geison (1995), Gradmann (2001).
17   Sauerteig (2000).
18   Quoted by Rothman (1998), p. 52.
19   Bernard (1949), p. 18.
20   McCullough (1998).
21   Tröhler (2000a), p. 130, Baker (1993).
22   Rothman (1998).
23   Maehle (1999b), Rabi (2002), Smith (1994).

Ethik (1902), he listed about 600 instances of non-therapeutic research from the medical press, cases that he considered unethical because of the damage inflicted, an unclear or evidently useless application, bad design and – most notably – absence of any form of information and/or consent by the patient-subjects. They had been published without further comment. This, Moll held, should no longer be considered as normal.[24]

The notion of informing a patient and obtaining consent did indeed exist but in the legal rather than the medical arena.[25] This holds particularly true for English law, which as early as 1830 was interpreted as insisting that the physician obtained the informed consent of a potential participant in experiments. "Otherwise, [the doctor] would be obliged to provide compensation for any injury that might arise from adopting a new method of treatment".[26] In the middle of the 19th century there were isolated criminal trials in France and Germany, and in the 1880s and 1890s in Norway and Austria, respectively. Doctors were condemned – mildly – for omitting to inform and not seeking consent. In the view of judges they had therefore inflicted physical injury on patients undergoing experimentation. Formal links between the doctors' ethos and administrative and legal practice were only established afterwards, in 1899, when Albert Neisser, professor of dermatology and venerology at the University of Breslau (and discoverer of the gonorrhoea bacillus), was condemned by the Royal Prussian Disciplinary Court for his actions. This was a tribunal concerned exclusively with the civil service, i.e. neither an ordinary criminal court nor a professional court of honour.

Neisser had injected cell-free serum from syphilitic patients into eight patients, some being minors and others prostitutes, without informing them or obtaining their consent. He wanted to test whether this might provide immunity against contracting syphilis. This and similar cases were exposed by the liberal press, highlighting the abuse of the poor in favour of finding a cure to hide the double standards of the wealthy. This raised public and even heated parliamentary debates, causing widespread consultations with medical and legal authorities by the Minister in charge. After the Neisser trial, official administrative regulations were introduced.

In December 1900 the Prussian Minister of Religious, Educational and Medical Affairs issued a specific Directive (*Anweisung*).[27] It was addressed to all heads of state clinics, policlinics and other hospitals in the country. The physicians and surgeons-in-chief were advised that intervention with other than diagnostic and therapeutic aims or for the purpose of immunisation were excluded under all circumstances in minors and otherwise legally not fully competent persons and unless the potential participant had consented unambiguously after relevant explanations of possible adverse consequences. These conditions and the precise circumstances of the study had to be documented in the case notes. This administra-

---

24   Moll (1902), pp. 504-590 .
25   Maehle (2000).
26   Perley et al. (1992), p. 150.
27   Minister (1901).

tive Directive was the first explicit, albeit legally weak, regulation of human experimentation. But it must be stressed that it concerned only non-therapeutic research, designed to advance (patho-)physiological knowledge. Even the frequent immunisations then prevalent were not considered: it was taken for granted that "patients in a public hospital submitted regularly [...] to new methods of treatment and diagnostic experiments".[28] In 1906 the Austrian Ministry of Education issued a nearly identical Directive.[29] Paul Ehrlich, when introducing his *Salvarsan*, the world's first chemotherapeutic agent, was certainly aware of the 1900 Directives and acted cautiously to avoid public scandal.[30]

Concerns and debates continued in interwar Germany, also in Parliament.[31] A generation later, in 1931, the 1900 Directive was further elaborated as Guidelines (*Richtlinien*) for Novel Therapeutic Trials and for Performing Scientific Experiments in Humans.[32] Issued by the Reich's Minister of the Interior, they included, as indicated by the title, both therapeutic and non-therapeutic research. As the Directive had done, the Guidelines required giving information and obtaining consent by participants and documenting these procedures. As administrative measures, they had no standing in criminal law. The question of the wider practical significance of these two regulatory measures remains unresolved, but practices in some places clearly worsened.[33] Although never revoked, they were certainly ignored during the period of National Socialism, particularly during the Second World War.

In the USA as well, before World War II, some doctors were aware of the moral dimensions of human research, the possible conflict between scientific advance and potential harm to patients and the recognised responsibility of physicians for their patients,[34] but it does not seem that any (inter)national entity discussed the subject.

III. "Never Again": Regulations in the Post-World War II Phase

As a reaction to the international public outcry against the atrocities of German researchers, which was made public at the end of the Second World War, the Nuremberg Code was drawn up during the trial against Nazi medical war criminals in 1946-47.[35] In ten principles, the Code specified the prerequisites that must be met for human experiments to be morally acceptable.[36] The Code could be interpreted as emphasising non-therapeutic studies only, as it did not mention

---

28   Quoted by Elkeles (1996), p. 209.
29   Elkeles (1996).
30   Sauerteig (2000).
31   Sauerteig (2000), Eckart/Reuland (2006).
32   Vollmann/Winau (1996), Eckart/Reuland (2006).
33   Frewer (2000), Eckart/Reuland (2006).
34   Lederer (1995).
35   See also the contribution by Ulf Schmidt in this volume.
36   Annas/Grodin (1992).

IV. The Wave of Codification of Ethics: A New Phenomenon

Around 1960, due to revelations about practices and scandals, human research again came under professional and public scrutiny in various countries.[52] The recognition that new drugs might have, albeit rarely, devastating effects, such as the limb abnormalities caused by *thalidomide*, made regulation more urgent. Thalidomide made international headlines. Local and national bodies such as the Harvard Medical School (1961), the British Medical Association (BMA) and the MRC (1963) reacted by issuing appropriate ethical guidelines. Academic and professional organisations of other European countries such as Germany and Switzerland followed suit. Indeed, in the 1960s many European governments passed formal acts which tightened up or introduced the licensing of new pharmaceutical products. Such was the case also in the United States, while the issue was avoided in France.[53] On an international level, as from 1960, various WMA organs dealt repeatedly with the issue leading in 1964 to the Recommendations Guiding Physicians in Biomedical Research involving Subjects. They were adapted by the General Assembly in Helsinki and published in the World Medical Journal, the Association's "house journal". This document, now known as the WMA Declaration of Helsinki (I), was an example of the ongoing regulation of moral issues arising in health care fields: both inter-governmental and non-governmental organisations (IGOs and NGOs, respectively) authored such documents. The latter did so partly in order to prevent "the enactment of criminal or legislative measures" in a field which doctors clearly considered their own province.[54] Albeit not legally binding, the Declaration had considerable impact on all five continents, both as a salient example and in terms of its contents.[55]

The wave of codification up to 2000 is illustrated in Figure 1. It shows the international guidelines, declarations, recommendations, etc., here summarised by the term "Ethics Codes", issued annually since 1947. The total number, as listed by S. Fluss, amounts to 326 variants. Eleven IGOs, ranging from the United Nations (1966) and its sub-organisations (UNESCO, WHO, UNAIDS), via, for example, the Council of Europe (CoE), the European Commission (EC), the Organisation of African Unity, to the World Labour Organisation (1999), have issued 107 such codes.

52   See various chapters in Eckart (2006).
53   Maio (2001).
54   Arnold/Sprumont (1998).
55   Human/Fluss (2001).

International Ethics Codes 1947 – 2000

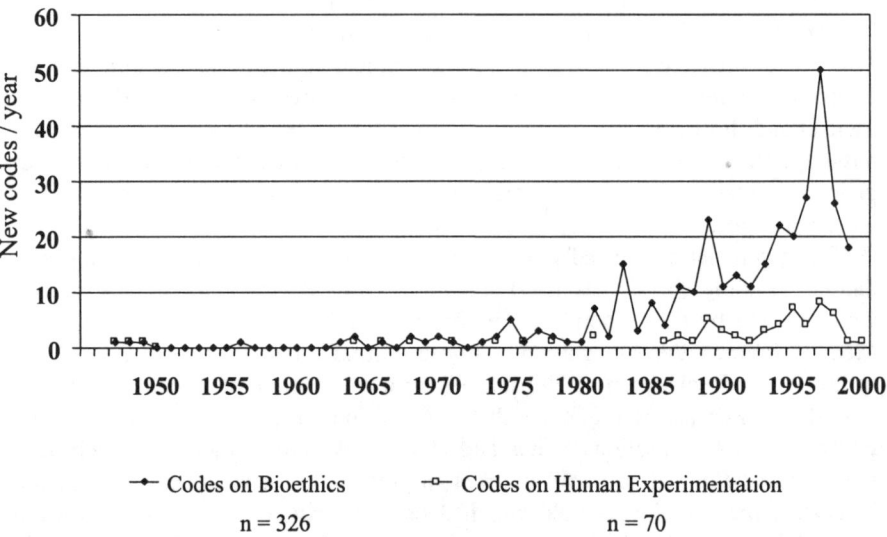

Figure 1: The number of international ethics codes (i.e., guidelines, recommendations, resolutions, conventions) issued by Inter-Governmental (IGO) and Non-Governmental Organisations (NGO) as well as miscellaneous international texts issued each year (from 1947 to 2000) is represented. Each amended version of a given code was counted individually. Drawn from data collected by S. Fluss (1999a) and my own research. n = Total number of codes of the respective category.

Thirty-six NGOs, ranging from the WMA (1948), via – to quote just a few – Amnesty International, the Council for International Organisations of Medical Sciences (CIOMS), the European Forum of Good Clinical Practice (EFGCP), the International Council of Nurses, the Human Genome Organisation, to the International Bar Association (2000), have produced 186 documents; the Governmental Entity of the Vatican six and miscellaneous bodies more than twenty. The number of national codes can only be estimated. Between 1969 and spring 2001 the Swiss Academy of Medical Sciences (SAMW) alone published twenty-seven versions in thirteen fields, including five versions of two codes regarding research on human beings; by March 2006 there were thirty-six versions in eighteen fields, and the process continues. In 2002, a Physician Charter, which represented a kind of Hippocratic Oath for the new millennium, was published simultaneously in the European *Lancet* and the US-American *Annals of Internal Medicine*. It was subsequently endorsed by dozens of professional bodies and certifying boards.[56]

This chapter cannot analyse the contents of such an enormous amount of source material.[57] Rather, I will suggest some of the reasons for this new phenomenon. Internal, scientific as well as external, socio-cultural reasons play a part. Taboos were being broken in specific fields. In reproductive medicine, for instance, Louise Brown, the first apparently healthy baby stemming from in vitro fertilisation, was born in the UK in 1978. In 1985, for the first time in history, a pregnancy was brought to full term by a surrogate mother; in 1990 the ova of aborted foetuses were marketed; 1998 featured, still in the UK, the successful cloning of the sheep Dolly, and, in 2000, the Parliament in Westminster engaged in a serious discussion of human "therapeutic" cloning (and approved it). In the early 1960s, euthanasia became an issue in many countries because of the availability of life-sustaining technologies. These were also a prerequisite for the criterion of brain death, which was sometimes discussed together with organ transplantation routines.[58] Most recently, xenotransplantation and tissue engineering raised moral concerns. Modern genetics, too, questions the basic concepts of society as well as of health care policies.

Since no progress in these areas is possible without human experimentation, one-fifth of all international codes have dealt with issues related to this major single field of concern in the aftermath of Nuremberg. More and more NGOs and IGOs have become active in related moral concerns in the 1990s (Figure 2). Further scandals in research have evidenced the inadequacy of the principle of subsidiarity, particularly in Germany and the United States.[59] National governments have intervened increasingly and in various ways in a field which had previously been regulated by the medical community.[60] France was the first country, in 1983, to establish, by presidential decree, a national bioethics committee as a consultation body (*Comité Consultatif National d'Ethique de la Médecine et des Sciences de la Vie*). It proposed moral norms and practical recommendations which "contaminated" subsequent laws, e.g. the Laws of Bioethics (*lois de bioéthique*) of 1994, including a regulation of human experimentation.[61] This political process did not fail to become internationalised, and the IGOs' involvement reflects the growing attention of international legislative bodies. But had this not been the intention of the Nuremberg Code forty years earlier?

56 Tröhler (1999), SAMW (2001a), SAMW (2001b) Tröhler (2002), Blank et al. (2003).
57 For an analysis respecting ethical issues see e.g. Sass (1988) and Veatch (1995).
58 Schöne-Seifert (1999), Bellanger/Steinbrecher (2006).
59 Baker (1998), Verdun-Jones/Weisstub (1998), Lemmens (1999).
60 Winslade/Krause (1998).
61 Mathieu (1998).

For example, the CoE, and later the European Union (EU) have developed activities with respect to research on human beings (Figure 2). It is a little known fact that there is a European Commissioner of Health and Consumer Protection, and that the decision-making on EC health programmes has hitherto not been transparent. Recently it has been recognised that it is important, democratically speaking, that NGOs, such as the International Alliance of Patients' Organisations be represented.[62] Indeed, moral issues in medicine have been increasingly seen from the perspective of moral rights.

As there are civil rights, human rights, and consumer rights, rights of minorities and of "vulnerables", such as of the mentally ill, the elderly, the physically handicapped, children, and prisoners – there are indeed patients' rights. The "rights approach" towards moral issues also takes account of race and gender. It can further be related to the new ecology and the womens' and students' movements of the 1960s, of which the patients' rights movement can be seen as an extension and continuation. Altogether these movements are an expression of deep socio-cultural changes in the Western world. The basic document behind all of them has been, of course, the Universal Declaration of Human Rights by the UN General Assembly in 1948. This was followed by the European Human Rights Convention signed in 1950 within the framework of the CoE in Rome, to which forty-eight states have signed up since. The latter is important in that it entailed, in 1952, the establishment of the European Human Rights Court in Strasbourg. This Court developed an unforeseeably dynamic and expansive jurisdiction, increasingly being used.

It is noticeable that, in the 1990s, besides the notion of human rights, the concept of human dignity has effectively emerged, marking yet another cultural shift (see below).

The next section will attempt a typology of the international ethics codes resulting from these scientific and cultural developments. It will focus on the reasons for, and the mechanisms involved in, their genesis by looking more closely at two typical codes from the perspective of an NGO and an IGO, respectively. This will highlight some of their distinguishing features.

62   Van der Zeijden (2000).

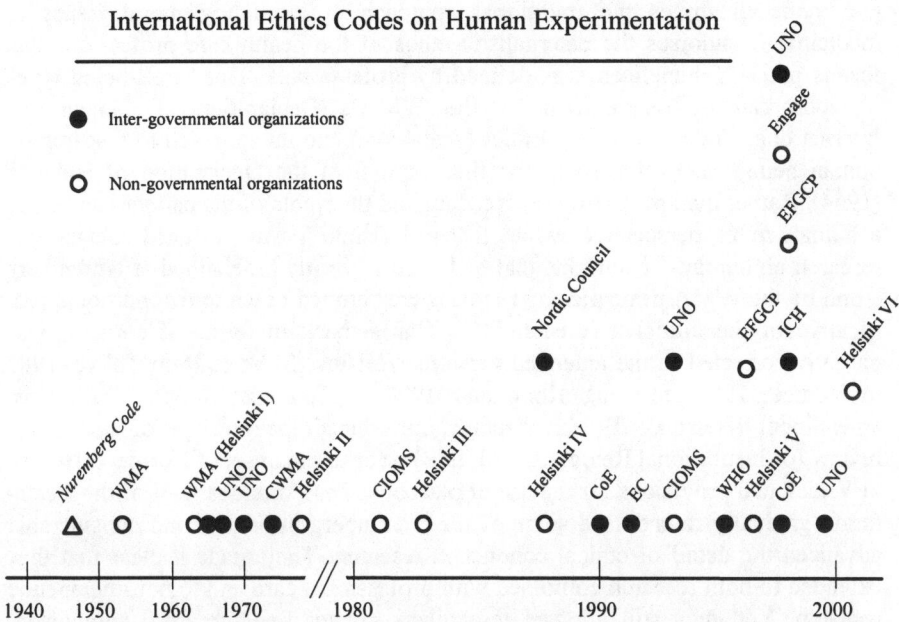

Figure 2: Twenty-five (versions of) international codes (guidelines, recommendations) regulating human experimentation are listed in order of the dates of publication. Drawn from data collected by S. Fluss (1999a), and my own research. The UN codes (Resolutions) deal only in part with human experimentation. Further explanations are contained in the text.

Abbreviations

WMA	World Medical Association
CWMA	Commonwealth Medical Association
CoE	Council of Europe
EC	European Commission
UNO	United Nations (Resolution on Human Rights and Bioethics)
CIOMS	Council for International Organizations of Medical Sciences
WHO	World Health Organization
EFGP	European Forum for Good Clinical Practice
ENGAGE	European Network of Good Clinical Practice (GCP) Auditors and Other GCP Experts
ICH	International Conference on Harmonization of Technical Requirements for Registration of Pharmaceuticals for Human Use

V. The WMA Declarations of Helsinki I - VI

One code illustrates the traditional approach at regulating moral issues in medicine. It endorses the paternalistic ethos of the health care professions that fosters patients' beneficence as defined by professionals. This "well-being type" of code can be exemplified by the WMA's Declaration of Geneva, its International Code of Medical Ethics (see above) and its approach to research on human beings as expressed in the first version of the Declaration of Helsinki (1964). Rather than protecting the freedom and the rights of the patient-subject, as a human rights perspective would foster, Helsinki I was designed to facilitate research on humans. The rights that had been so firmly proclaimed at Nuremberg – and by the WMA principles of 1954 – were "eroded down to a conditional pre-rogative of the clinician researcher".[63] This setback in terms of contents was partially corrected in the amended versions (Helsinki II–V; 1975 in Tokyo, 1983 in Venice, 1989 in Hong Kong and 1996 in Somerset West). The Tokyo amendment (Helsinki II), for instance, introduced the concept of committee review (or Institutional Review Board, IRB) prior to the onset of a project: Helsinki V included provisions for the use of placebo. These versions II–V of the Declaration gradually re-endorsed some of the Nuremberg principles and considerably advanced the detail of ethical conduct in research. They made it clear that they extended to both research combined with professional care and to non-therapeutic research. Yet, they still allowed researchers greater freedom from compulsory consent obligations.[64] While consent could be avoided in certain conditions, those legally or otherwise incapable were especially protected. Furthermore, the personal, non-transferable responsibility of the researcher to assure the ethical quality of the patient-subject's consent, and the right to leave the experiment if his or her personal condition seems to demand it (Markers 11 and 12 of Table 1), were not incorporated in any of the versions of the Helsinki Declaration.[65]

In this context it must be stressed that the WMA as a private organisation represents the interests of the national professional bodies, which it reunites (one per member country only). Its General Assembly has so far voted seventy-six ethics codes, i.e. declarations, statements, recommendations and resolutions, most of which are hardly known – as for instance the Declaration of Lisbon on Patients' Rights.[66] They have no legal force *per se*. But such "soft law" may become "hard law" when integrated into legal documents. The WMA has no democratic legitimacy either, for only a part of a nation's doctors is actually represented. The number of national delegates voting at the General Assembly depends on the number announced as paying the membership fee to the WMA. This number is arbitrary in that it depends on the financial commitment a national professional organisation is willing to make. The German Federal Medical Association (*Bundesärzte-*

---

63   Baker (1998), p. 322.
64   Baker (1998), Winslade/Krause (1998), Fluss (1999b).
65   Herranz (1998).
66   Declaration of Lisbon on Patients' Rights 1981, updated 1995; Fluss (1999a).

kammer), for instance, pays for some 30 per cent of its members which equals ten votes in the WMA General Assembly, whereas the USA have twelve votes and France seven. The Netherlands did not pay for some time and Switzerland once formally left the WMA and thus both countries temporarily had no vote.[67] The BMA resigned in the 1970s to protest against the admission of South Africa. It was re-admitted only in 1994. In that year, the membership numbered sixty-four countries.[68]

It is not clear how and by whom the WMA's ethics codes are formulated.[69] Certainly they do not follow a consistent philosophical concept of ethics. Rather they reflect compromises arrived at among doctors. An exception was the proposal for a completely new form of the Helsinki Declaration presented by the American Medical Association (AMA), led by Yale professor Robert Levine.[70] While the amended versions II–V corresponded to some extent to a rebirth of the Nuremberg Code from the mid-1970s to the mid-1990s, this proposal for Helsinki VI seemed to reflect a tendency to deregulation in view of commercial interests in the new biotechnologies.[71] It generated an extensive, compassionate debate within the profession and the WMA itself, unprecedented in the history of the WMA, involving numerous symposia and contributions to the leading medical and ethical journals. At stake were the use of placebos, the need to distinguish between therapeutic and non-therapeutic research and whether research should be related to social benefits for the price of, yet again, reducing the rights of the individual participating.[72] This would be contrary to a number of ethics codes issued by other NGOs and by non-professional IGOs such as the CoE. And such a hierarchy of values, calling to mind 18th and 19th century attitudes, is certainly not shared throughout the present-day world.

In 1999, the WMA opted for amendments of the latest version (V), that of Somerset West (1996). Finally, in October 2000, the General Assembly at Edinburgh adopted a version in which the fundamental distinction (introduced in the 1964 Helsinki I version) between diagnostic or therapeutic and non-therapeutic biomedical research (i.e., without implying direct value to the person subjected to it) was abolished. In the specific paragraphs allowing medical research to be combined with medical care "only to the extent that the research is justified by its potential prophylactic, diagnostic or therapeutic value *to the patient*", the last three words were deleted.[73] This meant that social benefit had become uppermost.

In agreement with this outlook, the critical point – formerly listed under "non-therapeutic research" – stating "the interest of science and society should never take precedence over considerations related to the well-being of the subjects" – was subtly changed to "considerations related to the well-being of the human

---

67   Doppelfeld (2000b).
68   Bulletin of Medical Ethics (1994).
69   Doppelfeld (2000a).
70   See also Levine (1999).
71   Angell (2000), Weatherall (2000), Tröhler (2000b).
72   Klinkhammer (2000).
73   WMA (2000a) and WMA (2000b).

subject should take precedence over the interests of science and society".[74] This was due to a considerable extent to the intervention of the German Federal Medical Association alarmed by the results of recent scholarly research on medicine during National Socialism.

Indeed, a new form of democracy was practised by having the Levine and subsequent amendment proposals published and circulated to the national medical associations who then reported to a Workgroup of the WMA.[75] Reflecting the growing connection between industrial interests and clinical research, this new version of Helsinki (VI) includes the obligation to adequately inform "each potential [...] subject of the [...] sources of funding, [about] any possible conflict of interest, [and] institutional affiliations of the researcher".[76] These are clear indications of a reorientation of the medical profession to contradictory, yet inevitable economic constraints.

Major state regulatory agencies such as the US Food and Drug Administration and the European Union's bodies (see below) showed negative reactions and disregarded Helsinki VI for different motives. In fact, discussions resumed. In two Notes of Clarification, the WMA relativised its strict position regarding placebo-controlled trials in 2002 and post-trial access to procedures identified as beneficial in the study (the best current therapy or a proven therapy?) in 2004. It is also contested who should rule research on emergency situations.[77] In practice, underlying ideas and principles of the Declaration are being referred to nowadays by researchers without specifying the version. In general, the legally binding force of this private medical code has varied between countries and changed within one and the same country, depending on whether or not it has been included in the professional deontological code. However, during the last decade, national laws as derived from international conventions have been enacted that may be either more restrictive or more permissive than certain "markers" of the Declaration of Helsinki or other codes.

In the next section, therefore, examples of ethics codes issued by IGOs will be analysed. Their perspective has, either surprisingly or not, changed remarkably as one looks back on the past.

VI.   The Council of Europe and its Ethics Codes

From a European perspective, the Council of Europe (CoE), founded in 1949 and reuniting today over fifty member states, for instance, has a long-standing history in matters of human rights, particularly in relation to medicine and biology. Until 1999 the Parliamentary Assembly voted a Recommendation and Resolution on the Rights of the Sick and Dying in 1976 followed by one on the Situation of the

---

74   Ibid., § 5.
75   WMA (2000a).
76   WMA (2000b), § 22.
77   WMA (2006).

Mentally Ill in 1977 and further eleven recommendations; the Committee of Ministers voted twenty-one resolutions, recommendations and protocols.[78] In contrast to the well-being type of code, which addresses scientists' duties, they stress the participants' rights. They thus represent the "rights-type" approach to moral issues in medicine.

As genetic engineering became possible around 1975, the Ministers of Justice of the member states created the *Comité ad hoc des experts en bioéthique* (CAHBI) three years later (1978). Each member state had one vote, but a free number of delegates (usually academics and/or civil servants) depending on a state's political and financial commitment were included. The CAHBI worked many years on a Convention on Human Artificial Procreation, which collapsed in the end because of the uncompromising attitude of one member country, Liechtenstein. It was finally published as principles by the CAHBI in 1989. As other problematic ethical fields in medicine were being debated in some of the member states, the Ministers of Justice in 1990 replaced the CAHBI by a standing Steering Committee on Bioethics (Comité Directeur de Bioéthique, CDBI). Again, all member states are represented with one vote, with Canada, the Holy See, the International Federation of Scientific Societies, Israel, Japan, Mexico and the USA having observer status at various levels. The CDBI has also installed task forces working on specific fields such as organ transplants and human genetics. But the main task desired by the ministers was the elaboration of a convention on ethical issues in medicine and biology. The aim was to promote informed consent, considered a patient right, in human research and in daily medical practice. They also wanted to bring order to the array of national and international codes. The committee of ministers soon realised that this was too restrictive an issue for successful political campaigning and insisted on including human rights and human dignity as issues. This led to a change in the title which now reads as the Convention on the Protection of Human Rights and Dignity of the Human Being with Regard to the Application of Biology and Medicine (HRBM) or in shortened form Convention on Human Rights and Biomedicine. Thus, in terms of contents, the document is a hybrid. A philosophically stringent system could not be implemented.

The Convention was drafted according to the conventional methods for arriving at such international agreements: they end up as compromises, sometimes consciously formulated in abstract, even incomprehensible terms – which do not, in the end, serve legal purposes. In the specific case of the HRBM Convention, the work of the CDBI was not very efficient, since many of the sixty to eighty delegates were neither particularly knowledgeable in international law nor in human rights issues and, as usual, the various legal systems had to be taken into account. Many points necessitated tough negotiations and the readiness to compromise.[79] The Convention was finally modelled upon that on human rights. Core paragraphs have a commentary to help interpretation. Additional protocols

78 Fluss (1999a).
79 Reusser (2000).

allow a rapid response to new issues. The political nature of this document is evident in the proviso that any country with its own legal regulations for a given issue need not to follow the Convention in this respect. In consequence some countries introduced laws prior to signing or ratifying the Convention.

The core paragraphs concern the following:

1. the formulation of the Convention's aim, namely the protection of the dignity of the human being "as soon as life begins" (which is nowhere defined), equal access to health care and the prioritising of the interests of the individual over those of society – an important statement in the context of human experimentation
2. the requirement of informed consent
3. the protection of the private sphere
4. the regulation of the human genome, forbidding discrimination, choice of sex, intervention in the germ line, etc.
5. the regulation of human research including points 1-3 above.
6. administrative directives, notably for updating the Convention, e.g. a complete revision foreseen five years after it takes effect.[80]

In 1994 a first draft was ready for national hearings, and in 1997 the final version, having been voted through by the Committee of Ministers, was presented for signing by governments and prepared for ratification according to national constitutions. So far, forty-three countries have signed, with the notable exceptions of Germany, for the Convention being too lax, Russia and the United Kingdom, for it being too restrictive, twenty-eight have ratified it, signifying that it is effective and that the ratifying countries, but not the others, must take appropriate legal measures.[81] The national hearings were a new feature. Previous international conventions were drawn up without this democratic instrument. The hearings evidenced serious concerns about research on persons not able to consent and research which is not in their own interest but in that of the population represented. These plus the main issues contested in Helsinki VI (see above) were regulated differently (in general more restrictively) in the Additional Protocol to the Convention [...] Concerning Biomedical Research in January 2005. It has so far been signed by eighteen and ratified by two member states.[82] While the CoE's Conventions need two active steps by member countries (signature and ratification) in order to enter into force, the Directives of the European Union are legally binding model bills that must be implemented as national laws by its now twenty-five member states who have to comply by a given deadline. This procedure has to be applied for human research in the case of the EC's Directive 2005/28/EL of 8 April, 2005 "laying down principles and detailed guidelines for

80   Council of Europe (2006a).
81   Ibid.
82   Council of Europe (2006b).

good clinical practice as regards investigational medicinal products for human use...". It refers to the earlier Directive 2001/20/EC "for the design, conduct and reporting of clinical trials on human subjects" involving such products. The latter "deliberately" quotes the 1996 version of the Declaration of Helsinki (Helsinki IV!) while confusingly, some (not binding) EU Guidelines rely even on Helsinki III (1989).[83]

In the 1990s time was ripe for a first wave of legislation. This is known in the history of law as a periodical phenomenon. Consequently, private codes, such as Helsinki have since gradually forfeited their formal significance – in those countries where legislation has been interfering in an ever more detailed way in matters of medicine, science and human rights.

VIII. Summary and Conclusion

Research on human beings gives an indication of the slow progress which was made in relation to the awareness and acceptance of the moral need in western-style medicine, namely that for protection of the participants. Moral issues such as the notion of not neglecting safety "for the sake of experiment" and of "benefit for the patient" were discussed by some members of the profession as early as the 18th century. These issues have, however, often been misconstrued by doctors and the public alike. Many people have thought that a therapeutic experiment, lest it constitute an abuse, should guarantee a successful outcome for the well-being of every patient. This is not what "benefit for the patient" means. Rather the benefit of a therapeutic trial lies, indirectly, in the reduction of uncertainty about a beneficial, harmful or non-effective intervention. A directly favourable outcome for an individual patient can, therefore, not be predicted, otherwise the experiment need not be performed. This fact must not be confounded with the requirement of taking appropriate measures to diminish potential harm in an experiment – "for the benefit of the patient".

A legal tradition took some shape in Germany around 1900 and 1930 and, with the Nuremberg Code, on an international level from 1947 onwards. The Code was hardly met with a positive response, even in the United States immediately after its inception. In 1964 the WMA changed the formerly protective attitude of its 1954 Principles when issuing the "paternalistic" Declaration of Helsinki (I). This was a compromise in reaction to serious abuses, exemplified by the thalidomide case, at a time of optimistic expectancies for the therapeutic yield of biomedicine fuelled by the success of, say, antibiotics, cortisone and new surgical procedures. It allowed research to proceed besides serving another purpose, i.e. it prevented legislative curtailment, at least for some time. In this vacuum, Helsinki I aimed at setting standards for the WMA's main concern, i.e. doctors' attitudes and behaviour, but not exclusively so: Ten years later, with the amended Helsinki Declaration (II), trial subject protection was improved, to be relativised again

83   European Union (2006).

twenty years later, towards the end of the twentieth century, in the updated Helsinki Declaration (VI). As in the 1960s this must be seen in the light of a wave of new hopes, induced this time by the expectancies from the "molecularisation" of medicine.

This adaptation stands in contrast to the "human rights and human dignity" approach of IGO codes, most particularly of the Convention of Human Rights and Biomedicine of the CoE (1997). It focussed on patients and other participants of the medical research enterprises, not least because new research scandals in the 1990s and the possibility of exporting research to developing countries,[84] had proved the irrelevance of the WMA's and many other international "soft law" ethics codes. The Universal Declaration on Bioethics and Human Rights, adopted by the General Assembly of the UNESCO in October 2005, is another response to this development and aims to internationalise the human rights approach through the field of "bioethics".[85] The historical review of the relation between "soft law" codes and legal regulations shows that, beyond their legal status, the impact of both codes and laws has been defined by their relevance to contemporary thought, whether they addressed conflicts perceived by society and whether they offered any means of solving them.

Incontestably, however, besides their input of principles and ideas, the "soft law" codes have offered other positive features in the political process of drawing up international conventions and national laws, namely specificity and rapid adaptability to new scientific and societal developments. However, their legitimacy, in contrast to democratically passed laws, was, by the 1990s, seen as problematic. As the example of the WMA codes has shown, the process of how they were conceived has come under scrutiny. Furthermore, the issue of international regulations raises the question of different ethical views and cultures, not only regarding the universality of conflicts, but also the means of solving them, for instance, via informed consent and other principles which need not necessarily be important everywhere.

If the purpose of an NGO-code or an IGO-document is to contribute to legal liability, their success in judging the validity of human research in view of continuous abuses over the past fifty years must be pondered. The future looks more optimistic for codes fostering patient rights and perhaps human dignity in daily medical practice.[86]

But ethics codes have had and still do have other purposes, namely the articulation of idealistic aspirations. They can play the role of symbols,[87] "express fundamental values, such as respect for persons and scientific integrity [...] set standards for moral criticism of medical practices or policies that may violate the rights of human subjects".[88] Their general nature has, in certain cases, actually

---

84   Lurie/Wolfe (1997), Rothman (2006).
85   UNESCO (2005).
86   Reusser (2000).
87   Smith (1996), Leven (1997).
88   Winslade/Krause (1998), p. 140.

"dramatised the need for national and international documents with binding authority".[89] They are more readable for researchers than legal texts. On the other hand, they can also serve as moral cover-ups. Last but not least, codes may serve as teaching aids. With legislation intervening in an ever more detailed way in all matters of medicine, science and human rights, it is important that codes are being observed, whatever their legal status, in order that "Hippocrates" not *hypocrisia* reign in human research.

It has become clear by now for many of us that science and ethics are not separable, but intrinsically intertwined. For in order to be scientifically sound, research has to be ethical, and to be ethical it has to be scientifically sound. In actual research practice, the standards accepted at any given time, both scientific and ethical, have always been decisive in their ever-changing mutual relationship. Whose standards were they anyway?

89   Perley et al. (1992), p. 160.

Abbreviations for the Chapter

AMA   American Medical Association
BMA   British Medical Association
CAHBI   Comité ad hoc des experts en bioéthique
CDBI   Comité Directeur de Bioéthique
CIOMS   Council for International Organisations of Medical Sciences
CoE   Council of Europe
EC   European Commission
EFGCP   European Forum for Good Clinical Practice
EU   European Union
HRBM   Convention on the Protection of Human Rights and Dignity of the
           Human Being with Regard to the Application of Biology and
           Medicine
IGO   Inter-governmental Organisation
MRC   Medical Research Council
NGO   Non-governmental Organisation
SAMW   Swiss Academy of Medical Sciences
UNAIDS   United Nations Programme on HIV/AIDS
UNESCO   United Nations Educational, Scientific and Cultural Organization
WHO   World Health Organization
WMA   World Medical Association

References

Annas, G. J./Grodin M. A. (eds.) (1992): The Nazi Doctors and the Nuremberg Code. Human Rights in Human Experimentation. New York, Oxford: Oxford University Press.

Angell, M. (2000): Is Academic Medicine for Sale? New England Journal of Medicine 342 (2000), pp. 1516-1518.

Arnold, P./Sprumont, D. (1998): The "Nuremberg Code": Rules of Public International Law, in: Tröhler/Reiter-Theil (1998), pp. 84-96.

Baker, R. (1993): Deciphering Percival's Code, in: Baker et al. (1993), pp. 179-211.

Baker R./Porter R./Porter D. (eds.) (1993): The Codification of Medical Morality, vol. 1: Medical Ethics and Etiquette in the Eighteenth Century. Dordrecht, Boston, London: Kluwer.

Baker, R. (1998): Transcultural Medical Ethics and Human Rights, in: Tröhler/ Reiter-Theil (1998), pp. 312-331.

Bassiouni, M. C./Baffes, T. G./Evard, J. T. (1981): An Appraisal of Human Experimentation in International Law and Practice: The Need for International Regulation of Human Experimentation, Journal of Criminal Law and Criminology 72 (1981), pp. 1597-1666.

Bellanger, S./Steinbrecher, A. (2006): Addressing Uncertainties. The Conceptualisation of Brain Death in Switzerland 1960-2000, in: Schlich/Tröhler (2006), pp. 204-224.

Bernard, C. (1949): An Introduction to the Study of Experimental Medicine. Translated by Henry Copley Greene. New York: H. Schuman.

Blank, L./Kimball, H./McDonald, W./Merino, J. (2003): Medical Professionalism in the New Millenium: A Physician Charter 15 Month Later, Annals of Internal Medicine 138 (2003), pp. 851-855.

Blom, K. (1973): Armauer Hansen and Human Leprosy Transmission. Medical Ethics and Legal Rights. International Journal of Leprosy 41 (1973), pp. 199-207.

Bondolfi, A./Müller, H. (eds.) (1999): Medizinische Ethik im ärztlichen Alltag. Basel, Bern: Schweizerischer Ärzteverlag.

Brennan, T. A. (1999): Proposed Revisions to the Declaration of Helsinki – Will they Weaken the Ethical Principles Underlying Human Research? New England Journal of Medicine 341 (1999), pp. 527-530.

Bulletin of Medical Ethics (1994): World Medical Association is Reanimated (Editorial), Bulletin of Medical Ethics 101 (1994), pp. 3-4.

Bynum, W. F. (1988): Reflections on the History of Human Experimentation, in: Spicker et al. (1998), pp. 29-46.

Bynum, W. F./Porter, R. (eds.) (1993): Companion Encyclopedia of the History of Medicine. London, New York: Routledge.

Council of Europe (2006a): Convention for the Protection of Human Rights and Dignity of the Human Being with regard to the Application of Biology and

Medicine: Convention on Human Rights and Biomedicine, Oviedo (1997); European Treaty Series, no. 164.

Council of Europe (2006b): Additional Protocol to the Convention on Human Rights and Biomedicine concerning Biomedical Research, Strasbourg (2005). European Treaty Series, no. 195.

Currie, J. (1804): Medical Reports on the Effects of Water, Cold and Warm as a Remedy in Fever and Febrile Diseases, vol. 2. Liverpool, London: McCreery and Cadell.

Deutsch, E. (1998): The Nuremberg Code: The Proceedings in the Medical Case, the Ten Principles of Nuremberg and the Lasting Effect of the Nuremberg Code, in: Tröhler/Reiter-Theil (1998), pp. 71-83.

Doppelfeld, E. (1999): Generalversammlung des Weltärztebundes: Offene Fragen, ungelöste Probleme. Deutsches Ärzteblatt 96 (1999), pp. C-2297-C-2299.

Doppelfeld, E. (2000a): Weltärztebund – Probe für die Glaubwürdigkeit. Deutsches Ärzteblatt 97 (2000), pp. A-1587-A-1592.

Doppelfeld, E. (2000b): Paper read at the International Symposium: Das Menschenrechtsübereinkommen des Europarates – taugliches Vorbild für eine weltweit geltende Regelung? Heidelberg: Akademie der Wissenschaften [19 September 2000].

Drinan, R. F. (1992): The Nuremberg Principles in International Law, in: Annas/ Grodin (1992), pp. 174-182.

Eckart, W. U. (ed.) (2006): Man, Medicine, and the State. The Human Body as an Object of Government Sponsored Medical Research in the 20th Century. Stuttgart: Steiner.

Eckart, W. U./Reuland, A. (2006): First Principles: Julius Moses and Medical Experimentation in the Late Weimar Republic, in: Eckart (2006), pp. 35-47.

Elkeles, B. (1996): Der moralische Diskurs über das medizinische Menschenexperiment im 19. Jahrhundert. Stuttgart, Jena, New York: Gustav Fischer.

European Union (2006): Official Journal of the European Communities 9.4.2005 and 1.5.2001.

Fluss, S. (1999a): International Guidelines on Bioethics, EFGCP News (1999), supplement.

Fluss, S. (1999b): How the Declaration of Helsinki Developed. Good Clinical Practice Journal 6 (1999), pp. 18-22.

Frewer, A. (2000): Medizin und Moral in Weimarer Republik und Nationalsozialismus. Die Zeitschrift „Ethik" unter Emil Abderhalden. Frankfurt am Main, New York: Campus.

Frewer, A./Neumann, J. N. (eds.) (2001): Medizingeschichte und Medizinethik. Kontroversen und Begründungsansätze 1900-1950. Frankfurt am Main, New York: Campus.

Geison, G. L. (1995): The Private Science of Louis Pasteur. Princeton, NJ: Princeton University Press.

Glantz, L. H. (1992): The Influence of the Nuremberg Code on U.S. Statutes and Regulations, in: Annas/Grodin (1992), pp. 183-200.

Gradmann, C. (2001): Robert Koch and the Pressures of Scientific Research: Tuberculosis and Tuberculin, Medical History 45 (2001), pp. 1-32.

Guthrie, G. J. (1815): On Gun-Shot Wounds of the Extremities. London: Longman.

Herranz, G. (1998): The Inclusion of the Ten Principles of Nuremberg in Professional Codes of Ethics: An International Comparison, in: Tröhler/ Reiter-Theil (1998), pp. 127-139.

Howard-Jones, N. (1982): Human Experimentation in Historical and Ethical Perspectives, Social Science and Medicine 16 (1982), pp. 1429-1448.

Human, S./Fluss S. (2001): The World Medical Association's Declaration of Helsinki: Historical and Contemporary Perspectives. Unpublished manuscript.

Klinkhammer, G. (2000): Medizinische Forschung am Menschen. Abkehr von einheitlichen Standards, Deutsches Ärzteblatt 97 (2000), pp. A-2205-A2206.

Lederer, S. (1995): Subjected to Science. Human Experimentation before the Second World War. Baltimore, London: Johns Hopkins University Press.

Lemmens, T. (1999): In the Name of National Security: Lessons from the Final Report on the Human Radiation Experiments, European Journal of Health Law 6 (1999), pp. 7-23.

Leven, K.-H. (1997): Der hippokratische Eid im 20. Jahrhundert, in: Toellner/ Wiesing (1997), pp. 111-129.

Levine, R. J. (1999): The Need to Revise the Declaration of Helsinki, New England Journal of Medicine 341 (1999), pp. 531-534.

Lurie, P./Wolfe, S. M. (1997): Unethical Trials of Interventions to Reduce Perinatal Transmission of Human Immmunodeficiency Virus in Developing Countries, New England Journal of Medicine 337 (1997), pp. 853-856.

Macbride, D. (1764): Experimental Essays, London: Millar.

Maehle, A.-H./Geyer-Kordesch, J. (eds.) (2002): From Paternalism to Autonomy? Historical and Philosophical Perspectives on Biomedical Ethics. Aldershot,Brookfield, Singapore, Sydney: Ashgate.

Maehle, A.-H./Tröhler, U. (1990): Animal Experimentation from Antiquity to the End of the Eighteenth Century: Attitudes and Arguments, in: Rupke (1990), pp. 14-47.

Maehle, A.-H. (1999a): Drugs on Trial: Experimental Pharmacology and Therapeutic Innovation in the Eighteenth Century. Amsterdam, Atlanta, GA: Rodopi.

Maehle, A.-H. (1999b): Professional Ethics and Discipline: The Prussian Medical Courts of Honour, 1899-1920, Medizinhistorisches Journal 34 (1999), pp. 309-338.

Maehle, A.-H. (2000): Assault and Battery, or Legitimate Treatment? German Legal Debates on the Status of Medical Interventions without Consent, c. 1890-1914, Gesnerus 57 (2000), pp. 206-221.

Maio, G. (2001): Ärztliche Ethik als Politikum. Zur französischen Diskussion um das Humanexperiment nach 1945, Medizinhistorisches Journal 35 (2001), pp. 35-80.

Mathieu, B. (1998): Ethical "Norms" and the Law: Legitimacy of "Experts" or Democratic Legitimacy, in: Tröhler/Reiter-Theil (1998), pp. 163-184.

McCullough, L. B. (1998): John Gregory's Writings on Medical Ethics and Philosophy of Medicine. Dordrecht, Boston, London: Kluwer.

McLean, C. (1817-18): Results of an Investigation Respecting Epidemic and Pestilential Diseases. London: Underwood.

Medical Research Council (1953): Draft Statement (revised) on Clinical Investigations, 9 October 1953, signed by H. F. Hinsworth, Manuscript MRC.53/518/B.

Minister der Geistlichen, Unterrichts- und Medizinal-Angelegenheiten (1901): Anweisung an die Vorsteher der Kliniken, Polikliniken und sonstigen Krankenanstalten [dated 29 December, 1900]. Centralblatt für die gesamte Unterrichts-Verwaltung in Preußen (1901), pp. 188-189.

Moll, A. (1902): Ärztliche Ethik. Die Pflichten des Arztes in allen Beziehungen seiner Thätigkeit. Stuttgart: Enke.

Perley, S./Fluss, S. S./Zbigniew, B./Simon, F. (1992): The Nuremberg Code: An International Overview, in: Annas/Grodin (1992), pp. 149-173.

Rabi, B. (2002), Ärztliche Ethik – Eine Frage der Ehre? Die Prozesse und Urteile der ärztlichen Ehrengerichtshöfe in Preussen und Sachsen 1918-33. Frankfurt am Main: Lang.

Reich, W. T. (ed.) (1995): Encyclopedia of Bioethics, 5 vols. New York: Simon and Schuster-Macmillan.

Reusser, R. (2000): Paper read at the International Symposium: Das Menschenrechtsübereinkommen des Europarates – taugliches Vorbild für eine weltweit geltende Regelung? Heidelberg: Akademie der Wissenschaften [19 September 2000].

Rothman, D. (1995): Research, Human: Historical Aspects, in: Reich (1995), vol. 4, pp. 2238-2258.

Rothman, D. (1998): The Nuremberg Code in Light of Previous Principles and Practices in Human Experimentation, in: Tröhler/Reiter-Theil (1998), pp. 50-59.

Rothman, D. (2006): Back to First Principles: First World Research in Third World Countries, in: Eckart (2006), pp. 279-288.

Rupke, N. A. (ed.) (1990): Vivisection in Historical Perspective. London, New York: Routledge.

SAMW (Swiss Academy of Medical Sciences) (2001a): Ethische Richtlinien – Ethics Guidelines and Recommendations. Basel: Schwabe.

SAMW (Swiss Academy of Medical Sciences) (2001b): Ethische Richtlinien. www.samw.ch , accessed 26 March 2006.

Sass, H.-M. (1988): Comparative Models and Goals for the Regulation of Human Research, in: Spicker et al. (1988), pp. 47-89.

Sauerteig, L. (2000): Ethische Richtlinien, Patientenrechte und ärztliches Verhalten bei der Arzneimittelerprobung (1892-1931), Medizinhistorisches Journal 35 (2000), pp. 301-332.

Schlich, T./Tröhler, U. (eds.) (2006): The Risks of Medical Innovation. Risk Perception and Assessment in Historical Context. London, New York: Routledge

Schmidt, U. (2001): Der Ärzteprozeß als moralische Instanz? Der Nürnberger Kodex und das Problem „zeitloser Medizinethik", in: Frewer/Neumann (2001), pp. 334-373.

Schmidt, U. (2004): Justice at Nuremberg. Leo Alexander and the Nazi Doctors' Trial. Basingstoke: Palgrave.

Schöne-Seifert, B. (1999), Defining Death in Germany, in: Youngner et al. (1999), pp. 257-271.

Schuster, E. (1997): Fifty Years Later: The Significance of the Nuremberg Code. New England Journal of Medicine 337 (1997), pp. 1436-1440.

Smith, D. C. (1996): The Hippocratic Oath and Modern Medicine. Journal of the History of Medicine and Allied Sciences 51 (1996), pp. 484-500.

Smith, R. G. (1994): Medical Discipline: The Professional Conduct Jurisdiction of the General Medical Council, 1858-1990. Oxford: Clarendon Press.

Spicer, C. M. (1995): Nature and Role of Codes, and Other Ethics Directives, in: Reich (1995), vol. 5, pp. 2605-2612.

Spicker, S. F./Engelhard, H.T. Jr./Alon, I. (1988), The Use of Human Beings in Research. Dordrecht, Boston, London: Kluwer, pp. 29-46.

Starr, C. (1998): Blood. An Epic History of Medicine and Commerce. New York: A. Knopf.

Toellner, R./Wiesing, U. (eds.) (1997): Geschichte und Ethik in der Medizin. Von den Schwierigkeiten einer Kooperation. Jena: Fischer.

Tröhler, U./Maehle, A.-H. (1990): Anti-Vivisection in Nineteenth-Century Germany and Switzerland: Motives and Methods, in Rupke (1990), pp. 149-187.

Tröhler, U. (1993): Surgery (modern), in: Bynum (1993), vol. 2, pp. 984-1028.

Tröhler, U. (1998): From Rehn's Risky Cardiac Suture (1896) to Routine Cardiac Transplantation (1996): Historical and Ethical Perspectives, Journal of Cardiovascular Surgery 39 (1998), supplement 1 to no. 2, pp. 7-22.

Tröhler, U./Reiter-Theil, S (eds.) (1998): Ethics Codes in Medicine: Foundations and Achievements of Codification since 1947. Aldershot, Brookfield, Singapore, Sydney: Ashgate.

Tröhler, U. (1999): Das ärztliche Ethos und die Kodifizierung von Ethik in der Medizin, in: Bondolfi/Müller (1999), pp. 39-61.

Tröhler, U. (2000a): To Improve the Evidence of Medicine: The Eighteenth Century British Origins of a Critical Approach. Edinburgh: Royal College of Physicians.

Tröhler, U. (2000b): Asilomar-Konferenz zur Sicherheit in der Molekularbiologie von 1975: Rückschau und Ausblick, Schweizerische Ärztezeitung 81 (2000), pp. 1585-1587.

Tröhler, U. (2002): Human Research: From Ethos to Law, from National to International Regulations, in: Maehle/Geyer-Kordesch (2002), pp. 95-117.

UNESCO (2005): Universal Declaration on Bioethics and Human Rights, adopted 19 October 2005.

Van der Zeijden, A. (2000): Citizens and Patients as Partners in Decision-Making and Implementation, Issues in European Health Policy 3 (2000), p. 8.

Veatch, R. M. (1995): Medical Codes and Oaths II: Ethical Analysis, in: Reich, (1995), vol. 3, pp. 1427-1435.

Verdun-Jones, S. N./Weisstub, D. N. (1998): The Regulation of Biomedical Experimentation in Canada: Developing an Effective Apparatus for the Implementation of Ethical Principles in a Scientific Milieu, in: Weisstub (1998), pp. 328-354.

Vollmann, J./Winau, R. (1996): Informed Consent in Human Experimentation before the Nuremberg Code, British Medical Journal 313 (1996), pp. 1445-1447.

Weatherall, D. (2000): Academia and Industry: Increasingly Uneasy Bedfellows. Lancet 355 (2000), pp. 1574-1575.

Weisstub, D. N. (ed.) (1998): Research on Human Subjects. Ethics, Law and Social Policy. Oxford: Elsevier Science (Pergamon).

Winslade, W. J./Krause, T. L. (1998): The Nuremberg Code Turns Fifty, in: Tröhler/Reiter-Theil (1998), pp. 140-162.

WMA (World Medical Association, Inc.) (2000a): Documents WG/DoH, July 2000; 17.C/WW3/2000.

WMA (World Medical Association, Inc.) (2000b): The Declaration of Helsinki (revised version adopted 3 October, 2000 in Edinburgh), Bulletin of Medical Ethics, October 2000, pp. 8-11.

WMA (World Medical Association, Inc.) (2006): www.wma.net/e/ethicsunit/helsinki/htm, accessed 26 March 2006.

Youngner, S. J./Arnold, R. M./Schapiro, R. (eds.) (1999): The Definition of Death, Contemporary Controversies. Baltimore and London: Johns Hopkins University Press.

Dietrich von Engelhardt

The Historical and Philosophical Background of Ethics in Clinical Research

I. Introduction

In a time which is rich in opportunities and risks, and in which progress is fast, medicine and natural sciences play an important role. Modern society, with its emphasis on health and beauty, good or even eternal life, accepts and challenges these disciplines. Modern medicine offers society the prospect of new diagnostic and therapeutic technologies but, at the same time, produces feelings of unease and concerns about the potential and risks of modern biomedical research. This ambiguity and ambivalence of modern medicine and medical research deserve scholarly attention and analysis. This chapter will look at the historical and philosophical context of biomedical research ethics.

Basic principles of medical ethics existed in antiquity. The health and the wish of the patient or "salus aegroti suprema lex" and "voluntas aegroti suprema lex" characterised the different viewpoints up until the present time. The ethics of medical research has been grounded in the philosophy of medicine and in the nature of man; conversely, present day medical ethics or bioethics has its roots in European history.[1] These roots can be found not only in the natural sciences and in the various medical disciplines, but also in the arts and literature, theology and philosophy, and they are generally influenced by socio-economic conditions. Physicians and patients are a part of their culture and society; they depend, to a great extent, on the dominant concepts and social perception of health and disease.

The word "bioethics" has been used to propose a variety of norms which refer to the relationship between man and organic nature, to practices of biotechnology and medicine, to those of a religious-ethical nature, and norms relating to jurisprudence and philosophical ethics.[2]

The need for ethics in the field of medicine and in the relationship between man and nature is today indisputable. Its extent and direction, however, is the subject of diverse and sometimes controversial debates and interpretations that depend on the perspective of the patient and physician, and on the particular religious beliefs or philosophical convictions which are predominant in a given society. Medical ethics or ethics in medicine, in short, relates to particular situations in the life of species, like, for example, birth, illness, and death.

1   Beauchamp (1989), von Engelhardt (1997), Jonsen (1998), Frewer (2000), Bergdolt (2004).
2   Potter (1971), Reich (1995), Ach/Runtenberg (2002).

Ethics in medicine is not limited to the work of the physician but it also refers to the role of the patient, to his family and to society more generally. In this medico-ethical triangle, the doctor-patient relationship undoubtedly has a central significance. Each part of this triangle is linked, in one way or another, to the others and to itself; the patient is connected to other patients, to the doctor, to his family and to society; the physician is linked to the patient, to society, to medicine and to his colleagues; society is connected to the patient, to the physician, to social infrastructures and also to the society and people in other countries. Medical ethics is influenced by the theoretical and practical role of medicine and by different ideals and material factors: philosophy, theology, the arts, economy, laws and politics.[3]

Medical ethics has to be included in the broader perspective of "medical humanities"; the arts, literature and philosophy can provide a fruitful input into medicine, to the work of the doctor and to the patient, the family and the social and political environment. Medicine itself is a science ("scientia") and an art ("ars"), living with a disease and coping with death and dying can be regarded as a science as well as an art ("ars vivendi" and "ars moriendi" of former days).[4] Therefore, when reflecting this subject within the above context, the following issues are important considerations:

- The decisive beginning of medical research during the Renaissance.
- The central justification of medicine and research: understanding man and his position in the world.
- The consequences and implications of medical research: assisting the suffering of patients, overcoming diseases, relieving the process of dying.
- The dichotomy between basic research and applied research.
- The development of specific areas and conditions of research (diagnostics, therapy, common or rare diseases, objective evidence versus subjective judgments etc.).
- The issue of morally and legally informed consent of healthy and sick participants, and the ethics of the scientist and the participant in research.
- The issue of research with persons who are unable to give valid and informed consent.
- The scientific design, realisation, evaluation and publication of research findings.
- The examination of medical research through ethics committees.
- The cultural, scientific, and economical conditions that shape the formation of research standards and practice.

3   Pfetsch/Zloczower (1973), Engelhardt (1986), Beauchamp/Childress (1989), Rupke (1990), Wiesing et al. (2000).
4   Rainer (1957), Imhof (1991), von Engelhardt (1995).

II.   The historical background

For many centuries the history of medical ethics, or of ethics in medicine, was based on philosophy and theology. Research as experimental, statistical, and empirical research, with control and randomised groups, was not a characteristic of medicine and medical science in antiquity. Medicine had a tradition of its own and was a form of applied philosophy. The original unity of medicine, theology and law has largely disappeared in modern times, but it can sometimes be rediscovered in the diverse and most significant moments of medical theory and practice.

The Hippocratic Oath, ascribed to the Hippocratic school in the fifth or fourth century B.C., has been an essential part in medical ethics up until the present time. The Oath includes prohibitions against abortion, active euthanasia and stone surgery, addresses the duties of the physician and the role of confidentiality, the resistance to injustice, the moral respect for the patient, and the requirement to be devoted to the teaching of medicine and to keep medical knowledge confidential. Beneficence, non-maleficence, dignity and justice are the guiding principles of the oath, but not autonomy. Despite the fact that the Oath says nothing about human experimentation, its principles deserve respect and recognition in modern medical research.[5]

During antiquity, certainly not all doctors complied with the Hippocratic Oath; likewise today, the Oath no longer conforms in its entirety to the reality of medical research and practice, and with the self-understanding of physicians and patients. In the stoic tradition, for example, the doctor was allowed to actively help the patient in committing suicide when the rational awareness and moral behaviour of a person was hindered or impaired by physical or psychic disorders.

The *Corpus Hippocraticum*, of which the Oath is part, includes numerous passages which are concerned with medical ethics and etiquette, with medical prescriptions, and the ideal way of behaving, dressing, and talking by the doctor. The duty of the physician to inform the patient, which is not mentioned in the Hippocratic Oath, may have been less prescriptive in antiquity. Indeed, the physician was required to withhold an unpleasant prognosis from the patient.

Information and consent were thought essential by Plato and Aristotle, whose father was a physician: "no treatment is prescribed by the physician unless the patient has been convinced".[6] Renunciation of therapy was justified or extended to diseases which were fatal. There existed also an ethics of the patient. The doctor was permitted to expect active collaboration from the patient: "the sick person must fight against the disease together with the doctor".[7]

With regard to research, the famous hippocratic aphorism, which was to be accepted by the physician, the patient and his family, deserves attention today as well: "The art is long, the life is short, the right moment is hasty, the experiment is

5   Edelstein (1969), Lichtenthaeler (1984), Schubert (2005).
6   Plato (1977), p. 269 (=720d).
7   Müri (1938), p. 8.

deceptive, the decision is difficult."[8] The sentence has not lost much of its meaning in modern medicine and research, in particular within the context of evidence-based medicine.[9]

For antiquity, there are only few known examples of animal and human vivisections that were carried out by hellenistic physicians who justified these acts by arguing that one person is of less value than society and mankind as a whole.[10] It is one of those arguments which we find time and time again in the history of medical research and human experimentation, and which was criticised even then as a way to justify unethical medical conduct. One could mention here the research on poisons by King Mithridates Eupator (121-64 B.C.). Eupator used slaves and criminals for trials to find a protective drug because he feared that he might be poisoned. The so called "Antidotum Mithridaticum" (antidote of mithridatis) should generally help in all cases of poisoning.

During the medieval period, there existed no evidence-based, empirical research as we know it today, nor was it developed or recognised as being of importance at the time. Doctors and patients, sickness and therapy, were dominated by the religious belief system of the time and the idea of transcendence. The figure of Christ as a healer ("Christus medicus") stood behind every doctor, and behind every patient stood the figure of the suffering Christ ("passio Christi"). In contrast to modern concepts, sickness could be considered as being positive and good for one's health ("salubris infirmitas") and health as negative and harmful ("perniciosa sanitas").[11]

Throughout the medieval period, there was strict compliance with the Hippocratic Oath, and Asclepios was replaced by Christ. Assisting the sick and the dying was considered to be one of the basic duties of doctors, and their work did not end once they had cured a patient. The active ending or shortening of life was seen as a sin, and so was abortion. Sickness, pain and death, which were to be ultimately overcome by the final resurrection ("restitutio") in one's earthly life ("destitutio"), were seen as a consequence of having been banned from Paradise ("constitutio").

Therapy, in the sense of a truly effective cure, could not be achieved in one's earthly life. It did not merely consist of a cure, but included assistance as well. The Greco-Roman relation between health, beauty and morality was abandoned in the medieval period; every sick, suffering, or handicapped person had the right to receive medical treatment and care, and the individual person possessed an undeniable value.

The four cardinal virtues (prudence, justice, fortitude and temperance), and the three theological virtues (faith, hope and charity), were applied to the physician, to the patient and to society or the family and friends. Apart from the seven physical or corporal works of mercy, there existed the concept of the seven

8   Ibid.
9   Sackett et al. (1997), Perleth (1998).
10   Schelenz (1962), pp. 125-127, Ruisinger (2001).
11   Sudhoff (1914).

spiritual works of mercy, which required individuals to rebuke sinners, instruct the ignorant, counsel doubters, tolerate injustice, console the sad, and pray for the living and dead persons. These virtues and works of mercy were also of great importance in medical research and therapy (prudence, justice, charity, instruction, counsel, consolation etc.).

One of the few examples of medieval experimental research was carried out by Frederick II., who is said to have performed experiments e.g. with neonates in order to learn about the development of language in humans.[12] But these experiments were not typical for the time, and not an integral part of clinical research: The Arabian physician and philosopher Avicenna was another exception to the rule. He insisted that experiments had to be made with human beings, for "testing a drug on a lion or horse might not prove nothing about its effect on man".[13]

Research in the way in which we understand it today is only, or especially, a phenomenon and result of modern times: Vesal, Galilei, Harvey, Bacon, Descartes, and Haller are important figures in this development.[14] The conceptual separation of body and soul opened up the possibility for unrestricted medical research. Technical procedures were developed for the diagnosis and therapy of diseases; science and medicine were dominated by causal thinking, and integrated into scientific institutions which were established inside and outside the universities. Secularisation was conceived as the realisation of eternal life, youth and beauty during ones earthly existence. Man was considered as "maitre et possesseur de la nature."[15], his essential motto was "knowledge is power".[16]

Pico della Mirandola, a famous philosopher of humanism, defined the virtue of man (*De dignitate*, 1486) in a logic of production or secularised creation:

> "We have given to thee, Adam, no fixed seat, no form of thy very own, no gift peculiarly thine, that thou mayest feel as thine own, have as thine own, possess as thine own the seat, the form, the gifts which thou thyself shalt desire. A limited nature in other creatures is confined within the laws written down by Us. In conformity with thy free judgment, in whose hands I have placed thee, thou art confined by no bounds; and thou wilt fix limits of nature for thyself. I have placed thee at the center of the world, that from there thou mayest more conveniently look around and see whatsoever is in the world. Neither heavenly nor earthly, neither mortal nor immortal have We made thee. Thou, like a judge appointed for being honorable, art the molder and maker of thyself; thou mayest sculpt thyself into whatever shape thou dost prefer. Thou canst grow downward into the lower natures which are brutes. Thou canst again grow upward from thy soul's reason into the higher natures which are divine".[17]

The secularisation affected the interest in medicine and medical ethics in general. The involvement in science, technology and empirical research increased, whereas the dependency on theology, philosophy and the arts gradually diminished. Since the Renaissance, individuals from outside and inside the field of medicine and

---

12   Salimbene de Adam (1905-13), pp. 350-353; Stürner (2000), p. 449.
13   Tschanz (2003), p. 16.
14   Diemer (1975), von Engelhardt (1975), Gillispie (1981), Kuhn (1962), Ramon (1961).
15   Descartes (1637).
16   Bacon (1996 [1597]).
17   Pico della Mirandola (1985), pp. 4-5.

natural sciences responded and commented about the ethical implications of medical and scientific research. Famous and important examples of that time were the self experiments of Santorio Santorio, professor of theoretical medicine at the University of Padua, parmacological trials, and scurvy experiments by James Lind.[18]

Around 1800, in the period of German idealism and romanticism, the philosophical dimension of medicine reappeared. Writers such as Kant, Schelling and Hegel produced philosophical accounts about physical and mental disease, about the possibilities and limitations in restoring health, and about the autonomy of the individual and social morality. Many physicians and medical scientists based their thinking and behaviour on the spirit of these scholars.[19]

During the late 18th century, Kant introduced a specific concept of autonomy and responsibility, which still, in many ways, influences modern concepts of medical research and therapy. His "categorical imperative" from 1785 stressed the respect of each individual as an end in itself. He acknowledged that human beings use other humans for their own ends, quite apart from a fundamental respect for every individual, but pointed out that the end for which humans used humans could not be a selfish or casual one, but had to be one which was oriented towards humanity: "Act always so that you treat humanity, in your own person or another, never merely as a means but also at the same time as an end in itself".[20]

In the 19th century, a great number of studies on medical ethics appeared which contained very different views about natural science and medicine.[21] Some scholars discussed the ethics of experimenting with animals and men,[22] others debated the role and ethics of anaesthesia for painless childbirth; there were also some physicians who had difficulties in balancing their medical work with their religious beliefs. Many physicians were also engaged in self-experimentation.[23] 19th century physicians already made a distinction between clinical research, on the one hand, and experiments with healthy human subjects, on the other.[24]

At the end of the 19th century, Germany began to develop some of the most stringent and clearly defined medical ethics regulations. As early as 1891 the Prussian Ministry of the Interior issued a regulation that ensured that tuberculin would "in no case be used against the patients' will" for the treatment of tuberculosis. Three years later, in 1894, the German Supreme Court stressed that surgical and other potentially life-threatening treatments needed the consent of the patient. In 1900, the Prussian Ministry of Religious, Educational and Medical Affairs issued a legal directive that non-therapeutic interventions on humans were "absolutely prohibited" if the subject "has not declared unequivocally that he consents to the intervention" and if "the declaration has not been made on the

---

18   Winau (1971), Rupke (1990), Maehle (1999).
19   Poggi (2000), Riese (1976), Temkin (1950), Wiesing (1995).
20   Kant (1785), p. 61.
21   Brand (1977), Bergdolt (2004).
22   Von Engelhardt (1975), Tashiro (1991), Elkeles (1996).
23   Altman (1987), Karger-Decker (1975), Marchionini (1957).
24   Von Engelhardt (1975).

basis of a proper explanation of the adverse consequences that may result from the intervention".[25] The directive officially recognised the requirement for voluntary informed consent as "fundamental to ethically sound experimentation".

In March 1931, the Reich Health Council (*Reichsgesundheitsrat*) issued the Regulations Concerning New Therapy and Human Experimentation.[26] The directives were among the most comprehensive research rules by any standard at the time and some elements were even more elaborate than the principles of the Nuremberg Code. Contentious issues, such as individual autonomy, beneficence, informed voluntary consent or therapeutic and non-therapeutic research, were formulated to protect the rights and dignity of patients. In § 12, which is concerned with non-therapeutic research, the 1931 Reich Regulations stated that "experimentation shall be prohibited in all cases where consent has not been given".[27]

The history of modern medical ethics standards has to be integrated into a wider political and social history of medicine. The 20th century experienced the reign and the decline of two political systems and ideologies: Nazism and communism. With its eugenic programme and violation of human rights in experimental medical research, the Third Reich was a tragic period for medicine and medical science. In the field of racial hygiene and Nazi psychiatry, especially, medical ethics was denied any meaningful role and was subordinated to a particular racial and ideological vision.[28]

After the Second World War, the international medical community launched a great number of initiatives to expand the role of medical ethics in medicine and medical research. The definition of health by the World Health Organisation (WHO) in 1947, the resolutions of national and international medical organisations, such as the Helsinki Declaration from 1964, and the revised declaration from 1975, the creation of ethics committees for research and therapy, the establishment of academies for medical ethics and corresponding associations have all been part of this development. The Declaration of Helsinki has been revised many times, most recently in Tokyo 2004. Autonomy, justice, non-maleficence and beneficence are guiding principles, the safety of the research, insurance and data protection are important goals of this declaration. Apart from research ethics committees (institutional review boards), the field of medical and bioethics has seen, for example, the establishment and institutionalisation of clinical committees for therapy, of ethics committees in the pharmaceutical industry, and of ethics committees in medical organisations and associations.[29]

25   Preußisches Kulturministerium (1900), see Annas/Grodin (1992).
26   Reichsminister des Inneren (1931), see Sass (1983), Annas/Grodin (1992).
27   Reichsminister des Inneren (1931).
28   See the contribution by Ulf Schmidt in this book.
29   Levine (1986), Toellner (1990), Wiesing (2003).

III. Structure – Dimensions

Medical ethics is more than a set of basic principles to guide the conduct of medical research and practice; it is also a theory about the practical realisation of these ethical principles and obligations; biology, psychology and sociology should be taken into consideration, and the autonomy and freedom of the individual be respected.

Ethics and law are linked by overlapping areas of discourse. Within these fields of study, evidence can serve as empirical proof and as the material to make a judgement. Autonomy does not generally mean arbitrariness, but reasonable will in the moral sense of the word. The word "autonomy" itself derives from the words "autos" (self) and "nomos" (law). The realisation of ethical principles takes place in the world of emotions and social contacts. But ethics should be independent of biology, psychology and sociology. Kant rightly stressed that "empirical principles are nowhere meant to be the basis of human laws".[30] According to German law, medical scientists who perform experimental or therapeutic research without consent and full information risk being sued for bodily injury. The social interaction between the physician-scientists and the patient requires the former to inform the latter, and the latter to give consent. Medical research only becomes ethical through the principle of informed consent when physicians pay proper attention to the autonomy and dignity of the patient.

Today, there are many areas of discourse within this field of modern medical research which attract the attention of scientists and ethicists: preimplantation diagnosis or diagnosis of the pole body of the eggs, general reproductive medicine and predictive medicine, organ transplantation, xenotransplantation, intensive or emerging medicine, are all areas of debate which highlight ethical dilemmas.

The ethics of biomedical research also refers to the ethical conduct of the researcher and even the patient. The manipulation of scientific data, and in some cases the fraudulent behaviour of researchers in recent years has caused concern among health organisations and politicians as well as among national and international medical societies. There is a need for researchers to be virtuous; Arnold S. Relman, editor of *The New England Journal of Medicine*, noted in a 1983 editorial that there is no human activity other than medicine and medical research which depends so fundamentally on criticism and scepticism, and, at the same time, on trust.[31]

---

30 Kant (1785), p. 76.
31 Relman (1983), p. 1417.

Medical Morality and Medical Ethics

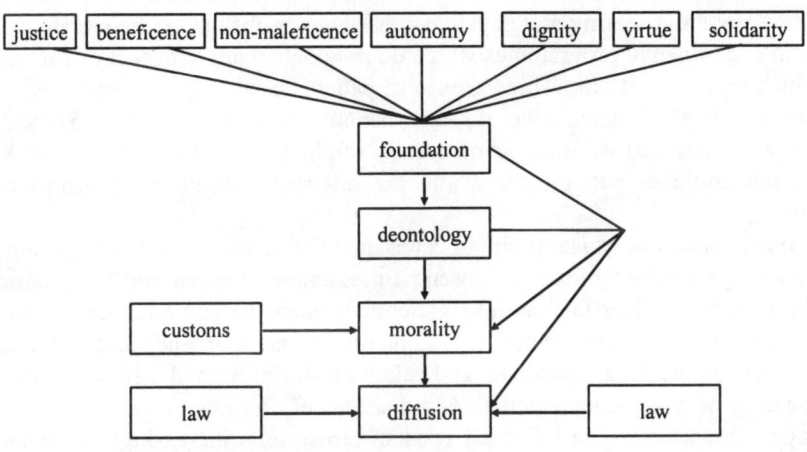

Figure 1: Medical Morality and Medical Ethics.

Structure of Medical Ethics

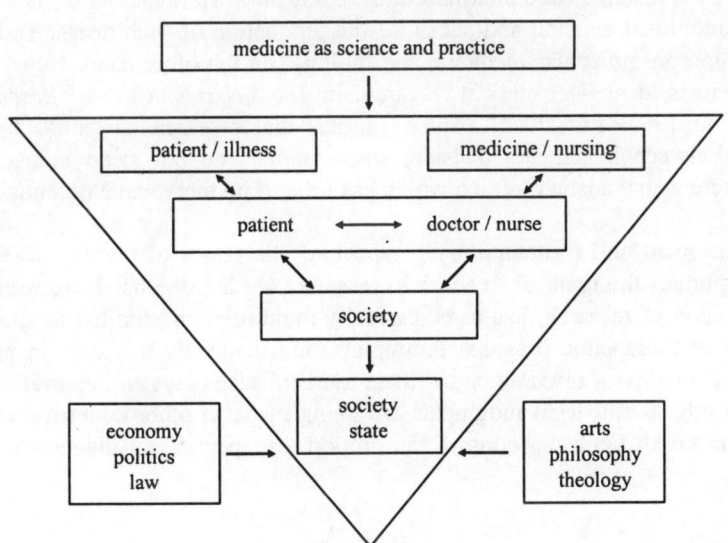

Figure 2: Structure of Medical Ethics.

The ethics of the patient is also an important part: his rights, his duties and his virtues. Some would go as far as to argue that the patient has a certain duty not to enter into a quasi-contractual research agreement without having been informed and having given consent. The patient has a right to refuse participation in human experiments without fearing any negative consequences for his treatment. He can enter into experimental programmes which do not contain any prospect of finding data which may benefit him. Three groups of patients need to be distinguished in this respect. First, patients who directly benefit from the research. Second, patients who, because of their involvement, might benefit from the research. Finally, the group of patients for whom the research contains no prospect of benefit.

Another important ethical problem is research that is carried out with persons who cannot give valid, informed consent, for example children and psychiatric patients, terminally ill or unconscious patients in intensive and emergency care, and, in some cases, elderly persons.[32] Contentious issues in such cases are as follows: the role of legal guardians and relatives, the presumed will, the living will, the issue of risk, personal benefit or at least benefit for other patients with the same age, disease, etc. The informed consent principle is increasingly accepted and recognised in a variety of medical specialities, for example in the field of paediatrics. If children do not consent to experimental research being carried out on them, then the decision has to be respected, unless, perhaps, the research is life-sustaining and therapeutic.[33]

Medical research has quite specific thematic orientations which depend on scientific, political and economic interests. Certain drugs, for example, are called orphan drugs. Given the limited profit potential of such drugs, they are often neglected by researchers and pharmaceutical companies. Here the State has a duty to create additional demand and subsidise the production of such drugs. Today's concentration on molecular medicine and biology, on the other hand, sometimes leads scientists to neglect clinical research. In *The Crisis in Clinical Research*, published in 1992, Edward H. Ahrens argues that researchers should find a "midway between bench and bedside, since animals do not sleep in beds".[34] Finally, there is diagnostic research which has little, if no therapeutic potential.

From a historical and contemporary perspective, the ethics of medical research also incorporates the issue of freedom in research. On the one hand, research, or the application of research, has to be carefully monitored and limited to specific diagnostic or therapeutic projects. Preimplantation diagnosis is a case in point. The internationality of research or "medical tourism" also plays an important role, given that ethical and legal judgments are being made in other countries which make it more difficult to control the import of specialised diagnostic and

32   Taupitz (1997), Maio (2001).
33   Burgio (1998 [1994]), Wiesemann et al. (2003).
34   Ahrens (1992), p. 236.

therapeutic procedures. On the other hand, research has to be free in order to benefit society in the future.

On the one hand, research or the application of research, – and it is known that in medicine research and therapy can not clearly or strictly be differentiated – has to be observed and limited. Preimplantation diagnosis is a good example. In this context one should discuss the internationality of research or "medical tourism" and the ethical and legal judgment and control of the import of diagnostic and therapeutical procedures which cannot be analysed or studied in one's own country.

On the other hand, research must be free – in the perspective of future benefits and especially in the perspective of better understanding man and nature. One has to accept that the progress of research cannot be totally foreseen and planned. The knowledge of nature and man and of his position in nature is the deepest justification of research and not only improving of man's life conditions. Research means freedom and rationality, modesty and pride; research has to acknowledge its limits and responsibility, but the ethics of the scientist also incorporates the defence of research and science in general against their enemies.

IV. Perspectives

Today's advances in medicine provide many new opportunities but also create many new ethical problems: artificial insemination, extra corporal fertilisation, prenatal diagnosis, gene therapy, the development of neonatology, etc. These developments raise the question of whether there is a need for new medical ethics standards. Certainly, there seems to be a need for ever new applications, ever new reflections on practice, and new judicial rules, but a new ethics does not seem to be necessary; many ethical principles of the past have not lost their importance and value in today's modern society.

Autonomy, dignity, integrity, and vulnerability as virtues seem essential from the historical and contemporary viewpoint. Autonomy, for example, is particularly relevant in the following areas: the explicit will of the patient, his supposed will, and the reasonable will of every man; dignity is important as far as the respect of the other is concerned and as an end in itself; integrity and vulnerability as beneficence and non-maleficence; virtue as man's capacity to realise ethical norms and moral obligations. Both the physician and the patient have rights and duties and can manifest virtues. One important factor in today's research and therapeutic practice is the exaggerated regard for legal liability issues. Physicians often make their decisions on the basis of legal considerations rather than on what is in the patients' best interest or what is needed in scientific research. The principle of informed consent is not in itself sufficient; what is needed is a certain understanding for the reality of the situation whether a person is ill or is dying, a process which transcends the logic of the law.

Given the various religious beliefs and ongoing changes in the political landscape, it is important to seek a minimum consensus as far as medical ethics is concerned. The ideals and experiences of the past can offer important lessons and guidance in this respect. Today's world is largely shaped by pluralism, but this must not necessarily mean that we renounce all theological or philosophical or metaphysical positions. On the contrary, it is important that universities and the media provide a platform for various ethical positions, and thus prepare physicians, patients and their families for the ethical dimensions and the corresponding needs and expectations.

A central need will be the development of a minimum consensus in medical ethics, whose violation would include potential legal consequences. The Declarations of Helsinki and Tokyo and all the subsequent versions were intended to provide such a minimum consensus. It can reasonably be argued that the progress in modern medicine in theory, therapy and research needs more than merely utilitarian, pragmatic and liberal principles, and their rather simplistic and positivistic solutions.

The history of medicine has witnessed many ethical problems, and medicine and medical progress have, at the same time, produced many new ones. The quest for a timeless and generally applicable set of ethical principles and standards in medicine and biology is repeatedly taken up by medical experts and philosophers. Despite the differences and divergences throughout the history of medicine, essential elements and fundamental principles such as dignity, autonomy, beneficence, non-maleficence, justice, virtue, freedom and responsibility have manifested themselves. It is probably a fair statement that mankind would not survive without medical and scientific research. But, at the same time, the law and medical ethics have to be respected. Research in medicine refers, after all, to human beings, to healthy and ill persons with a conscience and with language and social relationships.

The psychiatrist and philosopher Karl Jaspers defined the physician in the following way: "The doctor is neither a technician nor a saviour, but an existence for another existence, a transitory human being, who realised in the other, with the other and himself dignity and freedom, and recognises these principles as his rules".[35] This definition of the physician also applies to medical research.

---

35   Jaspers (1973 [1932]), p. 127.

References

Ach, J. S./Runtenberg, C. (2002): Bioethik: Disziplin und Diskurs. Zur Selbstauf-
klärung angewandter Ethik. Kultur der Medizin, Band 4. Frankfurt am Main,
New York: Campus.

Ahrens, E. H. (1992): The Crisis in Clinical Research. Overcoming Institutional
Obstacles. New York: Oxford University Press.

Altman, L. K. (1987): Who Goes First? The Story of Self-Experimentation in
Medicine. New York: Random House.

Annas, G. J./Grodin, M. A. (eds.) (1992): The Nazi Doctors and the Nuremberg
Code. Human Rights in Human Experimentation. New York, Oxford: Oxford
University Press.

Bacon, F. (1996 [1597]): Religious Meditations. Oxford: Oxford University Press.

Beauchamp, T. (1989): A History and Theory of Informed Consent. New York:
Oxford University Press.

Beauchamp, T./Childress, J. F. (1989): Principles of Biomedical Ethics. New
York: Oxford University Press.

Bergdolt, K. (2004): Das Gewissen der Medizin. Ärztliche Moral von der Antike
bis heute. München: Beck.

Brand, U. (1977): Ärztliche Ethik im 19. Jahrhundert. Freiburger Forschungen zur
Medizingeschichte, Neue Folge Band 5. Freiburg: Hans F. Schulz.

Brieger, G. H. (1982): Human Experimentation: History, in: Reich (1982.), pp.
684-692.

Burgio, G. R. (1998 [1994]): Primum Non Nocere Today, 2nd edn. Amsterdam:
Elsevier.

Diemer, A. (ed.) (1975): Konzeption und Begriff der Forschung in den Wissenschaften des 19. Jahrhunderts. Meisenheim am Glan: Anton Hain.

Descartes, R. (1995 [1637]): Discours de la Méthode. Paris: Flammarion.

Deutsch, E. (1999): The Protection of the Person in Medical Research in Germany, Medicine and Law 18 (1999), pp. 77-92.

Edelstein, L. (1969): Der Hippokratische Eid. Zürich: Artemis.

Elkeles, B. (1996): Der moralische Diskurs über das medizinische Menschenexperiment im 19. Jahrhundert. Stuttgart: G. Fischer.

Engelhardt, D. von (1975): Die Konzeption der Forschung in der Medizin des 19.
Jahrhunderts, in: Diemer (1975), pp. 58-103.

Engelhardt, D. von (ed.) (1997 [1989]): Ethik im Alltag der Medizin. Spektrum
der medizinischen Disziplinen, 2nd edn. Heidelberg: Springer.

Engelhardt, D. von (1995): Krankheit, Schmerz und Lebenskunst. München:
Beck.

Engelhardt, D. von (1997): Zur historischen Entwicklung der Ethik in der
Medizin. Prinzipien, Theorien, Methoden, in: Frewer/Winau (1997), pp. 37-
62.

Engelhardt, H. T. (1986): The Foundation of Bioethics. New York: Oxford University Press.

Frewer, A. (2000): Medizin und Moral in Weimarer Republik und Nationalsozialismus. Die Zeitschrift „Ethik" unter Emil Abderhalden. Frankfurt am Main, New York: Campus.

Frewer, A./Neumann, J. N. (eds.) (2001): Medizingeschichte und Medizinethik. Kontroversen und Begründungsansätze 1900-1950. Frankfurt am Main, New York: Campus.

Frewer, A./Winau, R. (eds.) (1997): Geschichte und Theorie der Ethik in der Medizin. Grundkurs Ethik in der Medizin, Band 1. Erlangen und Jena: Palm & Enke.

Galdston, I. (1946): The History of Research with Particular Regard to Medical Research, Ciba symposia 8 (1946), pp. 338-372.

Gillispie, C. C. (ed.) (1981): Dictionary of Scientific Biography. New York: Charles Scribners's Sons.

Grodin, M. A. (1994): Children as Research Subjects. New York: Oxford University Press.

Imhof, A. (1991): Ars Moriendi – Die Kunst des Sterbens. Köln: Böhlau.

Jaspers, K. (1973 [1932]): Ein Beispiel: ärztliche Therapie, in: Jaspers (1973), pp. 121-129.

Jaspers, K. (1973 [1932]): Philosophie, vol. 1, 4th edn. Berlin: Springer.

Jonsen, A. R. (1998): The Birth of Bioethics. Oxford, New York: Oxford University Press.

Kant, I. (1785): Grundlegung zur Metaphysik der Sitten. Riga: Hartknoch.

Kant, I. (1983): Grundlegung zur Metaphysik der Sitten, in: Werke, Bd. 6. Darmstadt: Wissenschaftliche Buchgesellschaft.

Karger-Decker, B. (1975): Ärzte im Selbstversuch. Ein Kapitel heroischer Medizin. Leipzig: Koehler & Amelang.

Kuhn, T. S. (1970 [1962]): The Structure of Scientific Revolutions, 2nd edn. Chicago: Chicago University Press.

Levine, R. (1986): Ethics and Regulation of Clinical Research, 2nd edn. Baltimore: Urban & Schwarzenberg.

Ley, A. (2001): Gewissenlos, Gewissenhaft: Menschenversuche im Konzentrationslager. Erlangen: Specht.

Lichtenthaeler, C. (1984): Der Eid des Hippokrates. Köln: Deutscher Ärzte-Verlag.

Loue, S. (1999): Textbook of Research Ethics. New York: Kluwer Academic.

Maehle, A.-H. (1999): Drugs on Trial. Experimental Pharmacology and Therapeutic Innovation in the Eighteenth Century. Amsterdam: Rodopi.

Maio, G. (2001): Zur Begründung einer Ethik der Forschung an nicht einwilligungsfähigen Patienten, Zeitschrift für Evangelische Ethik 45 (2001), pp. 135-148.

Marchionini, A. (1957): Selbstaufopferung im Dienste der praktischen und wissenschaftlichen Heilkunde. München: Hueber.

Müri, W. (1938): Der Arzt im Altertum. München: Heimeran.

Perleth, M. (ed.) (1998): Evidenz-basierte Medizin. München: Medizin-Verlag.

Pfetsch, F. R./Zloczower, A. (1973): Innovation und Widerstände in der Wissenschaft. Düsseldorf: Bertelsmann.

Pico della Mirandola, G. (1985): On the Dignity of Man. New York: Macmillan Publishing Company.

Plato: Nomoi. Gesetze (1977): Werke, vol. 8. Darmstadt: Wissenschaftliche Buchgesellschaft.

Poggi, S. (2000): Il genio e l'unità della natura. Bologna: Il Mulino.

Potter, Van R. (1971): Bioethics: Bridge to the Future. Englewood Cliffs, N.J.: Prentice-Hall.

Preußisches Kulturministerium (1900): [Regulations Concerning New Therapy and Human Experimentation], Centralblatt der gesamten Unterrichtsverwaltung in Preußen (1900), pp. 88-89.

Rainer, R. (1957): Ars moriendi. Von der Kunst des heilsamen Lebens und Sterbens. Köln: Böhlau.

Ramon, G. (1961): De la recherche scientifique en biologie et en médecine expérimentale hier et aujourd'hui, Biologie Médicale 50 (1961), pp. 1-26.

Reich, W. T. (ed.) (1982): Encyclopedia of Bioethics. New York, London: Free Press & Collier Macmillan.

Reich, W. T. (ed.) (1995 [1978]): Encyclopedia of Bioethics, vols. 1–5, 2nd edn. New York, London: Simon & Schuster Macmillan.

Reichsminister des Inneren (1931): Reichsrichtlinien zur Forschung am Menschen, Reichsgesundheitsblatt 6(1931), 55, pp. 174-175.

Reiser, S. J./Dyck, A. J./Curran, W. J. (eds.) (1977): Ethics in Medicine. Historical Perspectives and Contemporary Concerns. Cambridge, MA: MIT Press.

Relman, A. S. (1983): Lessons from the Darsee Affair, The New England Journal of Medicine 308 (1983), pp. 1415-1417.

Riese, G. B. (1976): "Philosophical" Medicine in Nineteenth-Century Germany: An Episode in the Relations between Philosophy and Medicine, Journal of Medicine and Philosophy 1 (1976), pp. 72-91.

Roelcke, V./Maio, G. (eds.) (2004): Twentieth Century Research Ethics: Historical Perspectives on Values, Practices and Regulations. Stuttgart: Steiner.

Ruisinger, M. M. (2001): Von Herophilos bis zum „Lübecker Totentanz". Anmerkungen zur Geschichte des Menschenversuchs, in: Ley (2001), pp. 10-34.

Rupke, N. A. (1990): Vivisection in Historical Perspective. London: Routledge.

Sackett, D. L./Richardson, W. S./Rosenberg, W./Haynes R. B. (1997): Evidence-Based Medicine: How to Practice and Teach EBM. New York: Churchill Livingstone.

Salimbene de Adam (1905-1913): Cronica, O. Holder-Egger (ed.), part 1-3. Hannover: Hahn

Sass, H.-M. (1983): Reichsrundschreiben 1931: Pre-Nuremberg German Regulations Concerning New Therapy and Human Experimentation, The Journal of Medicine and Philosophy 8 (1983), 2, pp. 99-111.

Schelenz, H. (1962): Geschichte der Pharmazie. Hildesheim: Olms. [Unveränderter reprografischer Nachdruck der Ausgabe Berlin 1904].

Schubert, C. (2005): Der hippokratische Eid: Medizin und Ethik von der Antike bis heute. Darmstadt: Wissenschaftliche Buchgesellschaft.

Smith, T. (ed.) (1999): Ethics in Medical Research. A Handbook of Good Practice. Cambridge: Cambridge University Press.

Stürner, W. (1992, 2000): Friedrich II, part 1-2. Darmstadt: Wissenschaftliche Buchgesellschaft.

Sudhoff, K. (1914): Eine Verteidigung der Heilkunde aus den Zeiten der "Mönchsmedizin", Sudhoffs Archiv 7 (1914), pp. 223-237.

Tashiro, E. (1991): Die Waage der Venus. Venerologische Versuche am Menschen am Menschen in der Zeit von 1885 und 1914. Husum: Mathiesen.

Taupitz, J./Fröhlich, U. (1997): Medizinische Forschung mit nichteinwilligungsfähigen Personen, Versicherungsrecht 22 (1997), pp. 911-918.

Temkin, O. (1950): Concepts of Ontogeny and History in Germany around 1800, Bulletin of the History of Medicine 224 (1950), pp. 227-246.

Toellner, R. (ed.) (1990): Die Ethik-Kommission in der Medizin. Stuttgart: Fischer.

Toellner, R./Wiesing, U. (eds.) (1997): Geschichte und Ethik in der Medizin. Von den Schwierigkeiten einer Kooperation. Stuttgart: Gustav Fischer.

Tschanz, D. W. (2003): A Short History of Islamic Pharmacy, Journal of the International Society for the History of Islamic Medicine 2 (2003), 1, pp. 11-17.

Wiesemann, C./Frewer, A. (eds.) (1996): Medizin und Ethik im Zeichen von Auschwitz – 50 Jahre Nürnberger Ärzteprozeß. Erlanger Studien zur Ethik in der Medizin, Band 5. Erlangen, Jena: Palm & Enke.

Wiesemann, C./Dörries, A./Wolfslast, G./Simon, A. (eds.) (2003): Das Kind als Patient. Ethische Konflikte zwischen Kindeswohl und Kindeswille. Kultur der Medizin, Band 7. Frankfurt am Main, New York: Campus.

Wiesing, U. (1995): Kunst oder Wissenschaft? Konzeptionen der Medizin in der deutschen Romantik. Stuttgart: frommann-holzboog.

Wiesing, U. (ed.) (2003): Die Ethik-Kommissionen. Neuere Entwicklungen und Richtlinien. Köln: Deutscher Ärzte-Verlag.

Wiesing, U./Simon, A./Engelhardt, D. von (eds.) (2000): Ethik in der medizinischen Forschung. Stuttgart: Schattauer.

Winau, R. (1971): Experimentelle Pharmakologie und Toxikologie im 18. Jahrhundert. Mainz, Habil.-Schr. [Maschinenschriftlich].

Winau, R. (1996): Medizin und Menschenversuch. Zur Geschichte des "informed consent", in: Wiesemann/Frewer (1996), pp. 13-29.

Ulf Schmidt

The Nuremberg Doctors' Trial and the Nuremberg Code

I. Introduction

Following the Second World War, the Allies decided to prosecute a number of doctors and scientist who were involved in Nazi medical atrocities. The Doctors' Trial, which lasted from December 1946 to August 1947, was the first of twelve subsequent American military tribunals. As an immediate reaction to Nazi medical crimes, and in order to distinguish between criminal physical injury, on the one hand, and permissible research on humans, on the other, the Nuremberg judges established a catalogue of ten principles which would protect the rights of experimental subjects and other vulnerable groups in the future. These principles are laid down in the so-called Nuremberg Code.[1] The aim of the Code was to find a solution to resolve one of the most fundamental conflicts in human experimentation: to balance the need for the advancement of medical science for the benefit of human society with the right of the individual to personal inviolability, autonomy and self-determination.

The judges in the Nazi Doctors' trial were all American nationals. The trial was nonetheless based on international law which had been outlined in the "London Agreement on the Punishment of the Major War Criminals of the European Axis" in 1945. This meant that the judgement – and thus the Code – was *de jure* international in character. The decision to include the Code into the judgement meant that, for the first time, written guidelines for permissible research on humans were incorporated into the canon of international law, although, in practice, the world medical community largely ignored the legal nature of the Code, stressing and criticising instead its relevance for modern medical ethics.[2] The Nuremberg Code was clearly the first international medical ethics code.

---

1   For a discussions about the origin, authorship and legacy of the Nuremberg Code see Annas/ Grodin (1992), Drinan (1992), Grodin (1992), Macklin (1992), Perley et al. (1992), Katz (1996), Maio (1996), Moreno (1996), United States Advisory Committee on Human Radiation Experiments (1996), Arnold/Sprumont (1997), Deutsch (1997), Katz (1997), Moreno (1997), Shuster (1997), Annas/Grodin (1998), Shevell (1998), Shuster (1998), Proctor (2000), Schmidt (2001b), Schmidt (2004).
2   Arnold/Sprumont (1997).

II. The Road to Nuremberg

Since the days of preparing the International Military Tribunal (IMT) the question
had arisen of whether the Four Powers should mount a second or even a third
international trial. During the London Conference in the summer of 1945 the issue
had appeared and reappeared when lists of potential defendants were produced
and discussed. Those standing on a separate list were likely candidates for a
second international trial, and the Charter later took due notice of this intention.[3]
The French and the Russians, in particular, pushed for a series of Nuremberg
Tribunals in parallel sessions. While the prosecutors were preparing one case for
trial, it was thought, they could prepare the evidence for a second. Defendants in
the second Tribunal were likely to include either further generals or, more probable, a trial against German industrialists and financiers for supporting and bene-
fiting from Germany's aggressive war. Robert Jackson, the United States Chief of
Counsel, opposed this approach and refused to commit the United States to a
second international trial, arguing that it was first necessary to see whether the
first trial could be successfully completed.[4] From the start the insistence by the
French and the Russians for more than one trial was essential in mounting the
subsequent Nuremberg proceedings. Ironically neither country would later be
party to them.[5]

One month after the formal opening of the IMT in November 1945, the Allied
Control Council in charge of overseeing Germany's occupation passed Control
Council Law No. 10 which introduced a uniform legal basis for the prosecution of
war criminals other than those dealt with by the IMT.[6] Law No. 10 provided the
legal framework for all subsequent military trials. Article III granted each of the
major Allies the right to try war criminals in their zone of occupation before an
appropriate tribunal. The law also allowed for the provision, if authorised by the
occupying authorities, that German courts could deal with crimes committed by
German nationals against German nationals or stateless persons. During the
Doctors' Trial, the latter part of the law became a major sticking point in the
debate on whether or not the prosecution should pursue "euthanasia" which had
been aimed at and conducted mostly on German nationals.[7]

Law No. 10 was in large parts based on broad precedents in terms of both
German criminal law and international laws and treaties, of which Germany had
been a signatory. It reflected the attempt by Allied legislators to prosecute and
punish German war criminals according to the nation's own existing law, and thus
counter from the start the charge that the tribunals stood in violation of the *ex post*

---

3   NDT-Records, London Charter, 8 August 1945.
4   NARA, RG 153/84-1, box 1, folder 2, Jackson to Patterson, 7 February 1946.
5   Tusa/Tusa (1995), p. 93, p. 138; for the position of the French and the Russians see NARA,
     RG 153/84-1, box 1, folder 2, Taylor to Petersen, 22 May 1946. The French were permitted
     to send trial observers to Nuremberg, but no French attorneys were allowed on the
     prosecution team; Weindling (2000b), p. 381.
6   Trials of War Criminals, vol. I, pp. XVI-XX; also Annas/Grodin (1992), pp. 317-321.
7   See also Weindling (2001b), pp. 311-333.

facto principle or that the proceedings were nothing but "victor's justice". Although international law had previously not codified specific war crimes, most of the offences with which the defendants were charged were illegal under German criminal law. The crimes specified in the London Charter and in Law No. 10 for the most part repeated the 1907 Hague Regulation on Warfare, which Germany had signed. Germany was also signatory to the Kellogg-Briand Pact of 1928, which condemned aggressive wars, and had signed the Geneva Convention a year later which laid out the rules for the protection of prisoners of war. It was in the tradition of staying close to existing German laws and regulations that the legal and medical experts of the US prosecution, like Leo Alexander, later drafted some of the elements of the Nuremberg Code. They wanted to show that almost all of the offences were not only crimes according to German law, but that the doctors had violated their own professional codes of conduct.

Although Law No. 10 obviated the necessity for a second international trial, several attempts were made to establish another four-power trial, some less half-hearted than others.[8] For the most part, a second IMT was lacking political support from the national governments which perceived Nuremberg as an increasingly antagonistic institution in the rapidly cooling climate between the four Allies. The planning of further trials in the American zone got under way with the establishment of the Subsequent Proceedings Division in the Office of Chief of Counsel for the Prosecution of Axis Criminality. Whereas a case against German finance and industry had encountered great obstacles from the start, a trial against the major medical perpetrators became all the more likely. A good deal of expertise had also been gathered in previous trials involving medical murder. From September to November 1945 the British had staged the Bergen-Belsen trial, and in March 1946 they had tried Bruno Tesch for his role in supplying Zyklon B to the concentration camps. From 18 March to 3 May 1946 the British had also established the first of a series of war crimes trials in the Curio-Haus in Hamburg, mostly against the guards and personnel of the Neuengamme concentration camp. In the course of the trial it became apparent that Nazi physicians had carried out tuberculosis experiments. Since the beginning of 1946, British prosecutors were also preparing a trial against the staff of the Ravensbrück concentration camp which included the indictment of key medical personnel from the nearby SS sanatorium in Hohenlychen. Finally, the IMT had drawn attention to the fact that a large number of doctors appeared to have been involved in crimes against humanity.

During the IMT a certain amount of evidence appeared to implicate Göring as the head of the German Air Force in the Dachau high-altitude research. When Göring called Field Marshall Milch as a defence witness, the prosecution realised that Milch was implicated more heavily than Göring.[9] Later in the trial, chance played once again into the hands of the prosecution. During the cross-examination of Wolfgang Sievers, the official of the SS-Ahnenerbe (Ancestral Heritage)

8   NDT-Records, fish 289 and 290, frames 460-560.
9   Taylor (1976), pp. 4-7.

Society who had been called as a witness to speak on behalf of the SS as an organisation, the British prosecuting lawyer, Lord Elwyn-Jones, produced the most damning documents which implicated Sievers in the "Jewish Skeleton Collection". This was a collection of heads and bodies of murdered Jews, compiled by the anatomist August Hirt at the Reich University of Strasbourg for anthropological purposes.[10] Both incidents shifted the attention of the prosecution to explore this area more closely and assess whether there was a systematic approach to the crimes. A trial against doctors appeared feasible from the American perspective, since many of the persons implicated in the crimes were in either British or American custody. A trial against German physicians was also seen as a means to re-educate and denazify German society.

Experts not officially charged with war crimes policies, like the representatives of FIAT (Field Information Agency, Technical), had also come across evidence that experiments on living humans had been performed under barbaric conditions. To explore this material further, however, was outside the agencies' jurisdiction. On 15 May 1946, nine British, four American and two French representatives of FIAT met for the first time at Hoechst in Wiesbaden to discuss how the material should be handled. No Russian representative had been invited. Among those present were the Canadian medical officer and wing commander John W. R. Thompson, the British forensic pathologists Sidney Smith and Keith Mant, as well as the bacteriologist Pierre Lépine from the Institute Pasteur in Paris. The meeting was chaired by the British Brigadier R. J. Maunsell, intelligence expert and head of the British section of FIAT. The conference attempted to co-ordinate the different war crimes branches and agencies whose responsibility was limited to the economic, technical and scientific exploitation of Germany. Although Britain and France disagreed over the extent to which medical war crimes should be morally condemned – with France wanting to condemn them more widely and more strongly – both nations agreed that further investigations should be undertaken by scientifically qualified experts.

As a result of the conference it was recommended that a four-power commission for the investigation of medical war crimes should be established which would involve both medical and legal experts. The proposal became the basis for an International Scientific Commission (for the Investigation of War Crimes of a Medical Nature), in short ISC (WC).[11] Although the meetings were important as far as discussions about the ethics of medical research on humans was concerned, the FIAT conferences and the ISC (WC) had almost no political weight.[12] For the Americans it was and remained a side-show, especially after August 1946, when the Doctors' Trial began to take shape. They were hardly interested in letting the initiative pass over to the French or the British once they had decided that they were going to prosecute German doctors in one of the Nuremberg trials. The Americans were also unimpressed by the unprofessional handling of witness

---

10   Taylor (1976), p. 4, Klee (1997), pp. 356-360.
11   NDT-Documents and Material, frames 460-525.
12   For a discussion about the importance of the meetings, see Schmidt (2004), pp. 124f.

testimonies by men like Mant. On 26 October 1946, Alexander G. Hardy told James McHaney, chief prosecutor in the medical case, that his "opinion of Major Mant's work is not too good" and that one could "readily see from reading his report on the Ravensbrück case that our hope of obtaining any real evidence from this source is dark".[13] The performance of the French was not much better, and by October the Americans thought that the French did not have much to contribute to the Doctors' Trial.[14] Yet the office of Telford Taylor, Jackson's successor as Chief of Counsel, monitored the activities by British and French war crimes experts, mainly because the British had amassed a considerable amount of incriminating evidence. Whether it could be used in a court of law was another matter. Most of the potential defendants were also in British custody which made continued collaboration necessary.

In mid-August 1946, it became clear that President Truman wanted to take an executive decision about the subsequent Nuremberg trials.[15] On 17 August, Taylor therefore proposed to the War Department that they establish six courts which would prosecute the representatives of certain segments of the German society in an expeditious fashion, including German physicians involved in medical murder. The proposed starting date for the first of the trials was 15 October 1946.[16] The original plan to mount eighteen zonal trials in the six courts in Nuremberg was later reduced to twelve; it involved the prosecution of representatives of the judiciary, of I.G. Farben, the *Einsatzgruppen*, the ministries and the German High Command. As a matter of expediency, the prosecution decided that a trial against German doctors was most likely to succeed, given the available incriminating evidence, and that it therefore was to become the first of the trials. Overall, the establishment of the Doctors' Trial was a matter of high politics decided by the US Office of Chief of Counsel for War Crimes in close coordination with Washington.

At the end of October 1946, the United States indicted twenty German doctors and three bureaucrats with war crimes and crimes against humanity. The indictment was issued only four weeks after the conclusion of the IMT and only one week after the Office of Military Governor of the United States (OMGUS) had issued the Ordinance No. 7, which gave American military tribunals the power to prosecute those indicted under Law No. 10. The Americans thereby signalled that they would go ahead with the establishment of the first of the subsequent Nuremberg proceedings, the Doctors' Trial.[17] All twelve subsequent

---

13 BAK, ZSg 154, box 72, Conference of International Commission on Investigation of War Crimes of a Medical Nature, Hardy to McHaney, 26 October 1946.
14 Ibid.
15 NARA, RG 153/85-1, box 2, folder 1, Jackson to Taylor, 16 August 1946.
16 NARA, RG 153/85-1, box 2, folder 1, Taylor to War Department, 17 August 1946.
17 The National Archives, London (TNA), WO309, file 468. On 6 September 1946 the British War Office informed the United Nations War Crimes Commission (UNWCC) about the plan by the United States to mount a trial against German doctors. The United States proposed that the trial should either be held by Anglo-American Military Government Courts under Law No. 10, or by American Military Courts in the American zone.

Nuremberg trials, which involved a total of 184 defendants, were to become American trials rather than four-power trials.[18]

III.   Planning the Prosecution

On 17 July 1946, one of Americas most distinguished medical scientists, the "conscience of US science", as some would call him, left Chicago to travel to Washington D.C. There he leafed through the files of the War Department on German medical war crimes for a couple of days before taking off for Wiesbaden, Germany, where he arrived on 27 July for what was originally designed as a fact-finding mission for the Secretary of War. Yet his involvement was to become crucial in the prosecution of Nazi physicians. The man who had left Chicago to advise the Nuremberg prosecution on its forthcoming medical case was Andrew Ivy, vice president of the University of Illinois, a respected professor of physiology and newly appointed Special Consultant to the Secretary of War.[19] Ivy's trip to Germany and France, which lasted from 18 July to 12 August 1946, shaped the strategy of the prosecution. His recommendations also ensured the recruiting of a German-speaking medical expert, limiting the potential damage to Allied – especially American – medical science, and called for written medical ethics guidelines on human experimentation.[20] Ivy's role, like that of Alexander, was central to the origins of the Nuremberg Code.

Throughout 1946, American attorneys had conducted preliminary investigations about the character of German experimentation. They wanted to know whether the experiments had really been necessary, adequately designed and carried out, and whether they had produced any valuable results. Since many of the experimental victims had allegedly been condemned to death, they feared that the use of such prisoners in human experiments could legally be sanctioned. If this was the case, it was likely to cause significant legal problems in the trial. Taylor's office had also received intelligence that American researchers had performed experiments on themselves and on human subjects during the war and thereafter. Of particular concern to the prosecution were a series of malaria experiments which had been conducted on hundreds of American prison inmates, reported in *Life* magazine in June 1945.[21] It also turned out that the British forces were

18   Annas/Grodin (1992), Taylor (1992), p. 611.
19   For Ivy's appointment, see Weindling (2000b), p. 376.
20   I am grateful to Michael Grodin, Boston University, for supplying me with a complete copy of Ivy's reports as a Consultant to the Secretary of War. It consists of three parts. Part One: A Report on War Crimes of a Medical Nature Committed in Germany and Elsewhere on German Nationals and the Nationals of Occupied Countries by the Nazi Regime During World War II, 26 Bl. + Appendix A on Rules for Animal Experimentation. Part Two: A Report on the Paris Meeting (31 July 1946) of the Representatives of the American, British and French Governments to Consider the War Crimes of a Medical Nature. Part Three: An Outline of the Itinerary. All three parts can also be found in NARA, RG 153/86-3-1, box 11, folder 4, book 3.
21   Anonymous (1945), pp. 43-46.

supporting Robert Alexander McCance (1898-1993) from the British Medical Research Council in carrying out experiments on infants suffering from meningomyelocele, a birth defect that is commonly known as spina bifida. McCance had asked the authorities "to make some tests on these children, which will not in their experience do them any harm, but which they do not feel quite justified in carrying out on perfectly healthy children".[22] These cases raised the question whether American and perhaps British researchers were likewise guilty of professional misconduct, and if not, why not. It appears that neither the prosecution nor the judges nor anyone else involved in establishing the trial had a clear idea at this point what the main legal and ethical issues were which the trial needed to address. "If we had been able to do it over again three years later", Taylor mused in 1976, "we would have done it in a much more sophisticated way ... with greater awareness of the implications of the positions we were taking".[23] Upon his arrival in Germany, Ivy found that the prosecution appeared to be "somewhat confused" about the legal, ethical and scientific dimensions in the forthcoming trial.[24] Taylor put it more diplomatically: "We were educated in large part by our opponents".[25]

For the experts who assisted the judges in formulating the Nuremberg Code, there was no question but that research on humans which involved risks to the subject could only be carried out on volunteers and only after informed voluntary consent had been obtained. During an inter-Allied conference in the summer of 1946 in Paris, Ivy laid down some of the "Principles and Rules of Experimentation on Human Subjects" which he saw as essential. He listed three principles:

"I. Consent of the subject is required; i.e., only volunteers should be used.
(a) The volunteers before giving their consent should be told of the hazards, if any.
(b) Insurance against an accident should be provided, if it is possible to secure it.
II. The experiment to be performed should be so designed and based on the results of animal experimentation that the anticipated results will justify the performance of the experiment; that is, the experiment must be useful and be such as to yield results for the good of society.
III. The experiment should be conducted
(a) so as to avoid unnecessary physical and mental suffering and injury, and
(b) by scientifically qualified persons.
(c) the experiment should not be conducted if there is [an] a priori reason to believe that death or disabling injury will occur".[26]

The requirements were far from specific. There was no mention of what "consent" meant, how it would be obtained and by whom, or what kind of information the subject was entitled to receive. There was also no reference to vulnerable groups

22   Quoted from Moreno (1999), p. 67.
23   Taylor (1976), p. 6; see also Moreno (1997), p. 348.
24   UWAHC, Andrew C. Ivy Papers (#8768), Box 6, Folder 12, Andrew Ivy, "Nazi War Crimes of a Medical Nature", talk presented to the Federation of State Medical Boards, Chicago, 10 February 1947; see also Ivy (1947) and Ivy (1948), pp. 5ff.
25   Taylor (1976), p. 6.
26   Andrew Ivy, A Report on the Paris Meeting (31 July 1946), Appendix D, in: NARA, RG 153/86-3-1, box 11, Folder 4, book 3; also Ivy (1947), pp. 133-146.

like the mentally handicapped and children, nor did the rules explain what "for the good of society" actually meant. Whilst claiming that the principles applied "in all countries of the world" which had contributed to the "progress of medical science" in the past, Ivy had kept them deliberately vague in order to allow room for interpretation for medical scientists in the future, a tendency which can be observed in subsequent medical ethics codes, including the Declaration of Helsinki.

On his return to the United States, Ivy submitted a comprehensive report which included his three ethics rules to the American Medical Association (AMA) Board of Trustees. These "inadequate" guidelines, as Jay Katz has called them, were subsequently adopted in a shortened and significantly modified form by the AMA House of Delegates on 10 December 1946, one day after the opening of the Doctors' Trial.[27] Ivy had probably realised that any future expert testimony by the prosecution would be strengthened if the witness could refer to some written, and indeed published, medical ethics rules. Ivy's ethics rules were written in anticipation of his own role as an expert witness in the Trial, something he only admitted during cross-examination by the defence.[28]

On 25 October 1946, the Chief of Counsel for War Crimes filed the indictment against the defendants in the Doctors' Trial. On 5 November the indictment was served to the defendants, giving them thirty days to prepare their defence.[29] It listed the accused according to the position that they had held in the Nazi medical hierarchy. The defendants were charged with a common design or conspiracy, with war crimes, crimes against humanity and membership of an organisation declared criminal by the IMT, particularly with criminal experiments in the concentration camps of Dachau, Sachsenhausen, Natzweiler, Ravensbrück, Buchenwald and others. In the course of the experiments hundreds of inmates had experienced extreme suffering, torture and death. Some experiments were carried out in order to study the limits of human endurance at extremely high altitudes, others to find an effective rewarming method for persons suffering from severe hypothermia. Malaria and mustard gas experiments had been performed to develop effective new treatments, sulphonamide drug experiments at the concentration camp of Ravensbrück to test the effectiveness of that drug, to name but a few.[30] Several of the defendants were also charged with murder, torture and maltreatment of people that were not related to medical experiments, for example with the 'euthanasia' programme. All of the twenty-three defendants pleaded not guilty to the crimes they were charged with, yet were soon about to come face to

27 Report of Reference Committee on Miscellaneous Business, Journal of the American Medical Association, 133 (1946), 33. The AMA guidelines stated: "In order to conform to the ethics of the AMA three requirements must be satisfied: (1) The voluntary consent of the person on whom the experiment is to be performed must be obtained; (2) the danger of each experiment must be previously investigated by animal experimentation; and (3) the experiment must be performed under proper medical protection and management", see Katz (1996), pp. 1663f.
28 Ibid.
29 NARA, RG 153/87-2, book2, box 14, Beals to Gunn, 21 November 1946.
30 United Nations War Crimes Commission (1948), p. 333.

face with the four men who had been seconded to Nuremberg to pass judgement on them.

Information about the judges in the subsequent Nuremberg trials is relatively scarce, particularly in the Doctors' Trial. Yet we know a little bit about the recruitment process. In August 1947, officials from the War Department noted that "the judges for the Zonal trials should be so far as possible of standing and prestige equal to that of the Nuremberg judges" and that therefore the selection process would "require exceptional care and review by the most responsible authorities in the department".[31] The recruitment of the judges was coordinated in the war crimes branch of the War Department. Legal consultants were delegated to "tour the country to interview persons who are selected as the judges whom the Secretary of War would like to nominate".[32] High ranking military persons, circuit and district court judges, state court judges and experts working in the judicial field such as "members of the bar and law school professors of high standing" were potential candidates. The law schools of Michigan, Chicago, California and Texas were regarded as the best places to recruit able judges. The lawyer Charles Horsky was appointed by the Secretary of War as an unpaid emissary to select and interview shortlisted candidates.[33] The War Department proposed its candidates to General Lucius Clay, who conferred with the Office of Chief of Counsel and the Legal Division of OMGUS.[34]

Almost all of the judges took up their Nuremberg appointments under considerable cost, both personally and professionally. Their own knowledge of the historic nature of the Tribunal, with its potential implications for the creation of new international law, found little support from legal colleagues in the United States. The American public was also beginning to lose interest in controversial military trials. Some federal judges were openly critical about the trials and questioned the underlying rationale of the war crimes programme. The appointment of the judges in the Doctors' Trial was eventually confirmed by executive order No. 9813, signed by President Truman on 20 December 1946.[35]

Since Jackson left Nuremberg the prosecution was under enormous time pressure. The Doctors' Trial was "an improvised affair", as Taylor later put it, neither carefully prepared nor thought-through.[36] Throughout the summer of 1946, Taylor tried to improve the quality of his legal staff, most of whom he regarded as ill-qualified. The Army's ban on bringing spouses to Nuremberg made it difficult to recruit the most able legal brains, and this rule was progressively loosened. As late as September 1946, Taylor complained to the Assistant Secretary of War that

31 NARA, RG 153/87-2, book3, box 14, Memorandum for Petersen, 5 August 1946; also book 1, box 13, Memorandum for Gunn, 7 August 1946.
32 NARA, RG 153/87-2, book 1, box 13, Memorandum for Gunn, 7 August 1946.
33 NARA, RG 153/87-2, book 1, box 13, Memorandum for Mr Petersen, Assistant Secretary of War, 21 August 1946.
34 See also NARA, RG 153/84-1, box 1, folder 3, Taylor to Petersen, 30 September 1946.
35 SCHST, Sebring papers, Clay to Sebring, 25 October 1946, Patterson to Sebring, 28 November 1946; Executive Order No. 9813, signed by President Harry S. Truman, 20 December 1946. For the appointment of the judges in the Doctors' Trial see Schmidt (2004), pp. 141ff.
36 Taylor (1976), p. 6; see also Marrus (1999), p. 110.

"with few exceptions" his men were "utterly vacuous political hacks. They are of no earthly use to us and if they aren't very unhappy already they are going to be very shortly".[37] Others were total eccentrics who thought they could sort out the war crimes cases in no time but literally fled from Nuremberg once they realised that it would involve a lot of work.[38] Taylor also desperately needed intelligent "German-speaking research people" who could organise and interpret the mass of incriminating evidence.[39] Even so, the number of Taylor's staff was impressive. Compared to the small working legal team of the British prosecution at the IMT headed by Sir Hartley Shawcross, the Americans favoured quantity rather than quality. From May to July 1946, Taylor's staff increased from 25 attorneys to 113. By the end of October, his team amounted to more than 400 American and Allied attorneys, interrogators, investigators and special agents of the Office of Chief of Counsel for War Crimes (OCCWC).[40] "The need for speed is the basic justification for employing a large staff to do this job", Taylor told Jackson.[41] In total the Americans employed a staff of 1,776 people. Officials in Washington were nonetheless aware of the lack of legal and medical expertise in Nuremberg which increased the potential pitfalls in the case against the doctors.[42]

At the beginning of November 1946, Taylor cabled to the War Department that he needed an

> "extensive paper on the history of medical experimentation on living human beings with particular emphasis on practice in US. Defendant Rose states that US doctors have extensively experimented on inmates of penal institutions and asylums, especially with malaria. Any truth in this? If so give us full facts".[43]

Taylor suggested to contact Ivy at the University of Illinois for further information whilst urging the military to fully explore this question, knowing that it was of vital importance in the forthcoming trial. In an encoded message from 16 November the War Department told Taylor that Ivy would be able to visit Nuremberg at the beginning of the trial and furnish the prosecution with all the necessary material about the history of human experimentation. The War Department had also recruited Morris Fishbein, editor of the *Journal of the American Medical Association* (JAMA), to support the Nuremberg staff. The material shows that a great amount of background work was being conducted behind the scenes by the American military authorities to ensure that German doctors would be held accountable. Yet the intricate connection between the US military and the Nuremberg Doctors' Trial also meant that the trial became of less relevance once the strategic and political priorities of the day moved in a different direction. As long as Washington saw the Nuremberg trials as part of the overall aim to create a new post-war order, the prosecution and indeed the judges had little to worry about

37   NARA, RG 153/84-1, box 1, folder 3, Taylor to Petersen, 30 September 1946.
38   Ibid.
39   Ibid.
40   For some of the staff, see NARA, RG 238, Entry 159, box 2.
41   NARA, RG 153/84-1, box 1, folder 3, Taylor to Jackson, 30 October 1946.
42   DUMC, Alexander diary (1946/47), p. 1, 13 November 1946.
43   NARA, RG 153/86-3-1, book 2, box 10, Taylor to War Department, 1 November 1946.

other than to establish the proper trial procedures. This naturally included the role of experts.[44]

IV.   Constructing the Doctors' Trial

In the weeks preceding the opening of the trial detailed discussions about the nature of German medical science and the principles of permissible and non-permissible experiments on humans emerged as a result of concerted efforts among the US prosecution to construct a legally viable prosecution case, and ultimately secure the conviction of as many of the accused as possible. The prosecution case was far from complete or satisfactory when Alexander and other senior members arrived at Nuremberg. The pressure for those on the ground was significant. To establish a trial with a shortage of qualified lawyers and staff, together with improvised organisational structures and communication facilities in an occupied zone where the population was more or less hostile towards the undertaking, was one thing; to constantly defend the rationale for the trials in a shifting political climate was quite another. While relations with the Soviet Union were deteriorating, support for war crimes trials was rapidly disappearing in Washington after the completion of the IMT. These factors contributed to a sense of emergency and need for improvisation among the prosecution team. Taylor and his staff knew that they had to "win" the medical case if they wanted to hold further war crimes trials. They also knew that they were creating a precedent for future trials. Although the IMT offered them some guidance as far as the rules of procedure was concerned, the US prosecution found itself on quite unfamiliar legal territory at the end of 1946.

Two interrelated factors triggered the debate about the nature of German medical science and the ethics of human experimentation in late November, early December 1946. First, the prosecution wanted to approach the medical case, as well as all the subsequent cases, as variations in the overall scheme of Raphaël Lemkin's principle of genocide, that is the intention and execution of murdering another people. Following lengthy discussions in the legal committee of the United Nations Assembly in November, it had become apparent that the genocide concept expressed not only the "specific criminal intent" with regard to large victim groups, but, like the concept of crimes against humanity, it called for "greater condemnation because it implied mass criminality and very great losses to humanity and civilisation".[45] In January 1947, Lemkin formally informed the War Department about the need to "develop the genocide concept in the doctor's case".[46] While conducting interviews with the victims of Nazi atrocities, he had

---

44   For the selection of experts for the defence see NDT-Documents and Material, fiche 296, frames 1045-1047.

45   NDT-Documents and Material, fiche 303, frame 1803.

46   Ibid., frames 1802-1804.

realised that the Nazis had not been interested in killing particular individuals, but in the systematic murder of ethnic and religious groups. The Nazis

> "did not know the names of the victims but handled them by numbers. They did not hate nor had any particular interest to kill Mr. X, Y, or Z, but their acts were motivated by the desire to eradicate the particular national or racial group to which Mr. X, Y, or Z happened to belong".[47]

Lemkin and other officials wanted to use the stigma of the genocide concept as a means of preventing the defendants to claim that their work had been scientific in nature, and therefore apparently not criminal.[48]

The second factor was that the prosecution was expecting the defence to use the *tu quoque* argument, that is that Allied medical scientists had conducted similar experiments, and that there was no grounds for the indictment. The defence was expected to argue that either doctors of both nations were guilty of violating principles of professional medical ethics, or none of the doctors were. Both factors convinced Alexander of the need for an explanatory framework which stressed the differences between Allied and German medical science. To back up the charges of genocide in the realm of medical science, and pre-empt the expected counter-attack by the defence, the prosecution invented and applied the concept of Thanatology. At the same time it was addressing issues which went beyond the immediate scope of the trial. These issues were concerned with permissible experiments on humans, and with wider questions as to what constituted ethical and non-ethical experiments. The debate about the ethics of human experimentation and about the concept of Thanatology were mutually interlinked. One stimulated the other and vice versa. The core arguments in both debates were formulated by Alexander on the same day, on 3 December 1946, after having completed the bulk of his interrogations.[49] "This dual focus", as Katz has pointed out, "led the prosecution and its expert witnesses, in what otherwise might have been a murder trial, to defend ethical research practices in the non-Nazi world in ways that tried to deny any past ethical transgressions".[50]

To understand the origins of the ten principles of permissible experiments on human subjects in the Nuremberg Code, one needs to look at how the debate developed at the beginning and in the course of the trial. Alexander's diary notes and memoranda are important in reconstructing this discourse, especially six of his unpublished papers which were directly related to both issues.[51] The Code evolved from these early debates and in stages throughout the trial.[52] Although there are still many gaps in the record in order to reconstruct the precise stages in its development and understand the forces which pushed the debate forward, we do have a good idea about how the origin of the Code did not develop. The Code

---

47   Ibid., frame 1802; see also Levi (1996), introduction, p. x.
48   Ibid., frame 1803.
49   DUMC, Alexander diary (1946/47), p. 79, 3 December 1946.
50   Katz (1996), p. 1662.
51   Schmidt (2004), pp. 162f.
52   See also Shuster (1998).

did not suddenly appear in the final judgement.[53] The Code was neither written on a particular day nor was it created by a particular commission, organisation or individual person. The idea that "medicine was not involved" in the drafting of the Code, as Rothman suggests, cannot be sustained.[54] On the contrary, a number of medical experts and medical organisations, including Alexander and Ivy, influenced the conceptual outline and textual formation of the Code. Elements of the Code were at first shaped within the relatively confined realm of the prosecution. Future guidelines on human experimentation were also debated in expert circles like the ISC (WC) in Paris.[55]

Once the trial started, however, the debate on medical ethics and human experimentation became a public debate, with journalists, lawyers, and medical representatives taking an active interest in expressing their particular views on the subject. Although the Tribunal had underestimated the importance of medical expertise in the trial, the judges quickly realised the centrality of research ethics. Throughout more than one-hundred-and-thirty trial days the judges frequently interrupted the witnesses or the prosecution to clarify specific points relating to medical ethics. The discussions among the prosecution staff as well as those in open court are crucial to understand the progress and character of the debate on human experimentation.

The suggestion that the Code evolved in stages throughout the trial proceedings is further corroborated if we look at the general Anglo-American court procedures applied in the Doctors' Trial.[56] As opposed to the German legal system, where judges studied all of the evidence for a particular case prior to the beginning of the proceedings, judges in the Anglo-Saxon legal system enter the trial proceedings with an open mind. Unlike their German colleagues, the judges will generally not have formed an opinion about the degree of culpability of the defendant. All this is to ensure the highest degree of impartiality towards the case in front of them. It is only during the actual trial that the judges begin to form their opinion about the issues at hand. Their opinion is being shaped by listening to what the witnesses say and by studying the trial transcript, by examining some of the witnesses themselves, and on the basis of the evidence introduced by both the prosecution and the defence. All this can sway the opinion of the judges, and it is only towards the end of the trial that they start to formulate the judgement.

The process in which the debate about permissible experiments on humans developed was multi-dimensional with many twists and turns, and shaped by unforeseen incidents. Discussions on medical ethics could be triggered or revived by a testimony of one of the medical experts. A letter by an outside medical organisation, requesting information on future medical ethics standards, could intensify reflections to draw up a more elaborate system of ethics principles. A strong and convincing presentation by one of the defendants could initiate plans to

---

53   Tröhler/Reiter-Theil (1997), introduction, p. 14.
54   Rothman (1997), pp. 75-87, p. 87.
55   Weindling (1996), see also Weindling (2000b) and Weindling (2001a).
56   See also Ebbinghaus (2001), p. 406.

bring in an expert rebuttal witness to counter the claims made by the defendant. All these "events" shaped the debate behind the scenes and in open court. In other words, a perceptive lay observer of the Nuremberg proceedings would have been able, and without great difficulty, to formulate all, or most of the principles which experts regarded as mandatory for permissible experiments on humans. The language of the principles might not have conformed to the actual Code, but the gist and content of the principles would have been there. In short, by the end of the trial, the ten principles of the Code were extant as an integral part of the courtroom discourse. What remained for the judges to do was to write them down to give them the force of law, like they do when they weigh the evidence for and against the accused in their attempt to formulate the judgement.

Arriving in Nuremberg, Leo Alexander, the medical expert of the prosecution, was promptly given the assignment to explore and point out the different characters of Allied and German medical science.[57] On 13 November, he wrote to Clifton T. Perkins, Commissioner for Mental Health in the Commonwealth of Massachusetts. He told Perkins that the war crimes authorities felt that it would be important in the forthcoming trial "to have evidence regarding the nature and procedural characteristics of the experimentation on human beings such as practised in institutions in this country including the State Institutions of the Commonwealth of Massachusetts in order to effectively contrast ethical with non-ethical experimentation on human beings".[58] In particular, Alexander wanted to know what the "conditions for approval of these experiments by the Research Council" were and how the voluntary character of the experiments was ensured. Alexander also approached officials at the Rockefeller Institute of Medical Research and a number of researchers at US universities and hospitals, asking them to send him an official statement which detailed

> "the general rules which govern such experimentation [on humans], any procedure for approval of particular experiments by a board of research scientists or officials of the hospital and the requirements laid down as to the need for consent of next of kin or guardian as well as for the consent and cooperation of the part of the patient".[59]

Thanatology was Alexander's answer to his assignment, a concept born out of practical necessity to counter the German defence and link the incriminating evidence in the medical case with the principle of genocide. On 21 November, Alexander mentioned the term "Thanatology" for the first time in his diary.[60] Throughout the following weeks he frequently referred to Thanatology in his reflections about the conduct of German scientists.[61] The origin of the concept of

---

57   DUMC, Alexander diary (1946/47), pp. 1f, 13 November 1946.
58   NARA, RG 153/86-3-1, book 2, box 10, Alexander to Perkins, 13 November 1946.
59   NARA, RG 153/86-3-1, book 2, box 10, Alexander to Cramer, 14 November 1946; Alexander to Overholser, 14 November 1946; Alexander to Taliaferro, 14 November 1946; Alexander to Rappleye, 14 November 1946; Alexander to Chesney, 14 November 1946; Alexander to Chairman, Board of Scientific Directors, Rockefeller Institute of Medical Research, 15 November 1946.
60   DUMC, Alexander diary (1946/47), pp. 11f, 21 November 1946
61   DUMC, Alexander diary (1946/47), p. 18, 22 November 1946; p. 19, 24 November 1946; p.

Thanatology thus stands in close connection with the preparation of the medical case by the American prosecution. Nazi medical experiments, some defendants argued, had been carried out to benefit the members of the German armed forces, to search for the most effective treatment of illnesses and offer solutions for aeronautical and naval combat and rescue problems. In its drive for 'living space' (*Lebensraum*), the German military had applied all means to achieve victory, irrespective of the countless loss of human lives. It was only when Alexander realised a marked discrepancy between the purpose of the experiments and their outcome that he approached the problem from a different angle. If one looked at the experiments from the perspective of "usefulness", he argued, in contributing new knowledge to a certain scientific problem, the result was almost always negative: "One cannot help feeling that the experiments were amateurish and poorly coordinated, that they failed to give the scientific information which was claimed to be desired, and that a unified policy was completely absent, except for the barbaric manner of their execution".[62]

For Alexander the study of Himmler's "field of science" warranted the conclusion that the main thrust of the research was aimed at finding methods to exterminate large populations by the "most scientific" and "least conspicuous" means. Experiments by the Ravensbrück physicians, like Fritz Fischer and Karl Gebhardt, exemplified the "callous disregard" for the lives of the victims. It was this context, Alexander believed, which was so markedly different from the experimental environment of the Allies. Nazi doctors developed a new field in which the main objective was not to search for methods of healing, but for methods of producing death. Only in one case, namely in the study of hypothermia, had the Germans discovered useful but non-original information. Yet even here "the only accurate statistical observation" concerned the length of time that was needed to kill humans by exposure to cold. On 3 December, six days before the start of the trial, Alexander recorded in his diary:

"Many of these so-called experiments are frankly and openly devoted to methods of destroying or preventing life, namely to 'euthanasia' and extermination methods, and to methods of sterilisation. But the preoccupation with methods of producing death runs also through many of the other investigations like a red thread, irrespective of the ostensible other purpose of the experiment. The frightful body of new methods of killing – the new lethal injections, the new gases, the poison bullets – constitute a formidable body of new and dangerous knowledge, useful to criminals everywhere, and to a criminal state if another one is permitted to establish itself again, so as to constitute a new branch, a destructive perversion of medicine worthy of a new name, for which thanatology had been suggested by our medical consultant. This thanatological knowledge supplied the technological methods for genocide, a

---

19, 25 November 1946; p. 34, 28 November 1946; p. 49, 29 November 1946; p. 78, 3 December 1946; p. 79, 3 December 1946; p. 107, 10 December 1946, p. 199, 1 March 1947, p. 199, 10 March 1947; p. 199, 11 March 1947; see also AP, Leo Alexander to Phyllis Alexander, 27 November 1946.

62   Alexander Paper 1, 30.11.1946; see also Alexander Paper 4, 15 January 1947; see also Schmidt (2004).

policy of the German Third Reich, which could not have been carried out without the active participation of its medical scientists".[63]

Taylor was the first to make use of the concept. On 30 November, Alexander told him that the indictment offered no discussion about the motives which inspired the accused in ordering, abetting or performing the experiments. In case Taylor wanted to include "such a discussion in the opening remarks of the prosecution", he might find the concept of Thanatology useful.[64] After having studied the experiments and Ivy's report on "War Crimes of A Medical Nature"[65], Alexander came to the following conclusion:

> "In the light of all these facts, it becomes obvious that the difference between the German human experimentation and ours is not only the voluntary character and the safety which was always maintained in our experiments, and which Dr. Ivy stressed in his report, but far more fundamentally the main object of the entire research. This German research was not research for methods of healing, but for methods, mechanics and time factors of producing death by various non-obvious and non-conspicuous means".[66]

But there were obvious problems with the approach adopted by the prosecution. The main legal problem with the concept of genocide was that it focused on the murder of *another* people, especially on the murder of European Jewry. Hence the concept of genocide not only excluded the persecution of gypsies and other groups deemed "asocial" but marginalised the issue of "euthanasia", where a state had implemented a programme to systematically kill one section of its *own* people.[67] The role of sterilisation was also neglected because it did not fall within the jurisdiction of the Tribunal. Although there was much to be said about linking the various crimes and show that the doctors had acted according to a common design,[68] the specific character, differences and stages of criminal medical conduct was likely to be glossed over. The judicial framework and the line of argument of the American prosecution explains why the War Department asked Alexander to "play down euthanasia" in his assessment of Nazi medical crimes.[69] To stress the murder of German adults and children with disability did not bolster the case of the prosecution, unless one could show that non-German nationals had been killed in the programme. Overall, the approach by the prosecution prevented,

63 DUMC, Alexander diary (1946/47), pp. 78f, 3 December 1946; also Alexander Paper 2, 5 December 1946; see also Schmidt (2001a), pp. 374f.
64 Alexander Paper 1, 30 November 1946.
65 BAK, ZSg 154, box 65, Andrew Ivy; Report on War Crimes of a Medical Nature Committed in Germany and Elsewhere on German Nationals and the Nationals of Occupied Countries by the Nazi Regime During World War II, 22 Bl., o.D. (1946).
66 Alexander Paper 1, 30 November 1946.
67 See Burleigh (1994), Friedlander (1995), also Schmidt (2002).
68 In the Doctors' Trial the legal concept of a "common design" was adopted instead of the concept of a "common plan" after it had become apparent that the latter was difficult to prove in open court during the IMT; for the debate within the prosecution, see NARA, RG 238, Entry 159, box 4, Memorandum, Subject: The Concept of "Common design", Ferencz to Heath, 17 July 1946.
69 DUMC, Alexander diary (1946/47), p. 4, 13 November 1946.

rather than facilitated, a full investigation of the first systematic mass murder of the Nazi regime during the Doctors' Trial.[70]

Thanatology was defined as being what Allied science was not, but like the principle of genocide, the concept of thanatology had substantial shortcomings; it was likely to gloss over the specific character and stages of criminal medical conduct in Germany. The concept overlooked processes of cumulative radicalisation, and massive changes in administration and centralisation of resources, or the relation between modern medicine and the industry of war. Thanatology was an overarching principle which left little room for issues of individual responsibility and moral dilemmas. The dichotomy between "human" Allied science and "inhuman" German science may have been helpful for the prosecution in bolstering their case against the German doctors. It also may have illuminated the specific character of certain kinds of Nazi science, but as a theory to explain the complicity of medical science as well as the complexity of Fascist science, at best the analytical potential of Thanatology is limited.

Yet, at the same time, the concept of Thanatology reached beyond the immediate objective of the trial by defining ethical and non-ethical experimentation more clearly. The indictment provided an accurate account of the murders and atrocities committed in the course of the experiments, a graphic image of medical cruelty. Its aim was to establish the links between allegations and crimes, words and deeds. However, the indictment did not offer a discussion about the motives of the accused and the reasons which inspired them.[71] The trial raised profound questions as to how and why physicians were able to commit medical crimes. How men and women devoted to the Hippocratic tradition, trained as professionals in one of the world's most advanced scientific cultures, could commit such crimes, and whether they actually understood that they were committing a crime. What did knowing and not knowing mean in this context, individual responsibility and responsibility as a group or as a profession? Most of these questions were outside the scope of the trial. Thanatology offered one of the first, albeit simplistic attempts to address these issues.

On 3 December, Alexander drafted a plan for a memorandum on "Ethical and Non-Ethical Experimentation in Human Beings".[72] The main question concerned the extent to which German experiments had been "non-crucial experiments", inadequately prepared, therefore inaccurate, misleading and unnecessary. His examples were high altitude and sea-water experiments.[73] On 7 December 1946, two days before the start of the trial, Alexander completed the first of two key texts on the ethics of human experimentation, which he addressed to Taylor. The second memorandum was completed in April 1947. Both memoranda contributed to the debate about human experimentation inside the prosecution team, and ultimately shaped parts of the Nuremberg Code.[74]

70 For a discussion about the shortcoming of the Doctors' Trial, see Marrus (1999).
71 Alexander Paper 4, 15 January 1947.
72 DUMC, Alexander diary (1946/47), p. 79, 3 December 1946.
73 Ibid.
74 DUMC, Alexander diary (1946/47), p. 105; 7 December 1946; NDT-Documents and

Alexander's concept of Thanatology and his first memorandum on human experimentation shows that, two days before the trial started, the prosecution had not only developed a theoretical model to address medical crimes under the umbrella of the genocide concept, but had also laid down a number of "conditions" which had to be met so that research on humans, if absolutely necessary, could be regarded as permissible. Most of the material had been haphazardly prepared and Alexander's theory was not fully thought-through. The aim was to distinguish Allied from German medical science. This became the central issue as the trial progressed, but it also blurred the essential nature of the case, namely that the defendants were on trial for murder. By drawing attention to the destructive energy of German medicine, the prosecution hoped to counter any attempts of *tu quoque* in the trial; and by establishing certain standards of professional conduct in experimental research on humans, preferably based on existing German regulations, they wanted to show that Nazi physicians had not only committed a criminal offence, but had also violated the professions' own code of ethical conduct. Whether both concepts would actually stand up in trial, and whether the dual strategy of the prosecution would work, was far from certain when on Monday, 9 December 1946, Military Tribunal I convened its first session.

During the opening statement, Taylor turned to the question of medical ethics as one of the most fundamental issues of the trial. Regardless of what they may have agreed to or signed at the time, none of the victims had been volunteers. Most of the victims had not been condemned to death, and those who had were not criminals, "unless it be a crime to be a Jew, or a Pole, or a Gypsy, or a Russian prisoner of war".[75] But most importantly, there had been no voluntary and informed consent prior to the experiments:

> "Whatever book or treatise on medical ethics we may examine, and whatever expert on forensic medicine we may question, will say that it is a fundamental and inescapable obligation of every physician under any known system of law not to perform a dangerous experiment without the subject's consent".[76]

All of the accused had departed from "every known standard of medical ethics". For the prosecution the case against the doctors was "one of the simplest and clearest", but it was also one of the most important because it epitomised Nazi thinking and Nazi way of life, the noxious merger of the German militarised state with Nazi racial policies.[77] Germany's leaders had failed to stand firm against the destructive forces of Hitler's party and their failure was the outcome of "that sinister undercurrent of German philosophy that preaches the supreme importance of the state and the complete subordination of the individual". In his concluding

Material, fiche 303, frames 1714-1724; also Alexander (1976c).
75   For Taylor's opening speech, see NDT-Records, frames 61-124; here frame 89.
76   Ibid.
77   New York Times, 10 December 1946.

remarks, Taylor noted that a nation in which the individual means nothing will find few leaders courageous and able enough to serve its best interests.[78]

Taylor's condemnation of the Nazi regime and its corrupted moral value system was widely acknowledged by American, German and French newspapers as an impressive example of legal rhetoric, in which judicial and moral argument had been skilfully woven together with graphic detail.[79] The *Philadelphia Record*, for example, noted that the prosecution had outlined its case "in sharp, bitter tones" and asserted that Nazi Germany had "died of its own poison".[80] Some observers also commended the thoroughness of the proceedings and the dispassionate way in which the prosecution was handling the material. The response by the world's media to the daily revelations in the trial was one of shock. George C. Putnam from the United Nations War Crimes Commission (UNWCC) described the opening of the trial as "showdown time" for the men of medicine who had ruled under Hitler's name: "Tales of deliberately wanton killings of so-called 'mercy killings' by torture – they're all on the record tonight".[81] An American physician expressed his anger over the lack of compassion and moral stature of the German doctors in a letter to the editors of the *New York Times*: "Not a single word of protest or of indignation was heard from the so-called outstanding men at the head of the German universities nor from the German Medical Association. Nothing of that sort is heard even today. They probably have the nerve to claim they did not know anything about it".[82] For David Willis from the UNWCC the demand to condemn the men as murderers was an "eminently reasonable proposal".[83] On 12 December the *New York Times* informed readers about a 50-page report on cold water experiments which was introduced as evidence by the prosecution as being "the most startling and succinct report on murder in the history of criminology".[84]

Many people were rather disconcerted when they first saw the defendants. The majority wore civilian clothes and those in uniforms had their decorations or insignia of rank taken off. Countess Alice von Platen, one of the three German trial observers, perceived "with horror the ordinary faces".[85] She found it difficult to come to terms with the fact that:

"no external features distinguished these twenty-three people from us ... The whole event would be easier to understand, if these were notorious sadists or psychopaths, but on the contrary they are men who for years filled the most responsible positions".[86]

---

78   NDT-Records, frame 119.
79   For newspaper responses about the opening of the trial, see NARA, RG 238, Entry 28, box 3, Daily Press Review; see also the reporting about the trial in *Die Welt*, in: NDT-Documents and Material, fiche 308, frames 2250-2257.
80   NARA, RG 238, Entry 28, box 3, Daily Press Review; Philadelphia Record, 9 December 1946.
81   NARA, RG 238, Entry 28, box 3, Daily Press Review.
82   FCLM, Beecher papers, box 11, folder 79.
83   NARA, RG 238, Entry 28, box 3, Daily Press Review.
84   New York Times, 12 December 1946.
85   Von Platen (1947a), pp. 29-31, p. 29.
86   Ibid., p. 29; also Von Platen (1947b), pp. 199-202.

The only woman on trial, Herta Oberheuser, attracted particular attention.[87] For many observers it was difficult to grasp that "a woman" could have been involved in such heinous and brutal acts. Other spectators were plainly outraged that not a single one of the accused had pleaded guilty to the charges, something many felt was nothing but "shameless and incredible arrogance".[88] These accounts shaped the public image of the otherwise insignificant looking men and the one woman in the dock.

For many observers and political analysts the extent of stomach-churning evidence introduced in court soon became repetitive. Yet for those exploring and exposing the evidence there was no end in sight to the stream of revelations about medical crimes. Archivists, researchers and translators who had been ordered to prepare the material for the prosecution sometimes had to interrupt their work in total disbelief of the content of the evidence. For many the work would haunt them decades after the trial was completed. On 31 December 1946, Alexander told his wife:

> "The mad old whirl is going on and more and more war crimes are unfolding. It sometimes seems as if the Nazis had taken special pains in making practically every nightmare come true. Some new evidence has come in where two doctors in Berlin, one a man and the other a woman, collected eyes of different colour. It seems that the concentration camps were combed for people who had slightly differently coloured eyes. That means people whose one eye had a slightly different colour than the other. Who ever was unlucky enough to possess such a pair of slightly unequal eyes had them cut out and was killed, the eyes being sent to Berlin. This is the carrying out into reality of an old gruesome German fairy tale which is included in the Tales of Hoffman, where Dr. Coppelius posing as the sandman comes at night and cuts out children's eyes when they are tired. The grim part of the story is that Doctors von Verschuer and Magnussen in Berlin did prefer children and particularly twins. There is no end to this nightmare, at least 23 are being tried now and, I trust, the others will follow later".[89]

News coverage about the trial was not restricted to Allied media or expert journals interested in the legal aspects of the trial. About two dozen German correspondents regularly reported the latest news from Nuremberg. The US zone radio station broadcasted fifteen-minute commentaries on the progress of the trial, and occasionally the odd Nazi would pay tribute to the former medical elite.[90] Frequent requests by medical students for passes were generally granted as part of the ongoing denazification effort. The German medical profession also sent a "commission of doctors" (*Ärztekommission*) as official observers to the trial. Led by the distinguished Heidelberg physician Alexander Mitscherlich, the commissions' objective was to report in medical expert journals about the extent of medi-

---

87   New York Times, 10 December 1946.
88   StaNü, KV-Prozesse, Generalia, P318, DANA papers, 9 December 1946; NARA, RG 238, Entry 28, box 3 Daily Press Review, 11 December 1946 and 13 December 1946.
89   AP, Leo Alexander to Phyllis Alexander, 31 December 1946; as to the role of Otmar von Verschuer and Karin Magnussen see Müller-Hill (1988); also Weindling (2000c), pp. 635-652.
90   FCLM, Beecher papers, box 11, folder 79.

cal misconduct during the Third Reich.[91] One of the problems for the commission was to get its articles published in expert medical journals, most of which feared that reports from Nuremberg would damage fragile post-war doctor-patient relationships or harm the reputation of the German medical profession.[92] More importantly, the trial raised the question about standards of existing and future medical ethics.

V. Leo Alexander and the Nuremberg Code

At the beginning of January 1947, questions about the ethics and quality of German medical science led to a controversy of whether one should publish the results of Nazi experiments. The debate was triggered in the British journal *Lancet* and followed up by the *British Medical Journal* (BMJ).[93] Although nothing had apparently been discovered which merited publication, the editors asked readers in January that if "facts of real value to medicine were still to emerge from the records of the experiments – should they be published or not?"[94] In the ensuing debate some argued that publishers would become "accessories to the crime" while others were adamant that scientists had a duty towards the victims to publish the results so "at least their suffering was of some benefit". Experts from the *BMJ* wanted to know if the Nazis had "discovered a cure for cancer would the rest of the world say that this information must be destroyed because of the manner in which it was obtained?"[95] Others thought that the controversy was unnecessary. Ivy, for example, believed that German medical science had made no significant discoveries during the war and that there was probably nothing "worth publishing".[96]

Unimpressed by some of the media hype and despite the constant need for improvisation, the prosecution was well aware that the trial was likely to make legal history. On 16 December, Alexander told his wife:

> "What a madhouse this is! I don't know what they would have done without me, the Snafu[97] is so terrific. I am working from 8.30 a.m. till 2.30 a.m. What a grind! But we'll come out with something really monumental, both historical and legal".[98]

---

91 Mielke (1948), pp. 29-31; also Platen-Hallermund (1993), p. I; for the controversy in the Göttinger Zeitung between Alexander Mitscherlich and Friedrich Hermann Rein about Nazi medicine, see NDT-Documents and Material, fiche 307/8, frames 2272-2284.
92 StUF, AMA, II2/115; von Platen to Mitscherlich, 10 January 1947.
93 Anonymous (1946), Mellanby (1946), Layton (1946), Hilton (1947), Herbert (1947).
94 DUMC, Alexander papers, box 1, folder 20, Office of Chief of Counsel for War Crimes, Public Relations Office, Special Release No. 99, 11 January 1947.
95 Anonymous (1947), p. 143, also Mellanby (1947), Rißmann (1947).
96 DUMC, Alexander papers, box 1, file 20.
97 The phrase "Snafu" refers to a an acronym which soldiers used to make a mocking comment about the military. It stands for "Situation Normal, All Fouled Up". Soldiers would also use an expletive instead of the word "Fouled". I am grateful to Jonathan D. Moreno for pointing this out.
98 AP, Leo Alexander to Phyllis Alexander, 16 December 1946.

Alexander was not alone in his assessment of the importance of the trial for future research ethics. The prosecution and the judges are likely to have realised at this point that general guidelines for future research on humans were needed and, perhaps, codified as part of the Nuremberg judgement. Yet up until mid-January 1947, Alexander does not seem to have spent much time reflecting about how such guidelines should look like in reality, mainly because he was tied up with interrogating defendants. The same appears to be true of the prosecution as a whole. Only after the meeting of the ISC (WC) at the Institute Pasteur in Paris on 15 January did the issue of medical ethics become a priority for the prosecution. The conference intensified international discussion about the formulation of ethics principles. As a member of the US delegation, Alexander was expected and well-positioned to make an impact on the debate.

Whereas some Allied countries were excluded, others did not want to partici-pate officially. The meeting was convened ad hoc, one day earlier as originally planned, thereby excluding the representative of the Danish medical profession, V. A. Fenger, who arrived too late to take part.[99] Both the Danish General Medical Association and French medical experts had proposed the creation of a scientific commission for the investigation of medical war crimes to the UNWCC earlier.[100] The decision by the French to move this crucial meeting forward was probably intended to confine membership in the Commission to the four Allied powers. By now the Commission had become a matter of national prestige and power politics. Unlike the Danish, who would have wished to participate, Taylor and Alexander had flown to Paris to take part as "unofficial delegates of the Nuremberg War Crimes Tribunal" because Washington was reluctant to boost the status of the Commission by despatching official representatives.[101]

The British commission was led by Lord Moran, Churchill's doctor and President of the Royal College of Physicians. In 1949, still sulking over the lack of American interest in the ISC (WC), Moran, considering the extent of medical war crimes, published a rather brief five-page report on the "Scientific Results of German Medical War Crimes" which concluded that the experiments were "not only ill-designed but were ill-conceived, and in many cases were unnecessary".[102] With no apparent scientific results identifiable from the experiments, and after having been snubbed by the Americans, the Commission felt unable (or perhaps unwilling) to come to any conclusions with regard to the moral issues involved. The British felt betrayed that the Americans had unilaterally established the Nuremberg trials as a forum to publicly condemn German atrocities and claim the moral highground. The initiative had by now clearly passed to the Americans.

Indeed, following the meeting of the ISC (WC), Alexander was homing in on the subject of medical ethics. He was determined to come up with a set of ethics

---

99   DUMC, Alexander papers, box 4, file 35.
100 United Nations War Crimes Commission (1948), p. 147.
101 BAK, ZSg 154, box 73, International Scientific Commission (War Crimes), 15 January 1947.
102 Foreign Office (1949), p. 3; see also United Nations War Crimes Commission (1948); also Weindling (2001c), p. 69.

guidelines which would supersede his own principles from December as well as those formulated by Ivy in the autumn of 1946 which had been adopted by the AMA in a modified version only a couple of weeks earlier. During the Paris conference Alexander had laid out his theory about the science of killing in his talk on "Ktenology as a Scientific Technique of Genocide" and had announced his intention to publish his theory in two articles.[103] Shortly before his departure to Paris, Alexander had also welcomed Ivy in Nuremberg who had just arrived from the United States. Both met again on 21 January after Alexander's return from Paris and continued their conversation about a future medical ethics code.[104] On 23 January, Ivy left Nuremberg to return to Chicago. A special press announcement from that day reveals that Ivy had recommended to the American military authorities that

> "an international, legalised Code of ethics should be published on the use of human beings as experimental subjects. Dr Ivy made this recommendation after spending the past ten days reviewing the record of the current war crimes trial of 23 doctors and scientists accused of conducting medical experiments on inmates of concentration camps".[105]

The discussions within the prosecution team throughout January as well as Ivy's public recommendations seem to have prompted Alexander into action. He wanted to become the author of Ivy's proposed medical ethics code. One day later Alexander recorded in his diary: "Sent off Ktenology article. Finished the additions to the article re[garding] ethical and unethical experimentation".[106] On or around the 24 January, Alexander therefore must have edited and expanded his three ethics-principles which he had outlined in December. Finally, on 25 January, he wrote: "Worked on Ethics article, drew up Affidavit".[107]

These diary entries are important in many respects. First, they tell us that Alexander's article on "Ethical and Non-Ethical Experiments on Human Beings" was formulated at the end of January. In the article, which has no date, and in the affidavit, which is dated 25 January, we find, word for word, Alexander's six ethics principles from April 1947.[108] The diary entries show that Alexander formulated these principles about three months earlier than scholars had previously assumed, because most concentrated on Alexander's memorandum from April 1947.[109] Alexander's principles stated the following:

> "1. Legally valid voluntary consent of the experimental subject is essential. This requires specifically:
> a) The absence of duress.
> b) Sufficient disclosure on the part of the experimenter and sufficient understanding on the part of the experimental subject of the exact nature and consequences of the experiment for which he volunteers, to permit an enlightened consent.

103 Alexander Paper 4, 15 January 1947; also BAK, Zsg 154, No. 73.
104 DUMC, Alexander diary (1946/47), p. 168, 21 January 1947.
105 Quoted from Weindling (2001c), p. 64.
106 DUMC, Alexander diary (1946/47), p. 174, 24 January 1947.
107 Ibid.
108 DUMC, box 4, folder 33.
109 Schmidt (2001a).

In the case of mentally ill patients, for the purpose of experiments concerning the nature and treatment of nervous and mental illness or related subjects, such consent of the next of kin or legal guardian is required; whenever the mental state of the patient permits (that is, in those mentally ill patients who are not delirious or confused) his own consent should be obtained in addition.

2. The nature and purpose of the experiment must be humanitarian, with the ultimate aim to cure, treat, or prevent illness, and not concerned with methods of killing or sterilisation (ktenology). The motive and purpose of the experiment shall also not be personal nor otherwise ulterior.

3. No experiment is permissible if the foregone conclusion exists, or the probability or the a priori reason to believe that death or disabling injury of the experimental subject will occur.

4. Adequate preparations must be made and proper facilities be provided to aid the experimental subject against any remote chance of injury, disability, or death. This provision specifically requires that the degree of skill of all those who are taking an active part as experimenters, and the degree of care which they exercise during the experiment, must be significantly higher than the skill which is considered adequate for the performance of standardised medical or surgical procedures, and for the administration of well established drugs. American courts are very stringent in requiring for the permissible use of any new or unusual technique or drug, irrespective of whether this use is experimental or purely therapeutic, a degree of skill and care on the part of the responsible physician which is higher than that required for the purpose of routine medical or surgical procedures.

5. The degree of risk taken should never exceed that determined by the humanitarian importance of the problem to be solved by the experiment. It is ethically permissible for an experimenter to perform experiments involving significant risks only if the solution, after thorough exploration along all other lines of scientific investigation is not accessible by any other means, and if he considers the solution of the problem important enough to risk his own life along with those of his non-scientific colleagues, such as was done in the case of Walter Reed's yellow fever experiments.

6. The experiment to be performed must be so designed and based upon the results of thorough thinking-through, of investigation of simple physico-chemical systems and of animal experimentation that the anticipated results will justify the performance of the experiment. That is, the experiment must be such as to yield decisive results for the good of society and should not be random and unnecessary in nature".[110]

Alexander's affidavit seems to have had no immediate effects among members of the prosecution throughout February and March 1947. It seems to have been produced as part of Alexander's "literary work" about ethically legitimate and illegitimate research on humans. It is not known what actually happened with the affidavit or who had access to it. Although the affidavit states that Alexander had been put under oath, this does not necessarily infer that he must have shared the information with others. As a member of the US prosecution he had been placed under oath anyway and had permission to draft legal documents, memoranda and affidavits. The affidavit therefore has to be treated with caution. It is quite possible that Alexander, after having made additions to his article, may have listed the six principles separately in the form of an affidavit in order to ensure that he would have to be credited with their authorship in the future. Alexander was

---

110 StUF, Alexander-Mitscherlich-Archiv, II 2, 106.7, Affidavit of Leo Alexander, 25 January 1947.

clearly not shy when it came to constructing an image of himself as a man of historical importance.

The same appears to have happened with Alexander's article about the ethics in human experimentation. He does not seem to have shown the article to anybody, except that he submitted it to the Public Relations Division of the War Department to receive clearance to publish it. Publication of the article was approved on 17 March 1947, when he was touring Holland to find further witnesses of medical atrocities.[111] Only after his return in April did Alexander revisited the subject of a medical ethics code. It is at that point that he himself created some confusion with regard to the precise origin of his medical ethics principles.

VI.   Werner Leibbrand and the Doctors' Trial

Prior to the presentation of the case for the defence the prosecution suffered a major setback when their medical expert witness, Werner Leibbrand, a psychiatrist and medical historian from Erlangen University, testified on 27 January 1947 on medical ethics – only two days after Alexander had formulated his six principles.[112] Leibbrand had been chosen for his immaculate credentials and because he was of German nationality. Allied legal advisers believed that a German medical expert might not only strengthen the case of the prosecution, but facilitate the process of denazification. Leibbrand's testimony was meant to convey that the Allied authorities saw only a *minority* of German doctors as having breached professional standards and as being guilty of crimes. It was an attempt at reconciling the medical profession with the Allied military government. However, the prosecution underestimated the power of cross-examination. Leibbrand's testimony backfired and left Allied medical science to appear almost in the same moral category as Germany medical science. Although this defence strategy had been foreseen, the actual ramifications and public relations impact came as a shock to Taylor's team.

The most embarrassing example introduced by Robert Servatius, Karl Brandt's lawyer, was evidence of large-scale malaria experiments on 800 American prisoners, many of them black, who had been selected from Federal penitentiaries in Atlanta, the Illinois State Penitentiary and New Jersey State Reformatory.[113] In June 1945 the magazine *Life* had given the story broad publicity in an article entitled "Prison Malaria" which revealed that the research was directed by the government-funded Office of Scientific Research and Development.[114]

111 NARA, RG 153/86-3-1, box 10, book 3, Leo Alexander, "Ethical and Non-ethical Experimentation on Human Beings. General Ethical, Medico-Legal and Scientific Considerations in Connection with the Vivisectionists".

112 NDT-Records, frames 2033-2100; see also NDT-Documents and Material, fiche 304, frame 1830; for the biography of Werner Leibbrand, see Seidel (2001), pp. 358f.

113 NDT-Documents and Material, fiche 307/8, frame 2252.

114 Anonymous (1945), pp. 43-46.

Human experiments had been conducted with malaria tropica, the most dangerous of malaria strands, to aid the war effort in the Asian theatre of operation. "Enemies of society are helping to combat other enemies", the article stated because "the experimenters ... have found prison life ideal for controlled laboratory work with humans".[115] Servatius read out the entire article in open court and described in meticulous detail each of the images and their captions; those referred to "violent chills" and "fever often as high as one hundred [and] six degrees". Some of the prison cases developed to "a considerable extent" before being treated with drugs. Then Servatius asked Leibbrand the obvious question: "Now, will you please express your opinion on the admissibility of these experiments?"[116] Leibbrand could not retract on his answer which he had previously given. American malaria experiments, he told the court, were likewise "excesses and outgrowths of biological thinking" because the consequences for the malaria infected prisoner could not be foreseen. Malaria is not "a mere cold", he said. Leibbrand also referred to the medical ethicist Albert Moll who had insisted that the morality of a physician is to hold back his "natural research urge in order to maintain his basic medical attitude that is laid down in the Oath of Hippocrates and which may result in doing harm to his patient".[117] "In consequence", Leibbrand concluded, "such experiments should be carried out on guinea pigs and not on human beings".[118]

The cross-examination of Leibbrand was a powerful condemnation of American wartime research in a court of American judges. It undermined the case of the prosecution by giving the impression to the Tribunal that German and Allied medical science was essentially the same. Although having anticipated this line of defence, the prosecution was caught off guard by the sheer force of the accusations against American medicine, not least because it came from their own medical expert. Beyond that, Leibbrand had been discredited as a trial expert, because as a medical historian and psychiatrist he showed himself unfamiliar with the literature and details of human experimentation.

From the perspective of the prosecution Leibbrand's philosophical discourse had become an unwanted delay in the conviction of the defendants. Inter-Allied frictions over questions about how to tackle medical war crimes, together with mounting political tensions in the American zone of occupation about war crimes trials generally, made the prosecution aware that any success by the defence was of potentially far-reaching consequences for all subsequent Nuremberg trials.

115 Ibid., p. 43.
116 NDT-Records, frame 2070.
117 Ibid., frame 2091; also Shuster (1997), p. 1438.
118 Ibid., frame 2071.

VII. The Nuremberg Code

Since Leibbrand's testimony it had become central to the prosecution to broaden the remit of the trial. The prosecution was under intense pressure to clarify what it considered to be ethical and non-ethical research on humans. In order to do so, they needed a medical authority on research physiology whose scientific work corresponded to that of the defendants.[119] Taylor and his staff had to convince the court that there were distinct differences in the methods and conduct between German and Allied experiments on humans during the war. The "Leibbrand incident" thus led to three interconnected initiatives by the prosecution: first, after his return to the United States, Ivy initiated the creation of a commission, the so-called "Green Committee", in order to investigate the ethics of malaria experiments which had been performed in American penitentiaries during the war. The findings of the commission were to serve as evidence to repudiate the accusation of the defence that American medical research had been unethical.[120] Secondly, Alexander modified and edited his article on ethical and unethical human experimentation and probably discussed his medical ethics principles with Telford Taylor.[121] And thirdly, to repudiate the claims made by the defence, the prosecution invited Ivy as a rebuttal witness to Nuremberg. Although active steps to recruit him as a rebuttal witness were not undertaken before April, the creation of the Green Committee stands in connection with Ivy's anticipated role to refute Leibbrand's testimony at the end of the trial. All of these steps were undertaken to ensure that the arguments put forward by the defence were repudiated. The Nuremberg Code originated in an environment of legal argument and counter-argument, pushed along, step by step, by internal and external initiatives.

During the trial the prosecution and the judges had realised that the formulation of a medical ethics code only made sense if the code was independent, at least in part, from the sphere of influence of the medical profession. In their view a medical ethics code had to be, if at all, part of the judgement to attain the status of law. The court probably saw this as the only guarantee that the interpretation and application of medical ethics standards would not solely remain within the power of the medical profession. Those formulating the Code did not consider, however, that the passage of time and developments in medical science might challenge the legal and ethical validity of the Code. They also may not have taken into account that the Code was issued by an American tribunal, rather than by an international court of law.

---

119 Shuster (1997), p. 1438.
120 See Harkness (1996).
121 DUMC, Alexander papers, box 1, folder 9, attached, handwritten note to Alexander Paper 6, no date and signature, which discusses Alexander's paper on ethical and non-ethical experimentation in human beings from 15 April 1947.

Ivy's testimony lasted four days, from 12 to 16 June 1947.[122] His appearance in court as the prosecutions' rebuttal witness sparked fierce controversy. The defence objected to the presentation of Ivy as "an expert on everything". Although his credentials read like a *Who's Who* of scientific organisations and medical associations, with more than 900 articles published, Ivy was less an expert on aviation medicine than he wanted the court to believe. In fact, he had written only two articles in this field. Both had been published after the war and after it had become clear that he would probably serve as a medical expert in the Doctors' Trial. It is quite possible that Ivy published the two papers in order to establish his credentials in yet another field.[123]

The suggestion that Ivy attempted to manipulate the outcome of the trial is further corroborated when we look at some of his policy initiatives in 1946 and early 1947. In his testimony, Ivy stated that the United States had specific research standards for research on humans which were laid down by the American Medical Association (AMA). He gave the impression that these rules were generally accepted research practice in America.[124] It turned out, however, that they were of a suspiciously recent origin and had been drafted by Ivy himself. Having studied the prosecution evidence in 1946, he had reported his views on permissible human experimentation to the AMA's trustees who adopted his recommendations.[125] During cross-examination, Ivy admitted that the principles had been published by the AMA on 28 December 1946, nineteen days after the opening of the trial. No such published principles had existed for the American research context before this time. Moreover, the publication of the AMA principles on experimental medical ethics had been made in anticipation of Ivy's testimony in the trial.[126]

The defence not only exposed the lack of international and published ethics standards on human experimentation, but also discredited Ivy's attempt at exonerating American medical research practice which had been criticised during Leibbrand's testimony in January. Ivy, after having returned to Chicago, had suggested to Illinois Governor, Dwight Green, in March that a committee be set up to examine the ethics of human experimentation, especially the malaria experiments which had been carried out at Stateville Prison.[127] He offered to serve as the chairman of the so-called "Green Committee". When Ivy finally gave his testimony at Nuremberg, he presented the findings of a non-existent and not-yet-functioning committee to the court. As the correspondence between the six members of the committee shows, by June 1947 the committee had not yet found

---

122 NDT-Records, frames 9196-9494; for a summery of Ivy's rebuttal testimony, see NDT-Documents and Material, fiche 304, frames 1952-1957; also fiche 307/8, frames 2224-2226; see also Moreno's groundbreaking analysis of Ivy's trial testimony; Moreno (1999), pp. 74-79.
123 NDT-Records, frames 9323ff.
124 Moreno (1999), p. 74.
125 NDT-Records, frames 9141ff.
126 Ibid., frames 9337f; also Moreno (1999), pp. 75f.
127 Harkness (1996), p. 1673.

"a convenient date and time" for its first session.[128] The final report of the committee exonerating American malaria experiments was not submitted before December 1947.[129] Pressed by the defence on the nature of the Green Committee, Ivy was coming close to perjury. When asked whether there had been discussions among the committee members whether coercion had been exercised in the experiments, he cautiously answered in the first person singular: "Yes, I was concerned about that question". Not satisfied with the answer, the defence queried again: "There were discussions about that?"[130] "Not necessarily with others, but there was always consideration of that in my own mind".[131] What Ivy was effectively saying was that discussions on the ethics of human experimentation had been carried out in his own mind; he, as the head of the "Green Committee" had come to certain conclusions as a result of discussions with himself.[132] When questioned about the origins of the "Green Committee" and about a potential link between the committee and the trial, Ivy appears not to have been entirely truthful. He told the court that the committee had been established "according to the best of his recollection" in December 1946. But he must have known that the committee was just three months old since he himself had proposed its creation. To the question whether the "formation of this committee" had anything to do with the fact that the trial was going on, he replied: "There is no connection between the action of this committee and this trial".[133] This is perhaps the point where Ivy came closest to perjuring himself.

Despite these momentary victories for the defence, Ivy's testimony served another, more important purpose. He helped to explain the boundaries between ethical and non-ethical human experimentation, and clarify some of the loose ends for the judges in shaping a code of medical ethics. In a series of probing questions by judge Sebring, the bench tried to extract what criteria had to be fulfilled to make human experiments ethical, and therefore legally permissible. Sebring's questions, however, were not directed towards the most important issues of human experimentation, like voluntary consent, nor did the bench interfere when Ivy read his three ethics principles into the record. We need to understand that by June 1947 the judges had, in all probability, laid down some if not most of the ethics principles as we later find them in the Nuremberg Code.

In contrast to the emotive nature of the witness' testimonies, the closing argument by the prosecution concentrated all minds on the role of the law which needed to be applied. Above all it was essential to merge Hippocratic medical ethics with patient-centred human rights. The prosecution made it unequivocally clear that the principle of voluntary informed consent stood at the centre of the case. For Taylor and his team it was of central importance that the judges would accept this principle, and would give it legal standing through the judgement. This

---

128 Ibid., p. 1674.
129 NDT-Documents and Material, fiche 303, frames 1756-1762.
130 NDT-Records, frame 9382.
131 Ibid.
132 Harkness (1996), p. 1674.
133 NDT-Records, frame 9389; Harkness (1996), p. 1674.

was seen as the only way to enforce, and indeed create, international as well as German law.[134] For the most part the prosecution maintained that the defendants were on trial for the crime of murder, crimes which had undoubtedly been committed, and with which the defendants were inextricably connected. The criminal nature of these experiments had been established by clear and public proof so that no one, as Taylor had previously put it, can ever doubt that they were fact and not fable. But at the very core of the trial stood the fact that the experimental subjects had not been volunteers:

> "That, of course, is the cornerstone of this case ... [I]t is the most fundamental tenet of medical ethics and human decency that the subjects volunteer for the experiment after being informed of its nature and hazards. This is the clear dividing line between criminal and what may be non-criminal. If the experimental subjects cannot be said to have volunteered, then the inquiry need proceed no further. Such is the simplicity of this case".[135]

For the prosecution the question of what exactly constituted a volunteer was of mere academic relevance since the doctors never had the slightest intention of using volunteers.[136] There were, of course, other conditions which needed to be satisfied so that experiments on humans were ethically and legally permissible. McHaney, as the representative of the prosecution, used the opportunity to read into the record a number of Ivy and Alexander's ethics principles to ensure that the judges could easily use this material in the judgement:

> "The experiment must be based on the results of animal experimentation and a knowledge of the natural history of the disease under study and designed in such a way that the anticipated results will justify the performance of the experiment.[137] This is to say that the experiment must be such as to yield results for the good of society unprocurable by other methods of study and must not be random and unnecessary in nature.[138] Moreover, the experiment must be conducted by scientifically qualified persons[139] in such manner as to avoid all unnecessary physical and mental suffering and injury.[140] If there is an a priori reason to believe that death or disabling injury might occur, the experimenters musts serve as subjects themselves along with the non-scientific personnel[141] [...] The person planning, ordering, supporting, or executing the experiment is under a duty, both moral and legal, to see to it that the experiment is properly performed. This duty cannot be delegated.[142] It is surely incumbent on the doctor performing the experiment to satisfy himself that the subjects volunteered after having been informed of the nature and hazards of the experiment. If they are not volunteers, it is his duty to report to his superiors and discontinue the experiment".[143]

---

134 NDT-Records, frames 10908ff.
135 Ibid., frames 10920ff; see also Shuster (1998), p. 974.
136 Ibid.
137 Ibid., frames 11568-69; see principle three of the Nuremberg Code.
138 Ibid., see principle two of the Nuremberg Code.
139 Ibid., see principle eight of the Nuremberg Code.
140 Ibid., see principle four of the Nuremberg Code.
141 Ibid., see principle five of the Nuremberg Code.
142 Ibid., see principle one of the Nuremberg Code.
143 Ibid., frames 10921-10924; also NDT-Records, frames 11568-11569; see principle ten of the Nuremberg Code.

McHaney's summary provided the judges with core elements of seven of the principles as they stand in the Nuremberg Code. Of central importance in formula-ting the Code were Ivy's three principles from the autumn of 1946, which had been adopted by the AMA in December, and which had also been read into the trial record. Then there were Alexander's six principles from January and April 1947 respectively, which, we must assume, were in the hands of the judges, and, of course, the summary of Ivy and Alexander's memoranda which had been read into the record. By comparing the bulk of this material with the Nuremberg Code it becomes clear that there are a total of eight principles that are almost identical to those in the actual Code. The evidence shows that the Nuremberg Code was drafted in stages and that those who formulated it used a great variety of material in the process. The creation of individual principles was part of an ongoing process for the judges to clarify the ethical issues which had arisen during the trial.

This raises the question of authorship. Both Ivy and Alexander claimed authorship of the Nuremberg Code in the mid-1960s. Their retrospective recollections have to be treated with caution, however, especially since they were written at a time when the issue of medical ethics violations was making national headlines in the United States and elsewhere. Both scientists were skilled operators when it came to promoting their professional image to a wider public. They knew that it could be beneficial for their own reputation to position themselves as the authors of the Code.

The most convincing argumentation to date has been put forward by Evelyn Shuster. She argues that "authorship was shared" between a number of persons including Ivy, Alexander and the judges, and that "the famous 10 principles of the Code grew out of the trial itself".[144] I fully agree with her view that the "key to Nuremberg is to understand the actual testimony of the witnesses at the trial", except that I would extend this point to the testimony of all participants, be this the defendants, the experts, or the prosecution, who were involved at any one time during the trial.[145] As we have seen, the origin of the Code needs to be assessed in the context of a specific evolutionary process which took place during the trial. In this sense the creation of the Code was a "joint solution" (*Gemeinschaftslösung*). Certain individuals contributed at different times important elements to the Code and drafted some of the principles which constituted the basis for the judges to write the Code. Without this material, supplied and annotated by the experts, and communicated to the judges directly or indirectly through the trial transcript, and other perhaps less formal channels, the creation of the Code in its existing form would hardly have been possible.

Yet the question remains as to whether authorship of the Code, in a strict sense of the term, can really be "shared" with the judges. The purpose of the

---

144 Shuster (1997), pp. 1436f; see also Michael Grodin's groundbreaking work on the historical origins of the Nuremberg Code. He was the first who examined the various personalities who shaped the formulation of the Code, Grodin (1992), see also Weindling (2001c).
145 Shuster (1998b), pp. 995f.

experts was to advise and inform the prosecution and the court in all questions of medical science and ethics. They undoubtedly shaped the opinion of the judges and influenced the actual wording of the Code. Yet can they really be considered joint authors of the Code? The Code is an integral part of the judgement. In that sense the author or authors of the Code have to be identical with the authors of the judgement. To write the judgement was the most important, intellectually challenging, legally and ethically complex endeavour of the entire trial. It was the sole duty of the four judges to do so. Their job was to apply the relevant legislation to the specific conditions of the trial and form an opinion on each of the defendants' guilt. No one can have a justified claim over the authorship of the judgement – and therefore the Code – other than the four judges.

That the judges considered the interpretation of the law their exclusive domain became apparent whenever the prosecution – or occasionally the defence team – transgressed into the legal and judgmental realm of the Tribunal. When, during Ivy's testimony, one of the prosecutors touched on legal questions about how scientists should act under certain situations, Sebring made it clear that the question was not for the witness to answer, but for the judges. They claimed the right to issue a legal opinion on medical ethics guidelines and professional medical conduct, and it was for no-one else to do so: "Isn't it possible", Sebring told the prosecution, "that this Tribunal will, in its opinion, answer that question in such a way [so that] scientists in the future will have some landmark to guide them".[146] The Nuremberg Code was meant to be exactly this landmark.

So who was the most influential force among the judges in writing the judgement and the Code? Did they write the judgement and the Code in a series of joint meetings, or was it a single judge, or perhaps two, who drafted the outline of the Code, and the others later commented on it? In the absence of sufficient documentation we need to be cautious in our assessment. Neither do we have precise information as to when the Code was formulated in its existing form, nor about the actual process of its formulation. We also have little knowledge about the communication between the prosecution and the judges, and it is uncertain if and when the judges may have had access to individual reports and memoranda of the medical experts. So far no draft version of the Code from the judges seems to have survived. Most of what can be said therefore remains somewhat speculative. The most likely sequence of events is that one of the judges wrote sections of the judgement in the later part of the trial before discussing it with the members of the bench. During these discussions, the others will have made corrections, suggestions, amendments and changes to the text. They could have formulated questions for individual defendants and witnesses in order to clarify specific points, and ultimately will have approved the judgement as the result of their joint endeavour. The judgement was meant to be the expression of the bench rather than of one individual judge, unless, of course, there was a dissenting opinion. For the Nuremberg Doctors' Trial there is no dissenting opinion.

146 NDT-Records, frame 9277.

According to Tom Sebring, the son of Sebring, who had accompanied his father to Nuremberg, the judges had a gentlemen's agreement that one of them would write the judgement.[147] Justice Beals was already quite old and suffering from arthritis – he died in 1952, five years after the trial – and Justice Crawford was apparently sick during 1947.[148] This left Swearingen and Sebring with the main task of writing the judgement. We can safely rule out Swearingen, not only because he was a junior member of the bench, but because he had not been a judge before coming to Nuremberg but a prosecuting attorney. He asked not a single question of any of the witnesses or defendants throughout the entire trial, and was excluded from reading out the judgement in court. By taking these factors into consideration, whilst being careful not to put too much weight on the oral testimony of interested parties, there is reason to believe that the judge who drafted most of the opinion, and therefore the Nuremberg Code, was probably Harold Sebring.

Since the beginning of the trial Sebring had turned out to be the most meticulous, intellectually able, and legally minded of the Tribunal. He would frequently point to some of the far-reaching legal and procedural problems during the planning period of the trial. Although Beals had been elected presiding judge because of his seniority, he would always consult with Sebring during the executive sessions in November 1946 before presenting a motion to the Tribunal. Questions asked by the bench came for most of the time from either Beals or Sebring. Only once, on 7 May, did judge Crawford question the defendant Georg August Weltz.[149] Otherwise he appears to have remained mostly silent, like his colleague judge Swearingen.[150] Beals only examined a witness on eleven occasions, Sebring did so in a total of thirty-one cases, starting with Karl Brandt on 6 February and concluding with the witness Constantyn Johan Broers on 30 June 1947.[151] Sometimes Sebring would also interrogate a witness more than once.[152] Even more significantly, almost all questions relating to medical ethics and professional standards of practice were asked by Sebring, particularly during the testimonies of Brandt, Handloser, Hartleben and Rostock in February, and during those of Sievers, Hielscher, Ruff, Romberg and Weltz at the end of April and beginning of May, and also during Beiglböck and Hoven's testimony in June 1947 and, of course, during Ivy's rebuttal testimony in the same month. In marked contrast to this, Beals rarely touched on issues of medical ethics.[153] Sebring was

---

147 Interview with H. L. (Tom) Sebring, Tallahassee, March 1998; Tom accompanied his father to Nuremberg as an adolescent. According to Tom Sebring, Nuremberg was one of the most stressful experiences in his fathers' life.
148 NARA, RG 153, 87-2, book 5, box 14.
149 NDT-Records, frames 7284-7285.
150 The trial transcript does not seem to record that Swearingen ever questioned any of the witnesses or defendants individually throughout the trial. Those instances where the tribunal questioned a witness jointly were not taken into consideration.
151 Schmidt (2004), pp. 249f.
152 Ibid.
153 See Gebhardt, 7 March 1947, NDT-Records, frames 4352-4353; Volhard, 3 June 1947, NDT-Records, frames 8639-8642.

not only the most actively involved judge during the second half of the trial, but also the one who seems to have been in charge of matters relating to professional medical ethics.

Sebring's biography reveals why he was so interested in upholding professional standards. Married to the daughter of a well-known physician of the Florida region, and an active member of the Baptist Church, Sebring enjoyed a reputation for adherence to professional ethics. He strongly believed in the responsibility of the doctor to society, whilst advocating the protection of the rights of the individual.[154] Colleagues described him as plain spoken and easy to work with, but extremely hard working and with a great sense of formality and protocol.[155] He once advised one of his younger colleagues: "When you accept the robe, remember it is like a clerical collar; don't do this unless you are willing to be a judge the rest of your professional life".[156] Sebring was also known for formulating lucid, intellectually flawless and convincing interpretations of the law. Many of his opinions later became landmarks in American law and were used for reference purposes by law students. It might not therefore be altogether surprising that the person with the greatest sense of professional legal standards appears to have been the driving force in devising a set of professional medical ethics standards.

There is, however, no evidence to substantiate this claim. Sebring was a modest man. If he wrote something on the subject he made sure that it could not be construed in such a way that it appeared that he had written the judgement or the Code. To do so would have meant not only to betray his Nuremberg peers, but also to act against the professional code of conduct of the legal profession. When during the IMT the British requested that either the ageing Gustav Krupp should be tried *in absentia* or his son Alfried should be added to the indictment, the Tribunal was shocked. One of the judges, while pacing up and down the park, told his aide: "Cap'n, if we were to grant this motion, there wouldn't be a lawyer in North Carolina that didn't think we had permitted substitution in a criminal trial".[157] For this judge the North Carolina Bar was the most important and trustworthy yardstick against which all principles and procedures would be have to be measured. Likewise the Florida Bar was the most important yardstick for Sebring.[158] He knew that for all Florida lawyers, and indeed for all members of the American Bar, it was an unquestioned principle that the judgement would be issued jointly, and not by any of the judges individually. If Sebring ever told someone about the origin of the Code, he will probably have done so in the strictest of confidence. For him it was important to follow the professional rules, far more important than any claim to fame.

---

154 SCHST, Sebring papers, Honorable Justice Harold L. Sebring; Fla.Cas. 86-89, So.2d, p. XLV.
155 SCHST, Sebring papers, Transcript of interview with Justice Roberts, 21 April 1980.
156 SCHST, Sebring papers, Remarks by Overton about Sebring, 2 November 1990.
157 Tusa/Tusa (1995), p. 139.
158 See also NARA, RG 153, 89-1, book 2, box 5, folder 2, Sebring to Young, 20 September 1948.

The actual formulation of the Code stands in close connection with the progression and development of the trial. The debates about, and proposals for the creation of a new international medical ethics code in the months before the start of the Doctors' trial, both within the US prosecution and as part of the ISC (WC), were important in drawing the attention of the judges to the issue of professional medical ethics. Yet it is during the trial that originally vague and broadly defined principles were being formulated into a code of legally binding, professional and moral-ethical guidelines for permissible research on humans which attained a universal status. These guidelines were pre-formulated in a collaborative environment between the US prosecution and the medical expert witnesses, and adopted by the judges in a partly identical or modified form in the judgement of the Tribunal. Moreover, the judges used the actual testimonies which were read into the record in order to formulate specific principles for research on humans. The authorship of the Nuremberg Code thus remains inextricably linked with the role of the judges, independent of whether parts of the Code were pre-formulated. Educated in the case law tradition it was not unusual for American judges to go significantly beyond the case in front of them if they believed that they were dealing with a precedent which needed the formulation of new law. In this case the new law constituted a code of medical ethics that was to serve as a guide to future research on human subjects. The decision of the judges to include the Code formally into the judgement also meant that, for the first time, written guidelines for permissible research on humans were incorporated into the canon of international law. This was a substantial achievement, irrespective of the limited effect which the Code had in the following decades for the protection of human and patient rights.

Sebring also read out the part of the judgement containing the Nuremberg Code which is, perhaps, another indication that he was most strongly involved in its formulation. Judged by the material which had been presented in court there were "certain types" of experiments on humans which, as long they would remain within "reasonably well-defined bounds", conformed to the ethics of the medical profession in the civilised world. The Tribunal acknowledged that scientists justified human experiments on the basis that they yield results for the good of human society which could not be produced by other means of study. "All agree, however, that certain basic principles must be observed in order to satisfy moral, ethical and legal concepts".[159] These principles were as follows:

"1. The voluntary consent of the human subject is absolutely essential.

This means that the person involved should have legal capacity to give consent; should be so situated as to be able to exercise free power of choice, without the intervention of any element of force, fraud, deceit, duress, overreaching, or other ulterior form of constraint or coercion; and should have sufficient knowledge and comprehension of the elements of the subject matter involved as to enable him to make an understanding and enlightened decision. This latter element requires that before the acceptance of an affirmative decision by the experimental subject there should be made known to him the nature, duration, and purpose of the experiment; the method and means by which it is to be conducted; all inconveniences and

159 NDT-Records, frame 11568.

hazards reasonably to be expected; and the effects upon his health or person which may possibly come from his participation in the experiment.

The duty and responsibility for ascertaining the quality of the consent rests upon each individual who initiates, directs or engages in the experiment. It is a personal duty and responsibility which may not be delegated to another with impunity

2. The experiment should be such as to yield fruitful results for the good of society, unprocurable by other methods or means of study, and not random and unnecessary in nature.

3. The experiment should be so designed and based on the results of animal experimentation and a knowledge of the natural history of the disease or other problem under study that the anticipated results will justify the performance of the experiment.

4. The experiment should be so conducted as to avoid all unnecessary physical and mental suffering and injury.

5. No experiment should be conducted where there is an a priori reason to believe that death or disabling injury will occur; except, perhaps, in those experiments where the experimental physicians also serve as subjects.

6. The degree of risk to be taken should never exceed that determined by the humanitarian importance of the problem to be solved by the experiment.

7. Proper preparation should be made and adequate facilities provided to protect the experimental subject against even remote possibilities of injury, disability, or death.

8. The experiment should be conducted only by scientifically qualified persons. The highest degree of skill and care should be required through all stages of the experiment of those who conduct or engage in the experiment.

9. During the course of the experiment the human subject should be at liberty to bring the experiment to an end if he had reached the physical or mental state where continuation of the experiment seems to him to be impossible.

10. During the course of the experiment the scientist in charge must be prepared to terminate the experiment at any stage, if he had probable cause to believe, in the exercise of the good faith, superior skill, and careful judgement required of him, that a continuation of the experiment is likely to result in injury, disability, or death to the experimental subject".[160]

The Nuremberg Code established fundamental human rights in medicine, and placed the welfare of the patients into the foreground of medical practice. In the Nuremberg Code neither medicine, nor science, nor society or any kind of collective or utilitarian ethics has priority over the protection of the individual to remain physically and psychologically unharmed. A persons' right to self-determination and inviolability cannot be calculated against some fictitious need for medical progress, or any other claim that society and science may or may not have towards its citizens. In a lucid and unambiguous language, the Code states that the rights and integrity of the research subjects have to be preserved at all times.

Of the ten principles, two principles – one and nine – specifically refer to the protection and rights of the experimental subject, and principle eight to their well being. Principle one of the Code has been of importance for the history of medical ethics which reaches far beyond Nuremberg. The principle links the experiment to the voluntary consent of the experimental subject. That means that the experiment can only be carried out after the "voluntary, personal consent" has been obtained, and only after the subject has been clearly informed about the risk involved in the best possible manner. The Code makes it unequivocally and categorically clear that the person involved in the experiment has to have the legal capacity to give a

160 Ibid., frames 11568-11569.

voluntary consent. Moreover, prior to obtaining consent, the exact nature, duration and objective of the experiment, the applied methods and means as well as all potential implications of the experiment for the health of the person have to be made clear. The experimental subject has to have sufficient knowledge of, and capacity to comprehend, the subject matter in order to make an enlightened and informed decision. This was meant to protect unconscious and mentally handi-capped persons or humans who, because of their specific illness, are unable to give voluntary consent. The Code made it clear that no experiments are legally and ethically permissible on the aforementioned patient groups. Since the late 19th century the status of the voluntary consent principle was greatly enhanced as a central element of medical research. The Code, for the first time, transferred this principle as part of the Nuremberg judgement onto international law.

Principle nine likewise deserves attention as another essential medical ethics' law: the right of the experimental person to terminate the experiment at any time. The principle was formulated as a right and not as a guideline, and thus constitu-ted another legal precedent. These innovative patient rights were given further weight through the formulation of unequivocal duties of the physician-researchers to act at all times responsible towards the patient-subject. The rights of the patient do not replace the duties of the researcher as outlined in principles two to eight. A person who has given his or her voluntary consent cannot be used for a random number of experiments; these experiments cannot violate professional medical ethics' standards because the person had consented to the research. That is why, according to principle ten of the Code, it is the duty of the scientist in charge to terminate the experiment on his or her own initiative, and at any stage, if there is reason to believe that the continuation of the experiment would, in all probability, result in injury, disability or death of the experimental subject.

The Nuremberg Code constitutes a particular, and in many ways unique, combination of human rights, which are part of international law, and the Hippo-cratic medical ethics. For the judges Hippocratic medical ethics was an important precondition to protect the welfare and lives of patient-subjects, but it appeared insufficient in protecting human lives in human experimentation. They realised that research subjects needed to have quite specific rights, if they were to be sufficiently protected from potential harm. That is why the conditions under which informed voluntary consent can be obtained in the Code are formulated in a much more comprehensive and legalistic fashion than in any other earlier medical ethics' codes. The principle of voluntary consent in the Code thus demands the status of an absolute, *a priori* principle. Moreover, the experimental subject is given the right to terminate the experiment at any time. The Nuremberg Code is therefore a legal code and, at the same time, a medical ethics' code. That is the Code's particular strength.

VIII. Conclusion

The judgement reflected the creation of new legal principles to cover the issues which had arisen from this precedent. The judges believed in the creation of an international legal and professional framework which would empower those who had suffered harm to claim their rights against those who had violated them. The Nuremberg Code was in many ways a visionary and innovative medical ethics' code. Its principles were designed to apply to all research involving human subjects. Even today, the Nuremberg Code has significant symbolic and, in many ways, an influential role in the field of medical politics, ethics and law.[161] It also serves as a major point of reference to assess whether or not scientists who conducted experimental research on humans complied with, or failed to observe, medical ethics standards during the Cold War period.

At first, though, people paid little attention to the Code. The German people were not interested in the Nuremberg judgement, nor was the international medical community keen to acknowledge the existence of the Code. Western medical scientists were unwilling to relate what had been discussed in Nuremberg to their own research practice. The Code, in other words, had come into this world by default, mostly hidden away from the public eye, known to a few experts and institutions, and applied by even fewer medical innovators. The medical ethicist Jay Katz poignantly captured the attitude of post-war Western medical researchers who felt that "it was a good code for barbarians but an unnecessary code for ordinary physician-scientists".[162] Others, such as David Rothman, have observed that "the prevailing view was that [the Nuremberg medical defendants] were Nazis first and last; by definition nothing they did, and no code drawn up in response to them, was relevant to the United States".[163] But as evidence from cold-war Allied research laboratories is beginning to emerge in no small measure, one can wonder whether it might have been wiser, perhaps, if Western scientists had not ignored, or simply dismissed, the new professional guidelines on human experimentation which their own experts had formulated at Nuremberg. It not only might have prevented much subsequent embarrassment by the authorities and ongoing compensation claims in Anglo-American courts, but, more significantly, may in fact have prevented serious injuries, disabilities and death of hundreds of experimental subjects, not to speak of the untold human suffering of the relatives involved.

161 See also the article by Ulf Schmidt in this book.
162 Katz (1992), p. 228; also Katz (1996), p. 1663.
163 Rothman (1991), pp. 62f.

References

Primary Sources

AP   Alexander Papers, Boston (in possession of Cecily Alexander-
                  Grable)
BAK   Bundesarchiv Koblenz, Zsg 154
DUMC   Duke University Archive, Alexander Papers, Depository for
                  Medical Center Records, Collected Papers and Documents 65th
                  General Hospital
FCLM   Beecher papers. Francis A. Countway Library of Medicine,
                  Boston, Mass.
MGP   Michael Grodin Papers (Boston University)
NARA   National Archives and Record Administration, Washington D.C.
NDT-Documents and Material. Nuremberg Doctors' Trial-Documents and Mate-
                  rial, in: Dörner/Ebbinghaus (1999)
NDT-Records   Nuremberg Doctors' Trial-Records, in: Dörner/Ebbinghaus
                  (1999)
SCHST   Supreme Court Historical Society Tallahassee, Florida
StUF   Archivzentrum der Stadt- und Universitätsbibliothek Frankfurt
                  am Main
TNA   The National Archives, London
UWAHC   University of Wyoming, American Heritage Center, Andrew C.
                  Ivy Papers (#8768)

Alexander Papers 1-6
(For the whereabouts of the papers see DUMC, Alexander papers, box 1, folder 9
and 12; box 4, folder 34; see also Alexander 1976).

Alexander Paper 1: The Fundamental Purpose and Meaning of the Experiments of
    the Experiments in Human Beings of which the Accused (Military Tribunal
    No. 1, Case No. 1) have been Indicted: Thanatology as a Scientific Technique
    of Genocide, 30 November 1946.
Alexander Paper 2: Suggestions for a Discussion of the Thanatology Genocide
    Angle, 5 December 1946.
Alexander Paper 3: Ethical and Non-Ethical Experimentation on Human Beings, 7
    December 1946.
Alexander Paper 4: One Major Aim of the German Vivisectionists: Ktenology as a
    Scientific Technique of Genocide, 15 January 1947.
Alexander Paper 5: Ethical and Non-Ethical Experimentation· on Human Beings,
    15 April 1947 (10 pages).
Alexander Paper 6: Ethical and Non-Ethical Experimentation on Human Beings,
    General Ethical, Medico-Legal and Scientific Considerations in Connection
    with the Vivisectionists Trial Before the Military Tribunal in Germany, no
    date (29 pages).

Secondary Literature

Alexander, L. (1948/49): War Crimes and their Motivation. The Socio-Psychological Structure of the SS and the Criminalization of a Society, The Journal of Criminal Law and Criminology 39 (1948/49), pp. 298-326.

Alexander, L. (1949): Science under Dictatorship, March of Medicine 14 (1949), pp. 51-106.

Alexander, L. (1966): Limitations in Experimental Research on Human Beings. Lex et Scientia, International Journal of Law and Science 3 (1966), pp. 8-24.

Alexander, L. (1976): Ethics of Human Experimentation, Psychiatric Journal of the University of Ottawa 1 (1976), pp. 40-46.

Ambroselli, C. (1997): Proces des medecins a Nuremberg 1946-1997, Journal de l' Association des medecins israelites de France 45 (1997), 459, pp. 1-51.

Annas, G. J. (1992): The Nuremberg Code in U.S. Courts: Ethics versus Expediency, in: Annas/Grodin (1992), pp. 201-222.

Annas, G. J./Grodin, M. A. (eds.) (1992): The Nazi Doctors and the Nuremberg Code. Human Rights in Human Experimentation. New York, Oxford: Oxford University Press.

Annas, G. J./Grodin, M. A. (1996): Medicine and Human Rights: Reflections on the Fiftieth Anniversary of the Doctors' Trial, in: Mann et al. (1996), pp. 301-311.

Annas, G. J./Grodin, M. A. (1998): Medizinische Ethik und Menschenrechte: Das Vermächtnis von Nürnberg, in: Kolb/Seithe (1998), pp. 244-259.

Anonymous (1945): Prison Malaria: Convicts Expose Themselves to Disease so Doctors can Study it, Life 18 (1945), 23, pp. 43-46.

Anonymous (1946): A Moral Problem. The Lancet, 30 November 1946.

Anonymous (1947): Doctors on Trial, British Medical Journal 1, p. 143.

Arnold, P./Sprumont, D. (1997): Der Nürnberger Kodex: Regeln des Völkerrechts, in: Tröhler/Reiter-Theil (1997), pp. 115-130.

Baader, G./Schultz, U. (eds.) (1983): Medizin im Nationalsozialismus. Tabuisierte Vergangenheit – Ungebrochene Tradition? Berlin: Verlagsgesellschaft Gesundheit.

Baker, R. (1997): Transkulturelle Medizinethik und Menschenrechte, in: Tröhler/Reiter-Theil (1997), pp. 433-460.

Baker, R./McCullough, L. B. (eds.) (2007): A History of Medical Ethics. Cambridge, New York: Cambridge University Press (in press).

Boyes, R. (2000): Nazi Doctor Killed 772 Children. The Times, 21 March 2000.

Burleigh, M. (1994): Death and Deliverance, 'Euthanasia' in Germany, 1900-1945. Cambridge, New York: Cambridge University Press.

Deutsch, E. (1997): Der Nürnberger Kodex. Das Strafverfahren gegen Mediziner, die zehn Prinzipien von Nürnberg und die bleibende Bedeutung des Nürnberger Kodex, in: Tröhler/Reiter-Theil (1997), pp. 103-114.

Dörner, K. (2001): "Ich darf nicht denken". Das medizinische Selbstverständnis der Angeklagten, in: Ebbinghaus/Dörner (2001), pp. 331-357.

Dörner, K./Ebbinghaus, A. (eds.) (1999): Der Nürnberger Ärzteprozeß 1946/47. München. Mikrofiche.

Douraki, T. (1997): Die Anerkennung der Patientenrechte, insbesondere der psychisch Kranken. Internationale Organisation und die Europäische Menschenrechtskonvention, in: Tröhler/Reiter-Theil (1997), pp. 321-342.

Drinan, R. (1992): The Nuremberg Principles in International Law, in: Annas/Grodin (1992), pp. 174-182.

Ebbinghaus, A. (2001): Strategien der Verteidigung, in: Ebbinghaus/Dörner (2001), pp. 405-435.

Ebbinghaus, A./Dörner, K. (2001) (eds.): Vernichten und Heilen. Der Nürnberger Ärzteprozeß und seine Folgen. Berlin: Aufbau.

Elkeles, B. (1997): Der moralische Diskurs über das medizinische Menschen experiment im 19. Jahrhundert. Stuttgart, Jena, New York: Gustav Fischer.

Ernst, E. M./Weindling, P. J. (1998): The Nuremberg Medical Trial: Have We Learned the Lessons, The Journal of Laboratory and Clinical Medicine 131 (1998), 2, pp. 130-135.

Faden, R./Lederer, S. E./Moreno, J.D. (1996): US Medical Researchers, the Nuremberg Doctors' Trial, and the Nuremberg Code: Findings of the Advisory Committee on Human Radiation Experiments, Journal of the American Medical Association 276 (1996), 20, pp. 1667-1671.

Faden, R./Beauchamp, T. L. (1986): A History and Theory of Informed Consent. Oxford/New York: Oxford University Press.

Fluss, S. S. (1999): How the Declaration of Helsinki Developed, Good Clinical Practice Journal (1999), 6, pp. 18-22.

Foreign Office (1949): Scientific Results of German Medical War Crimes. London: HMSO.

Frewer, A. et al. (eds.) (1999): Medizinverbrechen vor Gericht. Das Urteil im Nürnberger Ärzteprozeß gegen Karl Brandt und andere sowie aus dem Prozeß gegen Generalfeldmarschall Erhard Milch. Bearbeitet und kommentiert von U.-D. Oppitz. Erlangen, Jena: Palm & Enke.

Frewer, A. (2000): Medizin und Moral in Weimarer Republik und Nationalsozialismus. Die Zeitschrift "Ethik" unter Emil Abderhalden. Frankfurt am Main, New York: Campus.

Frewer, A./Eickhoff, C. (eds.) (2000): "Euthanasie" und die aktuelle Sterbehilfe-Debatte. Die historischen Hintergründe medizinischer Ethik. Frankfurt am Main, New York: Campus.

Frewer, A./Neumann, J. N. (eds.) (2001): Medizingeschichte und Medizinethik. Kontroversen und Begründungsansätze 1900-1950. Frankfurt am Main, New York: Campus.

Friedlander, H. (1995): The Origins of Nazi Genocide. From Euthanasia to the Final Solution. London: Chapel Hill.

Friedman, T. (1997): Lessons from Nuremberg: Ethical and Social Responsibilities for Health Care Professionals, Health Care Organisations, and Medical Journals, Journal of the American Medical Association 277 (1997), 9, pp. 710-712.

Gerst, T. (1996): 50 Jahre Nürnberger Kodex. Entwicklung, Wirksamkeit und künftige Bedeutung ethischer Kodizes in der Medizin, Deutsches Ärzteblatt 93 (1996), 22, pp. 1020-1021.

Glantz, L. H. (1992): The Influence of the Nuremberg Code on U.S. Statutes and Regulations, in: Annas/Grodin (1992), pp. 183-200.

Grodin, M. A. (1992): Historical Origins of the Nuremberg Code, in: Annas/ Grodin (1992), pp. 121-144.

Grodin, M. A./Annas, G. J./Glantz, L. H. (1993): Medicine and Human Rights: A Proposal for International Action, Hastings Center Report 23 (1993), pp. 8-12.

Harkness, J. M. (1996): Nuremberg and the Issue of Wartime Experiments on US Prisoners. The Green Committee, Journal of the American Medical Association 276 (1996), 20, pp. 1672-1675.

Herbert, D. (1947): A Moral Problem. The Lancet, 11 January 1947, pp. 84-85.

Herranz, G. (1997): Der Eingang der zehn Nürnberger Postulate in berufsständische Ethik-Kodizes. Ein internationaler Vergleich, in: Tröhler/Reiter-Theil (1997), pp. 171-188.

Hilton, S. H. (1947): A Moral Problem. The Lancet, 4 January 1947, p. 43.

Horner, J. S. (1999): Retreat from Nuremberg: Can we prevent unethical medical research?, Public-Health 113 (1999), 5, pp. 205-210.

Human, D. (2000): World Medical Association and the Declaration of Helsinki, The EFGCP News (2000), 4, pp. 1-2, p. 14.

Ivy, A.C. (1947): Nazi War Crimes of a Medical Nature, Federation Bulletin 33 (1947), pp. 133-46.

Ivy, A.C. (1948): Nazi War Crimes of a Medical Nature, Phi Lambda Kappa Quart 22 (1948), pp. 5-12.

Katz, J. (1992): The Consent Principle of the Nuremberg Code: Its Significance Then and Now, in: Annas/Grodin (1992), pp. 227-239.

Katz, J. (1996): The Nuremberg Code and the Nuremberg Trial: A Reappraisal, Journal of the American Medical Association 276 (1996), 20, pp. 1662-1666.

Katz, J. (1997): Human Sacrifice and Human Experimentation: Reflections at Nuremberg, Yale Journal of International Law 22 (1997), pp. 401-418.

Katz, J. (1998): Menschenopfer und Menschenversuche. Nachdenken in Nürnberg, in: Kolb/Seithe (1998), pp. 225-243.

Kaufmann, D. ed. (2000): Geschichte der Kaiser-Wilhelm-Gesellschaft im Nationalsozialismus. Bestandsaufnahme und Perspektiven der Forschung, 2 vols. Göttingen: Wallstein.

Klee, E. (1997): Auschwitz. Die NS-Medizin und ihre Opfer. Frankfurt am Main: Fischer.

Kolb, S./Seithe, H. (1998): Medizin und Gewissen: 50 Jahre nach dem Nürnberger Ärzteprozeß. Frankfurt am Main: Mabuse .

Koonz, C. (2003): The Nazi Conscience. Cambridge, Mass., London: Belknap Press.

Krause, T. L./Winslade, W. (1997): Fünfzig Jahre Nürnberger Kodex, in: Tröhler/ Reiter-Theil (1997), pp. 189-220.

Layton, T.B./Nelson-Jones, A. (1946): A Moral Problem. The Lancet, 14 December 1946, p. 882.

Lemkin, R. (1944): Axis Rule in Occupied Europe. Proposals for Redress. Washington D.C.: Carnegie Endowment for International Peace.

Levi, P. (1996): The Drowned and the Saved. London: Abacus.

Macklin, R. (1992): Universality of the Nuremberg Code, in: Annas/Grodin (1992), pp. 258-275.

Maio, G. (1996): Das Humanexperiment vor und nach Nürnberg: Überlegungen zum Menschenversuch und zum Einwilligungsbegriff in der französischen Diskussion des 19. und 20. Jahrhunderts, in: Wiesemann/Frewer (1996), pp. 45-78.

Mann, J. M./Gruskin, S./Grodin, M. A./Annas G. J. (eds.) (1999): Health and Human Rights. New York, London: Routledge.

Marrus, M. M. (1999): The Nuremberg Doctors' Trial in Historical Context, Bulletin for the History of Medicine 73 (1999), 1, pp. 106-123.

Matheiu, B. (1997): Die ethischen Normen und das Recht: Legitimation durch die "Weisen" und demokratische Legitimation, in: Tröhler/Reiter-Theil (1997), pp. 221-248.

Matheiu, B. (1998): From the Nuremberg Code to Bioethics: Follow-Ups to a Founder Text, International Digest of Health Legislation 49 (1998), 3, pp. 549-554.

Mattei, J. F./Moatti, J. P./Rauch, C. (1997): Zur Ethik in der Politik der gerechten Verteilung knapper Ressourcen in Frankreich, in: Tröhler/Reiter-Theil (1997), pp. 423-432.

Mausbach, H. (1998): Thesen zum Nürnberger Ärzteprozeß. Charakter des Prozesses, Nachwirkungen und seine Bedeutung für die Zukunft, in: Kolb/Seithe (1998), pp. 260-268.

Mellanby, K. (1946): A Moral Problem. The Lancet, 7 December 1946, p. 850.

Mellanby, K. (1947): Medical Experiments on Human Beings in Concentration Camps in Nazi Germany, British Medical Journal 1 (1947), pp. 148-150.

Mielke, F. (1948): Der Nürnberger Prozeß gegen SS-Ärzte und Wissenschaftler und der deutsche Arzt, Niedersächsisches Ärzteblatt 2 (1948), pp. 29-31.

Mitscherlich, A./Mielke, F. (eds.) (1995): Medizin ohne Menschlichkeit. Dokumente des Nürnberger Ärzteprozesses. Durchgesehene und neu gesetzte Ausgabe. Frankfurt am Main: Fischer.

Mitscherlich, A./Mitscherlich, M. (1967): Die Unfähigkeit zu trauern. Grundlagen kollektiven Verhaltens. München: Piper.

Moreno, J. D. (1996): "The Only Feasible Means": The Pentagon's Ambivalent Relationship with the Nuremberg Code, Hastings Center Report 26 (1996), 5, pp. 11-19.

Moreno, J. D. (1997): Reassessing the Influence of the Nuremberg Code on American Medical Ethics, Journal of Contemporary Health Law and Policy 13 (1997), 2, pp. 347-360.

Moreno, J. D. (1999): Undue Risk: Secret State Experiments on Humans. New York: Freeman.

Müller-Hill, B. (1988): Murderous Science. Elimination by Sientific Selection of Jews, Gypsies, and Others, Germany 1933-1945. Oxford: Oxford University Press.

New York Times, 12 December 1946. New York Times, 12 December 1946.

Perley, S./Fluss, S. S./Zbigniew, B./Simon, F. (1992): The Nuremberg Code: An International Overview, in: Annas/Grodin (1992), pp. 149-173.

Peter, J. (1994): Der Nürnberger Ärzteprozeß im Spiegel seiner Aufarbeitung anhand der drei Dokumentensammlungen von Alexander Mitscherlich und Fred Mielke. Münster: Lit.

Peter, J. (2001): Unmittelbare Reaktionen auf den Prozeß. Die Kontroverse in der "Göttinger Universitätszeitung", in: Ebbinghaus/Dörner (2001), pp. 473-475.

Platen, A. von (1947a): Ärzteprozeß Nürnberg', Hippokrates 1 (1947), pp. 29-31.

Platen, A. von (1947b): Der Nürnberger Ärzteprozeß II, Hippokrates 17 (1947), pp. 199-202.

Platen-Hallermund, A. v. (1948): Die Tötung Geisteskranker in Deutschland. Frankfurt am Main: Verlag der Frankfurter Hefte.

Platen-Hallermund, A. v. (1993): Die Tötung Geisteskranker in Deutschland, [Reprint], Mit einem Vorwort der Autorin und einem Geleitwort von Klaus Dörner. Bonn: Psychiatrie Verlag.

Proctor, R.N. (2000): Expert Witnesses take the Stand. Historians of Science can Play an Important Role in US Public Health Litigation, Nature 407 (2000), pp. 15-16.

Reich, W. (2000): Betrayal of Care: Medicine and the Long Shadow of Nuremberg, Biomedical Ethics 98 (2000), 1, pp. 7-9.

Rißmann, B. (1947): Begriffsverwirrung, Die Gegenwart 2 (1947), pp. 12-14.

Roelcke, V./Maio, G. (eds.) (2004): Twentieth Century Ethics of Human Subjects Research. Historical Perspectives on Values, Practices, and Regulations. Stuttgart: Steiner.

Rothman, D.J. (1991): Strangers at the Bedside: A History of How Law and Bioethics Transformed Medical Decision Making. New York: Basic Books.

Rothman, D. J. (1997): Der Nürnberger Kodex im Licht früherer Prinzipien und Praktiken im Bereich der Humanexperimente, in: Tröhler/Reiter-Theil (1997), pp. 75-88.

Sass, H.-M. (1983): Reichsrundschreiben 1931: Pre-Nuremberg German Regulations Concerning New Therapy and Human Experimentation, The Journal of Medicine and Philosophy 8 (1983), pp. 99-111.

Schmidt, U. (1997): German Medical War Crimes, Medical Ethics and Post-War Justice: A Symposium held at the University of Oxford to Mark the 50th Anniversary of the Nuremberg Medical Trial, 14 March 1997, German History 15 (1997), 3, pp. 385-391.

Schmidt, U. (1999): Reassessing the Beginning of the 'Euthanasia' Programme, German History 17 (1999), 4, pp. 541-548.

Schmidt, U. (2000): Kriegsausbruch und "Euthanasie": Neue Forschungsergebnisse zum "Knauer Kind" im Jahre 1939, in: Frewer/Eickhoff (2000), pp. 113-129.

Schmidt, U. (2001a): Die Angeklagten Fritz Fischer, Hans W. Romberg und Karl Brandt aus der Sicht des Sachverständigen Leo Alexander, in: Ebbinghaus/ Dörner (2001), pp. 374-404.

Schmidt, U. (2001b): Der Ärzteprozeß als moralische Instanz? Der Nürnberger Kodex und das Problem "zeitloser Medizinethik", in: Frewer/Neumann (2001), pp. 334-372.

Schmidt, U. (2002): Medical Films, Ethics and Euthanasia in Nazi Germany. Husum: Matthiesen.

Schmidt, U. (2004): Justice at Nuremberg. Leo Alexander and the Nazi Doctors' Trial. Basingstoke: Palgrave.

Schmidt, U. (2005): The Scars of Ravensbrück: Medical Experiments and British War Crimes Policy, 1945-1950, German History 23 (2005), 1, pp. 20-49.

Schmidt, U. (2007): Medicine and Nazism, in: McCullough/Baker (2007), forthcoming.

Schmuhl, H.-W. (2001): Die Patientenmorde, in: Ebbinghaus/Dörner (2001), pp. 295-328.

Seidel, R. (2001): Die Sachverständigen Werner Leibbrand und Andrew C. Ivy, in: Ebbinghaus/Dörner (2001), pp. 358-373.

Seidelmann, W. (1998): Mit Nürnberg abgetan. Gewissen und Erinnerung in der Medizin, in: Kolb/Seithe (1998), pp. 269-279.

Shevell, M. I. (1997): Neurology's Witness to History (Part 2): Leo Alexander's Contribution to the Nuremberg Code, Neurology 50 (1997), 1, pp. 274-278.

Shuster, E. (1997): Fifty Years Later: The Significance of the Nuremberg Code, The New England Journal of Medicine 337 (1997), 20, pp. 1436-1440.

Shuster, E. (1998a): The Nuremberg Code: Hippocratic Ethics and Human Rights, Lancet 351 (1998), 9107, pp. 974-977.

Shuster, E. (1998b): The Significance of the Nuremberg Code: Letter to the Editor, New England Journal of Medicine 338 (1998), pp. 995-996.

Taylor, T. (1976): Biomedical Ethics and the Shadow of Nazism, Hastings Center Report, Special Suplememt 6 (1976), pp. 4-7.

Taylor, T. (1992): The Anatomy of the Nuremberg Trials: A Personal Memoir. New York: Knopf.

Toellner, R. (1998): Der Blinde Spiegel. Über das Verhältnis der deutschen Ärzteschaft zum Nürnberger Ärzteprozeß in seiner epochalen Bedeutung, in: Kolb/Seithe (1998), pp. 288-304.

Trials of War Criminals before the Nuernberg Military Tribunals under Control Council Law No. 10, Nuremberg, October 1946 – April 1949. Washington, D.C.: U.S.G.P.O.

Tröhler, U./Reiter-Theil, S. (eds.) (1997): Ethik und Medizin: 1947-1997. Was leistet die Kodifizierung von Ethik? Göttingen: Wallstein.

Tusa, T./Tusa, J. (1995): The Nuremberg Trial. London: BBC Books.

United Nations War Crimes Commission (1948): History of the United Nations War Crimes Commission and the Development of the Laws of War. London: HMSO.

United States Advisory Committee on Human Radiation Experiments (1996): Advisory Committee on Human Radiation Experiments Final Report. New York, NY; Oxford: Oxford University Press

Vanderpool, H. Y. (ed.) (1996): The Ethics of Research Involving Human Subjects. Facing the 21st Century. Frederick, Md.: University Publishing Group.

Weindling, P. J. (1996): Ärzte als Richter: Internationale Reaktionen auf die medizinischen Verbrechen während des Nürnberger Ärzteprozesses im Jahre 1946-47, in: Wiesemann/Frewer (1996), pp. 31-44.

Weindling, P. J. (2000a): Epidemics and Genocide in Eastern Europe, 1890-1945. Oxford: Oxford University Press.

Weindling, P. J. (2000b): From International to Zonal Trials: The Origins of the Nuremberg Medical Trial, Holocaust Genocide Studies 14 (2000), pp. 367-389.

Weindling, P. J. (2000c): Tales from Nuremberg: The Kaiser Wilhelm Institute for Anthropology and Allied Medical War Crimes Policy, in: Kaufmann (2000), pp. 635-652.

Weindling, P. J. (2001a): Die Internationale Wissenschaftskommission für medizinische Kriegsverbrechen, in: Ebbinghaus/Dörner (2001), pp. 439-451.

Weindling, P. J. (2001b). Gerechtigkeit aus der Perspektive der Medizingeschichte: "Euthanasie" im Nürnberger Ärzteprozeß, in: Frewer/Neumann (2001), pp. 311-333.

Weindling, P. J. (2001c): The Origins of Informed Consent: The International Scientific Commission on Medical War Crimes, and the Nuremberg Code, Bulletin of the History of Medicine 75 (2001), pp. 37-71.

Weindling, P. J. (2001d): Zur Vorgeschichte des Nürnberger Ärzteprozesses, in: Ebbinghaus/Dörner (2001), pp. 26-47.

Weindling, P. J. (2004): Nazi Medicine and the Nuremberg Trials: From Medical War Crimes to Informed Consent. Basingstoke: Palgrave.

Wiesemann, C./Frewer, A. (eds.) (1996): Medizin und Ethik im Zeichen von Auschwitz. 50 Jahre Nürnberger Ärzteprozeß, Erlangen, Jena: Palme & Enke.

Wiesing, U. (1997): Der "Nürnberger Kodex 1997". Ein Kommentar, Ethik in der Medizin 43 (1997), 4, pp. 335-339.

Winau, R. (1996): Medizin und Menschenversuch. Zur Geschichte des "informed consent", in: Wiesemann/Frewer (1996), pp. 13-29.

Winau, R. (2001): Der Menschenversuch in der Medizin, in: Ebbinghaus/Dörner (2001), pp. 93-109.

Wunder, M. (1998): Bioethik – Eine Philosophie ohne Menschlichkeit, in: Kolb/Seithe (1998), pp. 313-319.

Wunder, M. (2001): Der Nürnberger Kodex und seine Folgen, in: Ebbinghaus/Dörner (2001), pp. 476-488.

Young, S. N. (1998): Risk in Research – From the Nuremberg Code to the Tri-Council Code: Implications for Clinical Trials of Psychotropic Drugs, Journal of Psychiatry and Neuroscience 23 (1998), 3, pp. 149-155.

Till Bärnighausen

Communicating "Tainted Science": The Japanese Biological Warfare Experiments on Human Subjects in China

I.   Introduction

Between 1932 and 1945, the Imperial Japanese Military pursued an offensive and defensive biological warfare programme. Under the leadership of General Shiro Ishii, the programme evolved in three stages, from a laboratory at the Army Medical University in Tokyo (1932) to a first research station in Beyinhe, China (1932-1936), and finally to a system of research centres in different Chinese cities (1936-1945).[1] These research centres included the following: the so-called Unit 731 in Harbin, Unit 1644 in Nanjing, Unit 1855 in Beijing, Unit 100 in Mengjiatung and Unit 8604 in Guanzhou. In order to develop biological weapons, Japanese researchers conducted experiments with a large variety of potential biological warfare agents, including *Vibrio cholerae*, *Shigella dysenteriae*, *Salmonella typhi*, *Salmonella paratyphi*, *Brucella melitensis*, *Yersinia pestis*, *Francisella tularensis*, *Corynebacterium diphtheriae*, *Bacillus anthracis*, *Mycobacterium tuberculosis*, *Rickettsia prowazeki*, as well as the yellow fever virus and the rabies virus. The experiments involved controlled laboratory studies investigating the lethality of different viruses or bacteria in biological warfare trials which tested the efficacy of weapon systems in infecting human beings in the field. In addition to the biological warfare experiments, the Japanese scientists conducted experiments to investigate the reactions of human beings to cold, heat, electroshocks, x-rays, bloodletting, hunger and thirst.

The headquarters of the biological warfare program, the Unit 731 in Harbin, was able to function both as a university research department and a concentration camp. Most of the experiments were conducted on Chinese prisoners. The victims of the experiments were routinely killed, autopsied and incinerated in the crematory of Unit 731.[2] Estimates of the number of victims killed by the Japanese scientists range from 3,000 to tens of thousands.[3]

---

1   In this text, wherever possible, Japanese names and Chinese names are written with the given name first and the surname second (as in the English language). Exceptions are citations that use the reverse order of the given names and surnames (as in the Japanese language and in the Chinese language).

2   Harris (1994), Bärnighausen (2002), Han/Xin (1991).

3   There are at least two reasons for the discrepancies in the numbers. First, different authors use different methods to estimate the number of victims. For instance, summing up the victims whose deaths are documented in publicly available records produces a relatively

At the height of the research activity, more than 3,000 people worked for Unit 731.[4] After World War II, a small number of largely low-ranking members of some of the Japanese units for biological warfare received prison sentences at the Khabarovsk War Criminal Trials. At the Tokyo War Criminal Trials, the human experiments of the Japanese biological warfare researchers were mentioned once, when on 17 November 1945 the American prosecutor David Sutton read the following statement from a summary report of the Chinese Committee for War Crimes in Nanjing:

> "The enemy's TAMA Detachment carried off their civilian captives to the medical laboratory, where the reactions to poisonous serums were tested. This detachment was one of the most secret organisations. The number of persons slaughtered by this detachment cannot be ascertained".[5]

The presiding judge, Sir William Webb, decided not to pursue the charges further because of a lack of evidence.[6] None of the leading scientists of Unit 731 or any of the other Japanese biological warfare units were ever prosecuted.

The history of the Japanese biological warfare programme has been chronicled in detail elsewhere.[7] The aim of this chapter is to describe the channels through which scientific data from the Japanese experiments entered public medical knowledge (largely from 1940 to 1970), while the barbaric nature of the experiments remained secret. An understanding of these channels may inform the design of policies aimed at identifying unethically obtained data. Furthermore, it may inform the debate about the use of data which is considered to be "tainted".

The experiments conducted by the researchers of the Japanese units for biological warfare grossly violated the basic principles of ethical research: for instance, those laid out in the Nuremberg Code and the World Medical Association's Declaration of Helsinki.[8] Most significantly, the scientists did not "protect the life, health, privacy and dignity of the human subject".[9] Data from such clearly unethical experiments may pose a dilemma, if their publication and use could benefit other people. The objections to the use of "tainted data" are numerous. Some raise fundamental objections by arguing that the use of "tainted data"

---

small estimate, while projecting the number of victims based on the number of prison cells in the biological warfare units, the time periods during which these prisons were used, and the average lengths of experiments yields larger estimates. Second, the scope of the estimation varies among authors (e.g. only those victims who were killed by the unit 731 in Harbin between 1939 and 1945 versus victims that were killed by any of the biological warfare units in China between 1932 and 1945). See Harris (1994), Bärnighausen (2002), Han/Xin (1991).

4   Han/Xin (1991), p. 36.
5   Brackman (1987), p. 196. "TAMA Detachment" is another name for Unit 1644 in Nanjing, Gao (1982), p. 3.
6   Brackman (1987), pp. 196-197.
7   Williams/Wallace (1989), Han/Xin (1991), Harris (1994), Bärnighausen (2002). A discussion of the primary and secondary sources available on the Japanese troops for biological warfare can be found in Bärnighausen (2002) and Bärnighausen (2006), pp. 169-198.
8   Nuremberg Military Tribunal (1947), p. 1691, World Medical Association (2004).
9   World Medical Association (2004), p. 2.

jeopardises the creation of a "symbolic memorial" to the victims.[10] Those who have practical concerns argue that the use of "tainted data" conveys the idea that unethical research is being rewarded and thus makes future unethical research more likely.[11]

Different positions on the use of "tainted data" have evolved (see below). One example is the 1998 declaration on "Information from Unethical Experiments" by the Council on Ethical and Judicial Affairs (CEJA) that "maintains and updates" the Code of Medical Ethics of the American Medical Association:[12]

> "Based on both scientific and moral grounds, data obtained from cruel and inhumane experiments, such as, data collected from the Nazi experiments and data collected from the Tuskegee Study, should virtually never be published or cited. In the extremely rare case when no other data exist and human lives would certainly be lost without the knowledge obtained from use of such data, publication or citation is permissible".[13]

> "Should editors and/or authors decide to publish an experiment or data from an experiment that does not reach standards of contemporary ethical conduct, a disclaimer should be included. [...] This disclaimer should:
> a. clearly describe the unethical nature of the origin of any material being published;
> b. clearly state the need for publication of the data;
> c. pay respect to the victims;
> d. avoid trivialising trauma suffered by the participants;
> e. acknowledge the unacceptable nature of the experiments; and
> f. endorse higher ethical standards".[14]

The CEJA states that for clearly defined exceptions (the data is unique and the data will save lives), "tainted data" may be published, but never without a disclosure of their unethical origins and a specific justification for the publication. Results from the inhumane Japanese experiments entered public medical knowledge without disclosure of their origins and without preceding deliberations as to whether the use of the results could be justified. The channels by which the results entered medical knowledge demonstrate that the safeguards that are currently in place to identify "tainted data" are insufficient, because the safeguards are only effective if two assumptions are met. First, editors and peer reviewers must be aware of the nature of the experiments that generated a specific dataset. Second, publication must necessarily precede the use of "tainted data".

The case of the Japanese troops for biological warfare shows that data obtained from inhumane experiments can become general medical knowledge, if either of these two assumptions is violated: "tainted data" from the Japanese experiments entered medical knowledge

- directly through publication, because the researchers misrepresented their methods (violation of the first assumption); and

---

10   Mostow (1993/4), pp. 403–431.
11   Angell (1986), pp. 413–419.
12   American Medical Association (1847).
13   Council on Ethical and Judicial Affairs (1998), p. 5.
14   Ibid.

- indirectly through channels other than publication: communication of findings to other scientists, citation of non-published results, and careers that allowed the scientists who had conducted the experiments to incorporate "tainted data" into ethical follow-up research after World War II (violation of the second assumption).

The "tainted data" generated by the Japanese scientists could enter medical knowledge through these channels because the scientists were not brought to justice and their experiments were never publicly condemned. In the following, I will describe how the Japanese scientists escaped prosecution. Then, I will use the examples of research on epidemic hemorrhagic fever and research on frostbite to show how "tainted data" entered medical knowledge through four different channels: publication, communication, citation and the subsequent careers of the scientists. Finally, I will extract some policy implications from these findings.

II. Escape from Prosecution

Between 1945 and the end of the Tokyo War Criminal Trials in 1948, US military scientists from Fort Detrick, the headquarters of the American biological warfare programme, investigated the activities of the Japanese units for biological warfare in China. The American scientists conducted a total of four investigations.

Murray Sanders, a microbiologist at Fort Detrick, conducted the first investigation from September to October 1945. Sanders discovered that the Japanese Army had tried to develop biological weapons, but probably did not realise that prisoners had been killed in the pursuit of this goal.

The veterinarian and biological warfare specialist lieutenant Arvo T. Thompson and the microbiologist Nobert Fell, who headed the department for Planning and Pilot Engineering at Fort Detrick, conducted the second and the third investigations from January to March 1946 and from April to May 1947, respectively. They concluded that the Japanese biological warfare programme had failed because it had not been able to recruit civilian researchers, "thus denying the project the best technical talent in the empire".[15] This conclusion was clearly wrong. Shiro Ishii had been able to recruit both the best military scientists and the best civilian scientists.[16]

The fourth and last investigation, in October 1947, finally revealed the scale of the experimental programme with humans. Edwin v. Hill, the head of the Department of Basic Sciences at Fort Detrick, and the pathologist Joseph Victor secured detailed descriptions of human experiments from twenty-four Japanese scientists who had worked in the Japanese biological warfare programme (referred to as "Hill and Victor report" in the following). In exchange for providing these accounts, the Japanese scientists received financial compensation.

---

15   Thompson (1946), p. ii.
16   Bärnighausen (2002).

"Evidence gathered in this investigation has greatly supplemented and amplified previous aspects of this field. It represents data which have been obtained by Japanese scientists at the expenditure of many millions of dollars and years of work. [...] These data were secured with a total outlay of ¥ 250,000 to date, a mere pittance by comparison with the actual cost of the studies".[17]

Hill and Victor promised the Japanese scientists that they would try to prevent their prosecution as war criminals. In a letter accompanying their report about the experiments to General Alden C. Waitt, they argued the following:

"Furthermore, the pathological material which has been collected constitutes the only material evidence of the nature of these experiments. It is hoped that individuals who voluntarily contributed this information will be spared embarrassment because of it and that every effort will be taken to prevent this information from falling into other hands".[18]

Hill and Victor emphasised that the data was interesting because it contained information about the "human susceptibility to these diseases as indicated by specific infectious doses of bacteria". They also offered an explanation as to why the data was so valuable to the United States: "Such information could not be obtained in our own laboratories because of scruples attached to human experimentation".[19]

Ethical questions about the use of data that had been obtained through such inhumane methods were not raised in the report.[20] The reasons that motivated the United States to grant the Japanese scientists freedom from prosecution can be reconstructed from the telegram texts, transcribed radio messages, and letters that were exchanged between the centre of the State-War-Navy Coordinating Committee (SWNCC) in Washington and its subdivision in Tokyo.[21] The human experiments conducted by the Japanese scientists posed a problem of consistency to the SWNCC, as they acknowledged the similarities of the Japanese experiments to those of Nazi war criminals:

"Experiments on human beings similar to those conducted by the Ishii BW [Biological Warfare] group have been condemned as war crimes by the International Military Tribunal for the trial of major Nazi criminals in its decision handed down at Nuremberg on 30 September 1946. This Government is at present prosecuting leading German scientists and medical doctors at Nuremberg for offenses which included experiments on human beings which resulted in the suffering and death of most of those experimented on".[22]

---

17   Hill/Victor (1947), pp. 38-41.
18   Ibid.
19   Ibid.
20   Ishii later claimed that he had handed over about 80 per cent of his data to the Americans. He kept the remaining 20 per cent hidden. Possibly, these 20 per cent included evidence about the most inhumane experiments conducted at the Japanese units for biological warfare, which, if shared with the Americans, would have carried the risk of prosecution as a war criminal. According to his daughter, Ishii also considered offering himself as a "scapegoat" to the Americans in order to save his subordinates from prosecution. Masanori (1982).
21   The SWNCC was responsible for the American occupation of Japan.
22   State-War-Navy Coordinating Subcommittee for the Far East (1947), p. 3.

To distinguish the Japanese experiments from those of the Nazis, the SWNCC argued that while the experiments were comparable in cruelty, they differed with regard to one important aspect: in contrast to the German experiments, the main objective of the Japanese experiments had been to develop offensive biological weapons. From a military perspective, the data obtained in the experiments by the Japanese scientists seemed far more "justified" than the data obtained by German researchers. The Japanese data promised to be an advantage in an emerging arms race between the Cold War powers; the German data did not. The SWNCC outlined their position with the following statement:

> "This Japanese information is the only known source of data from scientifically controlled experiments showing the direct effect of BW [Biological Warfare] agents on man. In the past it has been necessary to evaluate the effects of BW agents on man from data obtained through animal experimentation. Such evaluation is inconclusive and far less complete than results obtained from certain types of human experimentation".[23]

The prosecution of Japanese scientists would not only have interrupted the "flow of ... additional information of a technical and scientific nature", but would also have made a large proportion of the already obtained information public.[24] This would have destroyed its value to the US.[25] Given this situation, the SWNCC decided not to prosecute the Japanese scientists. This decision followed the advice of a joint army and air force commission that had analysed the trade-off between current military security and future ramifications faced by the US.

> "It is recognised that by informing Ishii and his associates that the information to be obtained regarding BW [Biological Warfare] will be retained in intelligence channels and will not be employed as war crimes evidence, this government may at a later date be seriously embarrassed. However, the Army Department and Air Force Members strongly believe that this information, particularly that which will finally be obtained from the Japanese with respect to the effect of BW on humans, is of such importance to the security of this country that the risk of subsequent embarrassment should be taken".[26]

III 'Tainted science': Four Channels to Medical Knowledge

In the following, I will show how "tainted data" from the Japanese experiments entered medical knowledge, using examples from research on epidemic hemorrhagic fever and research on frostbite. These two research topics are exceptions among the set of topics that the Japanese troops for biological warfare had pursued. Most of the research topics investigated by the Japanese scientists were aimed at developing biological weapons. In contrast, the experiments investigating frostbite and epidemic hemorrhagic fever had a more traditional military medical objective, i.e. to prevent morbidity and mortality among

---

23   Ibid., Appendix "B", p. 7.
24   Ibid.
25   Ibid.; Harris (1994).
26   Special Staff (1947), p. 1.

Japanese troops who fought on the Manchurian-Soviet border.[27] Due to the focus on preventing disease, data from these experiments translated more easily into results of interest to civilian medicine than data from experiments investigating means to wage a biological war. Hence, the data from these experiments offers greater insights into how "tainted data" can enter medical knowledge than the data from the biological warfare experiments.

Epidemic hemorrhagic fever

Epidemic hemorrhagic fever was endemic in the border regions between Manchuria, China and the Soviet Union during World War II.[28] In 1938, the first soldier of the Japanese Guandong Army fell sick from the disease.[29] In the course of the following year, three epidemic outbreaks of the disease occurred in China, the largest of which covered an area of 72,000 square kilometers in Northern Manchuria.[30] In 1942, a commission of scientists who worked on the biological warfare programme decided to investigate the disease, because its cause and mode of transmission were unknown, there was no effective therapy, and the symptoms and pathology were not well described.[31] The commission was led by Shiro Kasahara. In the same year, epidemic hemorrhagic fever had become a serious problem for the Japanese Army. At times, one out of ten soldiers was sick from the disease.[32]

---

27   Today, Hantavirus is considered to be a candidate for the development of biological weapons. Supposedly, Kitano considered employing the pathogen causing epidemic hemorrhagic fever as a biological weapon. This seems unlikely because Hantavirus is difficult to culture. Bronze et al. (2002), pp. 316-325. Han/Xin (1991), p. 113.

28   Epidemic hemorrhagic fever has a number of alternative names, including: hemorrhagic fever with renal syndrome, Nephropathia Epidemica, Korean Hemorrhagic Fever and Songo Hemorrhagic Fever. It is caused by the Hantaan virus (family Bunyaviridae). Rodents are the reservoir host for the Hantaan virus. Mites, mosquitoes, sandflies, fleas, lice and ticks transmit the virus among the natural hosts. Humans are only infected if they come into contact with infected rodents or their excretions (via inhalation, or through broken skin, conjunctiva or mucous membranes). After an incubation period of between 12 and 24 days, fever develops, followed by a proteinuric-hypotensive phase, an oliguric phase, and a diuretic phase. Death occurs most commonly during the proteinuric-hypotensive phase. Complications include kidney failure, pulmonary edema and disseminated intravascular coagulation. Mortality ranges from 5 to 15 per cent. Cohen (1982), pp. 992-995, Krüger/Ulrich/Lundkvist (2001), pp. 1129-1144.

29   "Naval Aspects of Biological Warfare" (1947), p. 96, Tsuneishi (1986), p. 85.

30   731 Butaiten (1993), p. 65.

31   "Songo – epidemic hemorrhagic fever", Interview with Tachio Ishikawa, in: Hill/Victor (1947), p. 48.

32   Wang (1987), p. 24.

Frostbite

The Japanese troops in Northeastern China regularly suffered from frostbite.
Temperatures in Manchuria routinely fell to -40 degrees Celsius during the winter
months.[33] The army leadership knew that frostbite and other freezing injuries
could significantly impede the combat strength of Japanese troops. This would
pose a problem should Japan start to wage war against the Soviet Union.[34]
Japanese military scientists had already started to conduct frostbite experiments
with Chinese prisoners at the research centre in Beyinhe. In 1943, a cold
laboratory was built on the premises of Unit 731 in Harbin in which temperatures
between 0 and -72 degrees Celsius could be generated and maintained. A group of
scientists led by Hisato Yoshimura conducted freezing experiments in this
laboratory.[35]

III.1.   Channel 1: Publication

"Tainted data" can enter medical knowledge through publications (without any
recognition of the nature of the experiments and the suffering of its victims), if
authors misrepresent those aspects of their research that would clearly mark the
studies as unethical.

Hemorrhagic fever with renal syndrome

During and after World War II, the scientists of Unit 731, who had investigated
epidemic hemorrhagic fever, published a number of articles about their experiments, including the following:

> S. Ishii, "Studies on Song-go fever", *Japanese Army Medical Journal* 355 (1942), pp. 1757-
> 1758.

> S. Kasahara, M. Kitano, "Studies on Pathogen of Epidemic Hemorrhagic Fever", *Japanese
> Journal of Pathology* 33 (1943), pp. 476-483.

> R. Honzin, Y. Kuratat, K. Ikeda, "Studies Concerning Inflamations (especially Epidemic
> Hemorrhagic Fever)", *Transactiones Societatis Pathologicae Japonicae* 34 (1944), pp. 10-
> 11.

---

33 Han/Xin (1991), p. 115. The Square Building of the Unit 731 was (and is) located on the 46.
    Northern parallel.
34 Han/Xin (1991), pp. 115-116. Since the incident of 18 September 1931, when Japan began to
    occupy Manchuria, the Japanese Army leadership had considered declaring war on the Soviet
    Union. Nishi Toshihide testified at the War Criminal Trials at Khabarovsk that "[Y]oshimura
    told me that these researches were being conducted with a view to future war against the
    U.S.S.R.". Foreign Languages Publishing House (1950), p. 289.
35 Yuan (1951), pp. 10-11, Morimura (1985), p. 103, .Han/Xin (1991), p. 116.

S. Kasahara, M. Kitano, "Determination of the Causative Agent of Epidemic Hemorrhagic Fever", *Transactiones Societatis Pathologicae Japonicae* 34 (1944), pp. 3-5.

M. Kitano, "A study of Epidemic Hemorrhagic Fever", *Japanese Army Medical Journal* 370 (1944a), pp. 269-282.

M. Kitano, "Research about Epidemic Hemorrhagic Fever", *Manchoukuo Medical Journal* 40 (1944b), pp. 191-209.

S. Ozawa, Y. Hamazaki, "Epidemic Hemorrhagic Fever", *Transactiones Societatis Pathologicae Japonicae* 34 (1944), pp. 5-7.

M. Kitano, "Research on Epidemic Hemorrhagic Fever", *The History of the Activity of the Army Medical Corps during the Great Asian War*, Part 7 (1969), pp. 186-7.

The two studies published by Kasahara and Kitano in 1943 and 1944 ("Studies on pathogen of epidemic hemorrhagic fever", "A study of epidemic hemorrhagic fever") are good examples of how "tainted data" from inhumane experiments can enter the medical knowledge base through publication because the scientists misrepresented their methods in order to make them appear ethical.[36] An excerpt from Kitano and Kasahara's 1944 article provides a description of the methods employed in the experiments. It closely resembles the description that the two researchers gave to Hill and Victor after World War II – with one significant exception: the word "man" in the Hill and Victor report is replaced by the word "monkey" in the article:

> "203 mites picked from field mice in the epidemic area were emulsified in 2 cc saline and injected s.c. [subcutaneously] in a monkey. After 19 days the first monkey suffered from E.H.F. with a fever of 39,4° C. Then, that is during the period of elevated temperature, the blood from the first monkey was injected s.c. into the second monkey. After 12 days the second developed fever with albuminuria. When we dissected the second, we observed typical hemorrhage in its kidneys".[37]

The description in the article reveals to the reader familiar with the subject that the "monkey" was a "man". First, as Keiichi Tsuneishi points out, monkeys do not develop fever as high as the fever attributed to the monkeys in the article (up to 40.2 degrees Celsius).[38] Second, against the scientific convention of the time, the "monkey" is not further specified in the article.[39] Third, the Hill and Victor report mentions that "Monkeys-Incubation period 5-14 days, develops fever but no lesions and does not die". The true nature of the experiments was disguised in the publication, allowing "tainted data" to enter our medical knowledge through publication.

---

36   Kasahara/Kitano (1943), pp. 476-83, Kitano (1944a), pp. 269-282.
37   Kasahara/Kitano (1944), p. 3, as cited in: Tsuneishi (1986), p. 90.
38   Tsuneishi (1986).
39   Ibid.

Publication of frostbite experiments

Throughout World War II, the research group led by Hisato Yoshimura conducted frostbite experiments on prisoners at the Unit 731 in Harbin. According to testimonies at the Khabarovsk War Criminal Trials, these experiments were particularly cruel:

> "Experiments in freezing human beings were performed every year in the detachment, in the coldest months of the year: November, December, January and February. The technique of these experiments was as follows: the experimentees were taken out into the frost at night, at about 11 o'clock, and compelled to dip their hands into a barrel of cold water. Then they were compelled to take their hands out and stand with wet hands in the frost for a long time. Or else the following was done: the people were taken out dressed but with bare feet and compelled to stand at night in the frost in the coldest period of the year. When these people had gotten frostbite, they were taken to a room and forced to put their feet in water of 5°C temperature, and then the temperature was gradually increased. In this way means for healing frostbite were investigated".[40]

For other experiments, the scientists forced prisoners to stand motionless for twenty to thirty minutes in temperatures of -30 to -40 degrees Celsius with a naked finger, hand, foot, arm, leg, nose or scrotum exposed to the cold.[41] The scientists used a ventilator to generate air currents of different velocities in order to accelerate the freezing process.[42]

The victims of the freezing experiments suffered frostbite, and often developed necrosis and gangrene. Army physicians amputated the frozen body parts of some of the experimental victims, while less skilled soldiers sawed off the legs or arms of others.[43] Master Sergeant Kurakazu, who had served as a military police officer at the Unit 731 from 1940 to 1941, described the suffering of experimental victims at Khabarovsk:

> "When I walked into the prison laboratory, five Chinese experimentees were sitting on a long form; two of these Chinese had no fingers at all, their hands were black; in those of three others the bones were visible. They had fingers, but they were only bones. Yoshimura Hisato told me that this was the result of freezing experiments".[44]

Despite the immense cruelty of the experiments, Yoshimura and his colleagues were able to publish some of their data in the English-language *Japanese Journal of Physiology* after presenting them at the 21st, 22nd, and 25th meeting of the Japanese Physiological Society in 1942, 1943, and 1948:

---

40 Foreign Languages Publishing House (1950), pp. 357-8. These experiments resemble, in part, the experiments that were conducted by Nazi physicians at the Dachau concentration camp between 1942 and 1943. Frewer/Wieseman (1999), p. 117, pp. 328-333.

41 Han (1986), pp. 20-21.

42 Ibid., Morimura (1985), p. 103.

43 Morimura (1985), pp. 103-104, Yuan (1951), pp. 10-11.

44 Foreign Languages Publishing House (1950), pp. 357-8. In this citation, the surname is written before the given name according to the grammatical rules of the Japanese language. Yoshimura Hisato (according to Japanese grammar) is Hisato Yoshimura (according to English grammar).

H. Yoshimura, T. Iida, "Studies on the Reactivity of Skin Vessels to Extreme Cold I. A Point Test on the Resistance against Frostbite", *Japanese Journal of Physiology* 2 (1952a), pp. 147-159.

H. Yoshimura, T. Iida, "Studies on the Reactivity of Skin Vessels to Extreme Cold II. Factors Governing the Individual Difference of the Reactivity, or the Resistance against Frostbite", *Japanese Journal of Physiology* 2 (1952b), pp. 177-185.

H. Yoshimura, T. Iida, "Studies on the Reactivity of Skin Vessels to Extreme Cold III. Effects of Diets on the Reactivity of Skin Vessels to Cold", *Japanese Journal of Physiology* 2 (1952c), pp. 310-315.

In these publications, the scientists do not explicitly mention some of the most inhumane aspects of their experiments, namely that all of the experimental subjects were forced against their will to participate and were killed after the completion of the studies. However, those who read the article should have been highly suspicious of the nature of the experiments. For one, the trial participants were "Chinese coolies" and "Chinese pupils", while the researchers were Japanese, and the experiments had been conducted during the Second Sino-Japanese War and World War II when Japan had invaded large parts of North-eastern China. Moreover, the participants included children below 15 years of age and a baby:

> "The temperature reaction in ice-water was examined on about 100 Chinese coolies from 15 to 74 years old and on about 20 Chinese pupils of 7 to 14 years. The results obtained were averaged on groups of every 5 years, and changes of the reaction index with progress of age were observed as seen in fig. 1. The maximum reactivity was found at the ages of 25 to 29 years, and, as the age became younger and older, the reactivity generally decreased more and more, except that in childhood it was higher than in puberty. Thus the general aspect of change of reactivity with age was similar to that of the other physiological functions. Though detailed studies could not be attained on children below 6 years of age, some observations were carried out on a baby. As is seen in fig. 2, the reaction was detected even on the 3rd day after birth, and it increased rapidly with the lapse of days until at last it was nearly fixed after a month or so".[45]

It should have further raised suspicion that the Japanese scientists were able to tightly control the lives of the participants. A subset of experiments was conducted "after keeping awake for a night", "after hunger for 24 hours", "immediately after heavy meal", "immediately after hot meal", "immediately after muscular exercise", "immediately after cold bath", and "immediately after hot bath". The scientists stratified participants by the type of food the participants had exclusively eaten over the past five days as characterised by its protein content ("high protein (of animal nature)", "Do (of vegetable nature)", "low protein intake", and "standard diet") as well as salt content (45 g NaCl per day, 15 g NaCl per day, no salt).[46] Such tight control over daily life choices would not have been possible unless participants were patients in a hospital or imprisoned.

---

45   Yoshimura/Iida (1952b), pp. 177-178.
46   Yoshimura/Iida (1952c), pp. 311-314.

The medically trained reader could have realised that the experiments had caused the participants considerable pain. During the experiments, a middle finger, a whole hand, a toe or a lower leg of a victim was immersed into water of 0 degrees Celsius for either 30 or 60 minutes. The water was regularly stirred in order to maintain 0 degree around the immersed body part and the skin temperature of the body part was measured every minute. The temperature curves show a fall from normal body temperature to around 5 degree Celsius in the first ten minutes and then an oscillation around 5 degree Celsius for the remainder of the experiment, i.e. up to either 30 or 60 minutes.[47] Exposure to such temperatures for these lengths of time causes enormous pain. For example, Shinichi Sawada, Shunichi Araki and Kazuhito Yokoyama (2000) – three researchers who are among the many who cite one of the three 1952 publications by Yoshimura and colleagues (see below) – describe the pain caused by Yoshimura's procedure as follows:

> "As mentioned above, Yoshimura et al. proposed a local cold tolerance test, because the CIVD reactivity is closely related to an individual's frostbite resistance. This test method has, however, consisted of 30-min immersion of fingers in ice water (0° C [Celsius]). Under this test condition, most of the participants have tended to feel much pain and distress, and some have either fainted or had to withdraw prematurely from the experiment. We, therefore, previously proposed a simplified and less painful test for evaluating local cold tolerance as a substitute for Yoshimura's method".[48]

Unlike follow-up studies, which used Yoshimura's local cold tolerance test, not one participant withdrew from the original study, suggesting that the participants did not have the choice to withdraw.

The publication of Yoshimura's studies demonstrates how "tainted data" can enter our medical knowledge, if the scientists fail to report certain information about the study that would clearly identify it as unethical. In this particular case, it seems that the information that the authors did provide should have led to inquiries by the editors and reviewers that could have unmasked the inhumane nature of the experiments.

III.2. Channel 2: Communication

"Tainted data" can enter medical knowledge if scientists share their findings with other scientists directly, i.e. without the intermediary step of publication. In the initial communication, the scientists who share "tainted data" have control over whom they communicate with. This initial group of data recipients may be quite small. The selective nature of this channel, however, does not imply that the "tainted data" cannot diffuse into general medical knowledge. First, "tainted data" can be spread much more widely in scientific communication networks of researchers who share an interest in a certain topic. Second, the relevant audience

---

47   Yoshimura/Iida (1952a), pp. 148-149.
48   Sawada et al. (2000), p. 85. CIVD stands for cold-induced vasodilation.

for "tainted data" about a specific research topic may, in fact, be quite small, if only a few scientists worldwide work on the topic. This means that knowledge of the data within this selected group is equivalent to knowledge of the data within any larger group, because the use of the data would not differ if a larger group had knowledge of it. Third, once "tainted data" has been communicated to other scientists, it can enter the scientific knowledge through other channels, for example through citations or in follow-up studies (see below).

Hemorrhagic fever with renal syndrome

In November 1942, Masaji Kitano and Kasahara Ishii conducted a series of experiments to identify the causal agent and the mode of transmission of epidemic hemorrhagic fever.[49] Kitano Masji had been the vice commandant of the Unit 731 in Harbin. At the time of the experiments, he had replaced Ishii as the commandant of the unit.[50] Kasahara Ishii worked at Unit 731 as a civilian scientist. He had been recruited by Shiro Ishii from the renowned Kitasato Institute in Tokyo.[51] In 1947, the two scientists described their experiments to Hill and Victor:[52]

> "203 mites picked from field mice in that area were emulsified in 2 cc [cubic centimeters] saline and injected s.c. [subcutaneously] in one man with positive results. Another emulsion containing 60 mites produced no effect in another subject. In this way, the subsequent human material was derived from the first case which had been injected with 203 mites. In general, the incubation period was between 2 and 3 weeks. Blood from the first experimental case was drawn during fever 20 days after injection of the mites. Ten cc were injected into a 3rd man as well as into white mice and monkeys. Subsequent cases were produced either by blood or blood free extracts of liver, spleen or kidney derived from individuals sacrificed at various times during the course of the disease. Morphine was employed for this purpose".[53]

Similar experiments in which ticks instead of mites were used did not produce infections in man.[54] Kitano provided Hill and Victor with fever curves of the first, second and fourth victims of their experiments. The curves had similar shapes: after twelve, thirteen and seventeen days, respectively, the victims' temperatures rose abruptly (to 39.7, 39.3 and 40.0 degrees Celsius, measured in the evenings). In the following two weeks the temperatures of all three victims remained high. The victims' temperatures dropped significantly at day twelve, sixteen and fifteen after the initial temperature rise (to 36.4, 35.9 and 36.6 degrees Celsius, respectively). On these days, Kitano and Kasahara – by their own account – injected their victims with morphine and then killed them with an injection of the

---

49 "Songo – epidemic hemorrhagic fever", interview with Shiro Kasahara and Masaji Kitano, 13 November 1947, in: Hill/Victor (1947), pp. 42-43.
50 Ishii regained the position of commandant of the Unit 731 after two years. During these two years, Ishii commanded the Unit 1644 in Nanjing. Williams/Wallace (1989), p. 258.
51 Tsuneishi (1986), p. 90.
52 Ibid.
53 "Songo – epidemic hemorrhagic fever", Kasahara/Kitano (1943), pp. 42-43.
54 Ibid.

nerve poison Methylchloride. They then performed autopsies on the three victims and passed the victims' organs to Ishikawa, who performed the pathohistological examinations. A "%" marked the death of the victims in the study protocols.[55]

In the interviews with Hill and Victor, Kitano and Kasahara summarised the results of another set of experiments on epidemic hemorrhagic fever that they had conducted (between 1942 and 1945).[56] *Inter alia*, they reported that healthy human beings can be infected with the disease by subcutaneous injection, if the blood, serum, plasma, thrombocyte concentrate, leucocyte concentrate or erythrocyte concentrates are filtered before injection. Because the filters employed in the experiments let small viruses, but not bacteria, pass through, the military physicians concluded that the infectious agent was not a Rickettsia (as they had previously hypothesised), but a virus.[57] Kitano and Kasahara further stated that the mortality of epidemic hemorrhagic fever could be reduced to fifteen per cent, using symptomatic treatment with electrolytes, glucose and insulin. "However, mortality in experiment was 100 per cent due to the procedure of sacrificing experimental subjects".[58] Overall, Kitano and Kasahara killed more than a hundred healthy human beings in their experiments. Most of the victims were Chinese.[59]

The detailed accounts which Kitano and Kasahara provided of their experiments in the Hill and Victor report made it possible for the "tainted data" to enter our medical knowledge. For instance, it is likely that data from the Japanese experiments was used during the Korean War (1950-1953). Epidemic hemorrhagic fever occurred among US Army personnel during the Korean War with incidence rates of 3.85 per 1,000 person-years, 3.72 per 1,000 person-years, and 1.76 per 1,000 person-years in 1951, 1952 and 1953, respectively.[60] As Colonel Arthur Long, MC, stated in April 1954:

> "[P]erhaps of all the conditions encountered in the Far East to date, hemorrhagic fever has posed the greatest single challenge of any problem in the field of epidemiology, microbiology and preventive medicine".[61]

In 1952, one year after the first fatalities from epidemic hemorrhagic fever had occurred among American troops in Korea, Lt Colonel R. Hullinghorst, MC, and Lt. Colonel Arthur Steer, MC, from the Department of Pathology of the 406th Medical General Laboratory in San Francisco, wrote an article about the "Pathology of epidemic hemorrhagic fever" in the *Annals of Internal Medicine*. In the article, they mention that they received histopathological specimens from Kitano, Kasahara and the Japanese Army scientist Tokoro, in order to reexamine

---

55   Ibid, pp. 45-48.
56   See Bärnighausen (2002), Bärnighausen (2006).
57   "Songo - epidemic hemorrhagic fever", Kasahara/Kitano (1943), p. 43.
58   Ibid.
59   Interview with Kozo Okamoto, in: Hill/Victor (1947), p. 32, Tsuneishi (1986), p. 86.
60   Long (1954), p. 265.
61   Ibid.

them.[62] In addition, the US Army physicians cite personal communication with both Kasahara alone and Kitano, Kasahara and Ishikawa together.[63]

These examples demonstrate not only that institutional knowledge about the experiments conducted by the Japanese scientists must have survived in the US Army, but that an institutional link must have been maintained between the US Army and former members of the Japanese biological warfare programme. Such a link would have been necessary to allow initiation of the contact that led to the exchange of information and medical specimens, both of which the Japanese scientists had almost certainly derived from their human experiments. It is also noteworthy that the US Army physicians had contact with the second highest ranking member of the Japanese warfare programme, Masaji Kitano.

Since Lt. Colonel Hullinghorst and Lt Colonel Steer had access to the perpetrators of the experiments, it seems unlikely that they and other military physicians did not have access to the written information contained in the Hill and Victor report. This would imply that "tainted data" had been selectively communicated, so that those military physicians working on epidemic hemorrhagic fever could use it in their practice and research.

III.3.   Channel 3: Citation

"Tainted data" may be cited from a number of sources, including journal publications, research reports, presentations or personal communication. Since citations rarely describe the methods that generated a certain set of data, "tainted data" can enter medical knowledge more easily through citations than through publications. If a primary source contains evidence that the data has been generated by unethical means, the citation may function as a "data laundering" device: Once the "tainted data" has been cited without description and condemnation of its methods, it continues to exist as if it were "untainted".

Epidemic hemorrhagic fever

Out of fifteen references cited in the 1952 article "Pathology of epidemic hemorrhagic fever" by Lt. Colonel Hullinghorst, MC, and Lt. Colonel Arthur Steer, MC, eleven refer to at least one of the Japanese scientists who had participated in the experiments on epidemic hemorrhagic fever at Unit 731. These citations include seven scientific publications and the following two reports:

> T. Ibuki, "Report of a Special Committee on the Investigation of Epidemic Hemorrhagic Fever", Japanese Army Publication (1943).

> H. Osuzu (ed.), "Epidemic Hemorrhagic Fever, Clinical Aspects of Military Medicine", Japanese Army Publication (1944).

---

62   Ibid, p.79.
63   Hullinghorst/Steer (1953), pp. 77-101.

Indeed, the authors begin their article by stating that previous knowledge about the disease is based on studies by "Russian workers" and "a group of Japanese workers":

> "Since the early 1930s there has been a continually developing awareness by Russian workers of the existence of a nosologic entity characterised by fever, hemorrhage and severe renal involvement. [...] A group of Japanese workers confirmed many of these facts in the study of an identical disease occurring in sharply defined areas of Manchuria during the period of 1939-1945".[64]

Lt. Colonel Hullinghorst and Lt. Colonel Steer go on to regret that "[The] sudden termination of World War II interrupted further activities by this group, with many factors yet unknown and some basic work not confirmed by repetition. The transmissible agent was lost at the time of surrender or shortly thereafter".[65] Given these citations and the personal communications (see above), it seems likely that Lt. Colonel Hullinghorst and Lt. Colonel Steer were aware of the inhumane nature of the experiments by the Japanese scientists when they wrote their article in 1952. Independent of their knowledge, however, their citations transmitted "tainted data" into our medical knowledge.

Frostbite

Hisato Yoshimura's three 1952 publications on frostbite fail to explicitly describe the inhumane nature of his experiments. However, the incomplete descriptions that he does provide are sufficient to arouse the suspicion among readers that the experiments were unethical (see above). In contrast, the articles that cite Yoshimura's 1952 publications contain little or no information that could raise the suspicion that the cited data was "tainted" (see Table 1). For instance, Yoshimura established a "resistance index of frost bite" based on the mean temperature five to thirty minutes after immersion, the value of the first rise in temperature after immersion, and the time until the temperature first rises after immersion.[66] A number of scientists later employed the same method or a modification to test the effects of different factors on resistance to frostbite (see Table 1).[67] Their publications cite Yoshimura's 1952 articles, but do not provide evidence that the method had been developed in inhumane experiments. The citation history of Yoshimura's three 1952 publications thus provides an example of how citation can "cleanse" data.

---

64   Ibid., p. 77.
65   Ibid.
66   Yoshimura/Iida (1952a), pp. 148-149.
67   Sawada et al. (2000).

Factor examined	Articles
Age	Sawada/Yamamoto (1983); Spurr et al. (1955)
Sex	Tanaka (1971a)
Occupation	Tanaka (1971a); Miura et al. (1977)
Body heat	Hirai et al. (1968)
Clothing	Tanaka (1971b)
Cold Acclimatization	Bridgman (1991); Nelms/Soper (1962)
Environmental Temperature	Tanaka (1971a)
Ambient pressure	Konda et al. (1981)
Season	Tanaka (1971a)

Table 1: Articles that cite at least one of Hisato Yoshimura's three 1952 articles on frostbite.[68]

III.4.   Channel 4: Careers

Members of the Japanese programme for biological warfare were able to continue their careers after World War II. Many rose to prominent positions.[69] The researchers who had conducted human experiments on epidemic hemorrhagic fever and frostbite are no exception to the post-war successes of former members of the units for biological warfare. Shiro Kasahara rose to the position of chief pathologist and later vice president of the renowned Kitasato Institute in Tokyo. Masaji Kitano founded a company producing vaccinations. After the company went

---

68 Spurr et al. (1955), pp. 551-555, Nelms/Soper (1962), pp. 444-448, Hirai et al. (1968), pp. 12-21, Tanaka (1971a), pp. 269-280, Tanaka (1971b), pp. 169-177, Miura et al. (1977), pp. 75-81, Konda et al. (1981), pp. 207-213, Sawada/Yamamoto (1983), pp. 116-117, Bridgman (1991), pp. 733-738.

69 Examples include the dean of the Faculty of Medicine at the University of Tokyo (Kozo Okamoto), dean of the Medical Faculty of the University of Osaka (Tabuko Yamanaka), dean of the Faculty of Medicine of Osaka City University (Hideo Tanaka), dean of the Medical University of Kanazawa (Tachio Ishikawa), professor at the University of Tokyo (Tokoro, Konji Ando), professor at the University of Kyoto (Kanau Tabei), professor at the University of Osaka (Tsunesaburo Fujino), professor at Nagoya Prefectural University of Medicine (Toru Ogawa), professor at Showa Pharmacological University (Masao Kusami), honorary professor at the University of Juntendo (Yoshi Tsuchiya), General Staff Physician of the Japanese Army (Enryo Hojo), scientist at the National Institute of Health (Shinpei Ejima), director of the National Research Center for Preventive Medicine (Saburo Kojima), department head at the National Institute of Health (Kiyoshi Asanuma), secretary of the Japanese Penicillin Society (Yukimasa Yagisawa), founder of the Japanese pharmacological company Green Cross (Ryoichi Naito), president of the Japanese Company S. J. (Hideo Futaki) and director of research of the Japanese company Takeda (Kenichi Kanazawa). Han/Xin (1991), pp. 347, 332-352, Hill/Victor (1947), Japanese Politics Economy Research Institute (1963), p. 155, Tsuneishi (1986), pp. 79-92, Williams/Wallace (1989), pp. 236-242.

bankrupt, he became the director of the Tokyo branch of the Japanese Blood Bank. Hisato Yoshimura became president of Kyoto Prefectural University of Medicine. He also served as scientific consultant to the Japanese Antarctic expedition and as president of the Meteorological Society of Japan.[70]

Yoshimura's post-war career provides a good example of how "tainted data" can enter our medical knowledge if scientists who performed unethical experiments continue to pursue similar research questions with ethical experiments. The difference in Yoshimura's research during and after World War II is one of methods, not scientific topic. A selection of his post-war articles shows that he continued to study cold tolerance:

H. Yoshimura, S. Shiomi, K. Makihata, S. Hiramathu, "Studies on the Nature of Hypothermia I. Studies on Resistance to Cold-Induced Death", *Journal of The Physical Society of Japan* 23 (1961), pp. 173-181.

H. Yoshimura, "Studies on Cold Tolerance in Man", *Nippon Seirigaku Zasshi (Japanese Physiological Journal)* 29 (1967), pp. 673-678.

K. Hirai, T. Inoue, H. Yoshimura, "Studies on Effect of Heat Content on the Vascular Hunting Reaction to Cold, and the Reaction of Women Divers", *Nippon Seirigaku Zasshi (Japanese Physiological Journal)* 30 (1968), pp. 12-21.

Y. Ito, I. Kunishima, Y. Katayama, T. Inoue, H. Yoshimura, "Studies on Effects of Dietary Composition on Acclimation to Heat and Cold with Rats", *Nippon Seirigaku Zasshi (Japanese Physiological Journal)* 30 (1968), pp. 815-830.

Y. Ito, I. Kunishima, Y. Katayama, T. Inoue, H. Yoshimura, "Cold Tolerance and Critical Temperature of the Japanese", *International Journal of Biometeorology* 13 (1969), pp. 163-172.

M. Yoshimura, H. Takeda, H. Yoshimura, "Effect of Dietary Composition on Thermal Acclimation", *Nippon Seirigaku Zasshi (Japanese Physiological Journal)* 31 (1969), pp. 178-179.

M. Yoshimura, H. Yoshimura, "Quality of Diet and Human Adaptability to Heat and Cold", *Nippon Rinsho (Japanese Clinical Medicine)* 28 (1970), pp. 1988-1993.

M. Yoshimura, S. Hori, H. Yoshimura, "Effect of High-Fat Diet on Thermal Acclimation with Special Reference to Thyroid Activity", *Japanese Journal of Physiology* 22 (1972), pp. 517-531.

Instead of using prisoners of war to investigate the "[e]ffects of diets on the reactivity of skin vessels to cold", he now studied the "effects of dietary composition on acclimation to heat and cold with rats". Instead of studying a "resistance index of frost-bite" in "Chinese pupils" and "Chinese coolies", Yoshimura now published on the "critical temperature of the Japanese". It seems

---

70 Williams/Wallace (1989), pp. 236-242. Late in his life, the past caught up with Professor Yoshimura. Student protests about a number of issues which included his involvement in human experimentation in China forced him to step down from the presidency of Kyoto Prefectural University of Medicine. Gold (1996), p. 83.

highly plausible that Yoshimura used what he had learned in his wartime experiments throughout his post-war career to try to replicate the results from unethical experiments with ethical methods, to formulate new research hypotheses, and to evaluate findings from ethical research. Moreover, Gold (1996) reports that Yoshimura made direct references to his human experiments in China during a meeting of the Japanese Physiological Society, during university lectures and in his memoirs (published in 1984).[71] Finally, as a consultant to the Japanese Antarctic expedition, he might well have offered advice that was at least partially based on results obtained in his frost-bite experiments in Manchuria.

IV. Recognition and Identification

There are three ethical positions on how "tainted data" should be treated.[72] One is the position of "strict non-use", which argues that "tainted data" should never be published and used.[73] The position of "conditional use", such as that of the 1998 declaration by the American Medical Association mentioned above, holds that "tainted data" may only be published under exceptional circumstances.[74] The position of "strict use" states that data of scientific value should always be published because there are no absolute ethics, and each individual scientist reading the publication should decide whether or not to use the data based on ethical grounds.[75]

---

71 Gold (1996), pp. 83-84.
72 See Bärnighausen (2006).
73 Beecher (1966), pp. 1354-1360, Gaylin (1989), p. 18, Angell (1990), pp. 1462-1464, Post (1991), pp. 42-44.
74 Neter (1980), p. 23, Moe (1989), pp. 5-7, Sheldon/Whitely (1989), pp. 16-17, Post (1991), pp. 42-44.
75 Singer (1980), p. 24. It may seem contradictory that an article which discusses the communi-cation of "tainted data" and the ethics of using "tainted data" should itself describe some of the unethical experiments. However, the description of "tainted data" in a text about the history and ethics of human experimentation is different from the publication of scientific data. The aim of the former is to draw attention to the suffering of the victims of unethical research and challenge the researchers who conducted the studies, so that similar abuses may be less likely to occur in the future. The purpose of the latter, on the other hand, is to share scientific results for practical application. Much of the debate about the use of data from unethical experiments has so far focused on their use in medical practice and science, with little attention to their use in showing the bestiality of the experiments (e.g. Moe (1989), pp. 5-7, Sheldon/Whitely (1989), pp. 16-17). Examples where experts have condemned the unethical use of human subjects in medical research include Henry Beecher's exposé in the *New England Journal of Medicine*, published in 1966 (Beecher (1966), pp. 1354-1360) and Robert Berger's account of the hypothermia experiments at the Dachau concentration camp (Berger (1990), pp. 1435-1440). In theory, a position of 'strict non-use' could be extended to include descriptions of experiments with the purpose of exposing their unethical nature or remembering the suffering of the victims. Strictly applied, such a position would exclude the description of detailed evidence of the experiments and allow only abstract memorials to the victims of the experiments. While such an extreme interpretation of the position of 'strict non-use' would be more consistent than a less extreme interpretation which allows for the

"Tainted data" from the Japanese experiments continue to exist in our medical knowledge in a form which is not acceptable under any of the three positions. Certainly, "strict non-use" is not satisfied because "tainted data" has entered our medical knowledge. "Conditional use" is not satisfied because "tainted data" entered medical knowledge without prior deliberations and without any form of condemnation of the methods that led to its generation. "Strict use" is not satisfied because, at least for a proportion of the accessible data from the experiments, the description of the methods is either false or incomplete. This means that readers lack sufficient information to judge whether or not the data is ethical.

The situation would be significantly improved if
- the Japanese government publicly condemned the experiments and named the individual scientists who had performed them;
- the US government acknowledged its role and ascertained that all documents regarding the exchange of data for freedom from prosecution were made public;
- the scientific institutions in which former members of the Japanese units for biological warfare continued their post-war careers investigated on how far data from the inhumane experiments informed follow-up studies; and
- scientific publications by researchers who had worked for one of the Japanese units for biological warfare were systematically examined in order to assess whether they contain information obtained in inhumane experiments.

Without such recognition, public information and investigation, "tainted data" will not be identified as such and will continue to be used as if it were ethically obtained scientific knowledge. More generally, the case of the Japanese experiments demonstrates that the safeguards in place to prevent the use of "tainted data" are insufficient, because they are based on two assumptions that may be violated, namely that scientists correctly represent their methods and that publication must precede the use of data. Scientists and policy makers may need to consider how to improve the mechanisms that identify "tainted data", so that deliberations about the publication and use of specific data can take place.

---

description of the experiments, the author of this text believes that such an extreme interpretation is not defensible. In order to apply an extreme interpretation of the position of 'strict non-use' to a particular experiment, the experiment must first have been judged as unethical; in order to arrive at that judgment, one first has to provide some form of description of the experiment.

V. Conclusion

The failure to prosecute scientists who had worked in the Japanese biological warfare programme as war criminals and to publicly identify their experiments as crimes against humanity allowed "tainted data" from the experiments to enter our medical knowledge at a time when the suffering of the victims of the experiments was hidden from public view. Not only did the Japanese scientists share their data with other scientists, but some data were published in scientific journals and reports, and some have been cited in publications. Furthermore, as the scientists continued their careers after World War II, "tainted data" is likely to have entered medical knowledge through ethical follow-up studies. Data from inhumane experiments will continue to be used as if it had been obtained by ethical means as long as the following conditions are not met: the Japanese government publicly condemns the experiments; the US government acknowledges its role in preventing crimes against humanity from becoming public; and scientific institutions and journals investigate how far "tainted data" has entered medical knowledge.

References

American Medical Association (AMA) (1847): AMA Code of Medical Ethics.

Angell, M. (1990): The Nazi hypothermia experiments and unethical research today, New England Journal of Medicine (1990), pp. 1462-1464.

Bärnighausen, T. (2002): Medizinische Humanexperimente der japanischen Truppen für biologische Kriegsführung in China 1932-1945 [Medical Human Experiments of the Japanese Troops for Biological Warfare in China 1932-1945], Frankfurt am Main: Peter Lang.

Bärnighausen, T. (2006): Barbaric Research – Japanese Human Experiments in Occupied China: Relevance; Alternatives; Ethics, in: Eckart (2006), pp. 169-198.

Beecher, H. (1966): Ethics and Clinical Research, New England Journal of Medicine (1966), pp. 1354-1360.

Berger, R. (1990): Nazi Science – the Dachau Hypthermia Experiments, New England Journal of Medicine (1990), pp. 1435-1440.

Brackman, A. C. (1987): The Other Nuremberg trial: The Untold Story of the Tokyo War Crimes Trials. New York: William Morrow and Company.

Bridgman, S. (1991): Peripheral Cold Acclimatization in Antarctic Scuba Divers, Aviation, Space, and Environmental Medicine 62 (1991), pp. 733-738.

Bronze, M./Huycke, M./Machado, L./Voskuhl, G./Greenfield, R. (2002): Viral Agents as Biological Weapons and Agents of Bioterrorism, American Journal of the Medical Sciences 323 (2002), pp. 316-325.

Cohen, M. (1982): Epidemic Hemorrhagic Fever Revisited, Review of Infectious Diseases 4 (1982), pp. 992-995.

Council on Ethical and Judicial Affairs (CEJA) (1998): Information from Unethical Experiments, CEJA Report 5 – A-98, 1998.

Eckart, W. U. (ed.). (2006): Man, Medicine and the State: the Human Body as an Object of Government-Sponsored Medical Research. Stuttgart: Steiner.

Foreign Languages Publishing House (ed.) (1950): Materials on the Trial of Former Servicemen of the Japanese Army Charged with Manufacturing and Employing Bacteriological Weapons. Moscow: Foreign Languages Publishing House.

Frewer, A. et al. (eds.) (1999): Medizinverbrechen vor Gericht. Das Urteil im Nürnberger Ärzteprozeß gegen Karl Brandt und andere sowie aus dem Prozeß gegen Generalfeldmarschall Milch [Medical crimes before the court. The sentence against Karl Brandt and others at the Nuremberg Nazi Doctors' Trial as well as from the case against general field marshal Milch]. Erlangen and Jena: Palm & Enke.

Gao, X. (1982): Riben junbu he di 731 xijun budui [The Japanese headquarters and the bacteria Unit 731], Minguo chunqiu 6 (1982), pp. 3-6.

Gaylin, W. (1989): Nazi Data: Dissociation from Evil, Hastings Center Report (1989), p. 18.

Gold, H. (1996): Japan's Wartime Human Experimentation Program Unit 731 Testimony. Tokyo: Yenbooks.

Han, X. (1986): Rijun 731 budui faxisi baoxing jilu [Collection of the fascist atrocities of the troops 731 of the Japanese Army]. Heilongjiang wenshi ziliao [Historical Sources of the Province Heilongjiang] (1986).

Han, X./Xin, P. (1991): Rijun 731 budui zui eshi [The history of the crimes of the Unit 731 of the Japanese Army]. Harbin: Heilongjiang chubanshe.

Harris, S.H. (1994): Factories of Death: Japanese Biological Warfare 1932-45 and the American Cover-Up. London: Routledge.

Hill, E. V./Victor, J. (1947): Summary Report on BW Investigation, 12 Dezember 1947, RG 395, Entry 6909-C, National Archives, Suitland Reference Branch, Maryland, USA.

Hirai, K./Inoue, T./Yoshimura, H. (1968): Studies on Effect of Heat Content on the Vascular Hunting Reaction to Cold, and the Reaction of Women Divers, Nippon Seirigaku Zasshi [Japanese Physiological Journal] 30 (1968), pp. 12-21.

Honzin, R., Kuratat, Y. and Ikeda, K. (1944): Studies Concerning Inflammations (especially Epidemic Hemorrhagic Fever), Transactiones Societatis Pathologicae Japonicae 34 (1944), pp. 10-11.

Hullinghorst, R./Steer, A. (1953): Pathology of Epidemic Hemorrhagic Fever, Annals of Internal Medicine 38 (1953), pp. 77-101.

Ibuki, T. (1943): Report of a Special Committee on the Investigation of Epidemic Hemorrhagic Fever, Japanese Army Publication, 31 January 1943.

Ishii, S. (1942): Studies on Song-go Fever, Japanese Army Medical Journal 355 (1942), pp. 1757-1758.

Ito, Y./Kunishima, I./Katayama, Y./Inoue, T./Yoshimura, H. (1968): Studies on Effects of Dietary Composition on Acclimation to Heat and Cold with Rats, Nippon Seirigaku Zasshi [Japanese Physiological Journal] 30 (1968), pp. 815-830.

Ito, Y./Kunishima, I./Katayama, Y./Inoue, T./Yoshimura, H. (1969): Cold Tolerance and Critical Temperature of the Japanese, International Journal of Biometeorology 13 (1969), pp. 163–172.

Japanese Politics Economy Research Institute (1963): Who's Who in Contemporary Japan. Tokyo: Japanese Politics Economy Research Institute.

Kasahara, S./Kitano, M. (1943): Studies on Pathogen of Epidemic Hemorrhagic Fever, Japanese Journal of Pathology 33 (1943), pp. 476-483.

Kasahara, S./Kitano, M. (1944): Determination of the Causative Agent of Epidemic Hemorrhagic Fever, Transactiones Societatis Pathologicae Japonicae 34 (1944), pp. 3-5.

Kitano, M. (1944a): A Study of Epidemic Hemorrhagic Fever, Japanese Army Medical Journal 370 (1944), pp. 269-282.

Kitano, M. (1944b): Research about Epidemic Hemorrhagic Fever, Manchoukuo Medical Journal 40 (1944), pp. 191-209.

Kitano, M. (1969): Research on Epidemic Hemorrhagic Fever. The History of the Activity of the Army Medical Corps during the Great Asian War, part 7 (1969), pp. 186-187.

Konda, N./Shiraki, K./Sagawa, S./Ohta, Y. (1981): Cold-Induced Vasodilation Reaction of Skin Vessels at 2 ATA, Journal of UOEH 3 (1981), pp. 207-213.

Krüger, D./Ulrich, R./Lundkvist, Å. (2001): Hantavirus Infections and their Prevention, Microbes and Infection 3 (2001), pp. 1129-1144.

Long, A. (1954): General Aspects of Preventive Medicine in the Far East Command. Unpublished paper presented on 29 April 1954 to the Walter Reed Army Medical Center, Washington, D.C.

Masanori, T. (1982): Daughter's Eye View of Lt. Gen. Ishii, Chief of 'Devil's Brigade', The Japan Times (August 1982).

Miura, T./Kimotsuki, K./Tominaga, Y./Suzuki Y. (1977): Effect of Environmental Conditions on the Cold-Induced Vasodilation of Office Workers and Forestry Workers, Journal of Science of Labor 53 (1977), pp. 75-81.

Moe, K. (1989): Should the Nazi Data be Cited? Hastings Center Report (1989), pp. 5-7.

Morimura, S. (1985): The Devil's Gluttony [Chinese translation of the Japanese original], part 3. Beijing: Qunzhong Publishing.

Mostow, P. (1993/4): 'Like Building on Top of Auschwitz': on the Symbolic Meaning of Using Data From the Nazi Experiments, and on Nonuse as a Form of Memorial, Journal of Law and Religion 2 (1993-1994), pp. 403–431.

"Naval Aspects of Biological Warfare", 5. August 1947, General Records of the Department of the Navy 1798-1947, Formerly Top Secret General Correspondence of the CNO/Secretary of the Navy 1944-47, CNO Top Secret, RG 330, Box 55, National Archives, Washington, D.C., USA.

Nelms, J./Soper, D. (1962): Cold Vasodilatation and Cold Acclimatization in the Hands of British Fish Filleters, Journal of Applied Physiology 17 (1962), pp. 444-448.

Neter, E. (1980): Ethics and Editors: Commentary, Hastings Center Report (1980), p. 23.

Nuremberg Military Tribunal (1947): The Nuremberg Code. Journal of the American Medical Association 276 (1996), p. 1691.

Osuzu, H. (ed.) (1944): Epidemic Hemorrhagic Fever, Clinical Aspects Of Military Medicine, Japanese Army Publication.

Ozawa, S./Hamazaki, Y. (1944): Epidemic Hemorrhagic Fever, Transactiones Societatis Pathologicae Japonicae 34 (1944), pp. 5-7.

Post, S. (1991): The Echo of Nuremberg: Nazi Data and Ethics, Journal of Medical Ethics 17 (1991), pp. 42-44.

Sawada, S./Yamamoto, S. (1983): Stability of Individual Difference of Cold-Induced Vasodilatation Response at Different Room and Water Temperature and Immersion Time, Sangyo Igaku [Japanese Journal of Industrial Health] 25 (1983), pp. 116-117.

Sawada, S./Araki, S./Yokoyama, K. (2000): Changes in Cold-Induced Vasodilatation, Pain and Cold Sensation in Fingers Caused by Repeated Finger Cooling in a Cool Environment, Industrial Health 38 (2000), pp. 79-86.

Schafer, A. (1989): On Using Nazi Data: The Case Against, Dialogue Canadian Philosophical Association 25 (1986), pp. 413–419.

Sheldon, M./Whitely, W. (1989): Nazi Data: Dissociation From Evil, Hastings Center Report (1989), pp. 16-17.

Singer, E. (1980): Ethics and Editors: Commentary, Hastings Center Report (1980), p. 24.

Special Staff, United States Army Civilian Affairs Division, "Interrogation of certain Japanese by Russian prosecutor", 26. September 1947, 17/18/B, Box 628, Entry 468, National Archives, Washington, D.C., USA.

Spurr, G./Hutt, B./Horvath, S. (1955): The effects of Age on Finger Temperature Responses to Local Cooling, American Heart Journal 50 (1955), pp. 551-555.

State-War-Navy Coordinating Subcommittee for the Far East (SWNCC Subcommittee), "Interrogation of certain Japanese by Russian prosecutor", 1. August 1947, Appendix "A", 17/18/B, Box 628, Entry 468, National Archives, Washington, D.C., USA.

Tanaka, M. (1971a): Experimental Studies on Human Reaction to Cold – Differences in the Vascular Hunting Reaction to Cold According to Sex, Season, and Environmental Temperature, Bulletin of Tokyo Medical and Dental University 18 (1971), pp. 269-280.

Tanaka, M. (1971b): Experimental Studies on Human Reaction to Cold – Different Vascular Hunting Reaction of Workers to Cold, Bulletin of Tokyo Medical and Dental University 18 (1971), pp. 169-177.

Thompson, A. T. (1946): Report on Japanese Biological Warfare, 31. May 1946, 57 4926 Cy 1, Library of Congress, Science and Technical Reports Section, Washington, D. C.

Tsuneishi, K. (1986): The Research Guarded by Military Secrecy – The Isolation of the E. H. F. Virus in Japanese Biological Warfare Unit, Historia Scientiarum 30 (1986), pp. 79-92.

Wang, S. (1987): Sunwure' de jinxi: Riben qinlüezhe zui'ede renti shiyan [Past and Present of the 'Sunwu Fever': the Criminal Human Experiments of the Japanese Invaders]. Sunwu wenshi ziliao [Historical Sources of the District of Sunwu] 2 (1987), pp. 22-29.

World Medical Association (WMA) (2004): World Medical Association Declaration of Helsinki – Ethical Priniples for Medical Research Involving Human Subjects, 9 October 2004.

Williams, P./Wallace, D. (1989): Unit 731: Japan's Secret Biological Warfare Unit in World War II. New York: The Free Press.

Yoshimura, H. (1967): Studies on Cold Tolerance in Man, Nippon Seirigaku Zasshi (Japanese Physiological Journal) 29 (1967), pp. 673-678.

Yoshimura, M./Hori, S./Yoshimura, H. (1972): Effect of High-Fat Diet on Thermal Acclimation with Special Reference to Thyroid Activity, Japanese Journal of Physiology 22 (1972), pp. 517-531.

Yoshimura, H./Iida, T. (1952a): Studies on the Reactivity of Skin Vessels to Extreme Cold I. A Point Test on the Resistance Against Frostbite, Japanese Journal of Physiology 2 (1952), pp. 147-159.

Yoshimura, H./Iida, T. (1952b): Studies on the Reactivity of Skin Vessels to Extreme Cold II. Factors Governing the Individual Difference of The Reactivity, or the Resistance Against Frostbite, Japanese Journal of Physio-logy 2 (1952), pp. 177-185.

Yoshimura, H./Iida, T. (1952c): Studies on the Reactivity of Skin Vessels to Extreme Cold. III. Effects of Diets on the Reactivity of Skin Vessels to Cold, Japanese Journal of Physiology 2 (1952), pp. 310-315.

Yoshimura, H./Shiomi, S./Makihata, K./Hiramathu, S. (1961): Studies on the Nature of Hypothermia I. Studies on Resistance to Cold-Induced Death, Journal of The Physical Society of Japan 23 (1961), pp. 173-181.

Yoshimura, M./Takeda, H./Yoshimura, H. (1969): Effect of Dietary Composition on Thermal Acclimation, Nippon Seirigaku Zasshi [Japanese Physiological Journal] 31 (1969), pp. 178-179.

Yoshimura, M./Yoshimura, H. (1970): Quality of Diet and Human Adaptability to Heat and Cold, Nippon Rinsho [Japanese Clinical Medicine] 28 (1970), pp. 1988-1993.

Yuan, C. (1951): Rikou xijunzhan baoxing [The Atrocities of the Bacterial War of the Japanese Bandits]. Shanghai: Shanghai tonglian shudian.

731 Butaiten, Zenkokujikkoiinkai [Exhibition about the Unit 731, Japanese action committee] "Exhibition about the Unit 731. July 1993–December 1994", Tokyo, 1993.

II.
The Helsinki Declaration
in an International Context

Susan E. Lederer

Research without Borders:
The Origins of the Declaration of Helsinki

I.   Introduction

In June 1964 the eighteenth assembly of the World Medical Association (WMA) endorsed a series of recommendations for the conduct of human experimentation. The Declaration of Helsinki, named after the city where the assembly was held, has been hailed as the "most influential international ethics document governing the conduct of clinical research".[1] The first international set of guidelines for human experimentation, the Declaration reflected the longstanding interest of the WMA in issues of medical ethics and the enduring shadow of the Nazi medical war crimes. But the road to the Helsinki Declaration was neither straight nor smooth; the development of the recommendations for human experimentation required more than a decade of active discussion and debate among WMA members before the Declaration was brought to the General Assembly for formal adoption in 1964.

The prolonged period of disagreement and discussion, noted Ronald Winton, an Australian physician-delegate to the WMA and a one-time president of the organisation, was not "due to procrastination or lack of concern on the part of the Council of the WMA or of its Committee on Medical Ethics, but to the desire to produce a truly useful and practical document".[2] This prolonged period resulted from more than philosophical differences and practical concerns. The Declaration reflected the organisational politics and financial structure of the WMA. Although the ostensible product of an international medical association, the Declaration of Helsinki, like the Nuremberg Code which it followed, bore a sturdy American stamp. This paper examines the winding road to the Declaration of Helsinki and the American issues that shaped its ultimate form in 1964.

---

1   Weijer and Anderson (2001), p. 19.
2   Winton (1976), p. 59.

II.   The Founding of the World Medical Association

In 1946, physicians representing thirty-two national medical organisations met in London to discuss an international association of doctors and national medical societies. Prompted by the suggestion of Polish physician George de Swiet, president of the Polish Medical Association in Great Britain, the 1946 meeting took place in London. Hosted by the British Medical Association (BMA) in conjunction with the Association Professionelle Internationale des Médicins (APIM), the assembled physicians sought to promote international medical relations and the advancement of medicine and its social and cultural aspects. Physicians from the recently defeated nations of Germany and Japan did not take part in the meeting. More surprising perhaps, American physicians declined to participate, although the American Medical Association (AMA) asked two British doctors to act as observers on its behalf.[3]

Representatives from the AMA were among those present at the first meeting in 1947 of the newly established WMA. The assembled physicians unanimously adopted a series of explicit policy objectives, ranging from the professional to the universal. These objectives included maintaining the honour and protecting the interests of the medical profession, assisting the people of the world to attain the highest possible level of health, and the promotion of world peace. In addition, delegates to the assembly unanimously agreed to establish relations with, and to represent the views of their profession, to the World Health Organisation (WHO), UNESCO, and other international bodies.[4]

The first meeting of the new organisation was held in Paris in September 1947, only one month after judgments had been rendered in the trial of twenty-three Nazi medical and administrative personnel (the case known as United States of America v. Karl Brandt et al. or the Nuremberg Doctors' Trial).[5] The "betrayal of medicine by German doctors" cast a lengthy shadow over virtually all activities of the WMA.[6]

One of the first acts of the fledgling association was the adoption of a statement about the dedication of the physician to his profession. In 1948, the General Assembly of the WMA formally endorsed the Declaration of Geneva or the Physician's Oath. The association recommended the oath to physicians of all nations, especially young physicians embarking on their professional career. The framers of the declaration self-consciously modified the Oath of Hippocrates, described by one representative as "obviously developed for physicians of Greece in the period of the School of Hippocrates [...] and not especially suited to such conditions as prevail today".[7] All references to the deity or deities were omitted, as well as the Hippocratic injunctions against surgery, abortion, and euthanasia. The physician who adopted the Declaration pledged not to allow considerations of

3   Pridham (1951).
4   Howard-Jones (1981); Lee (1997).
5   Weindling (2001); Schmidt (2004).
6   War Crimes and Medicine (1949), p. 8.
7   Dedication (1949), p. 4.

nationality, race, party politics, and social class to interfere with the professional responsibility for the patient's welfare.[8]

In 1949, the WMA proposed an International Code of Medical Ethics, which incorporated the Declaration of Geneva and other professional commitments of the physician. Finding appropriate language to reflect different national traditions created some discord among the delegates. For example, when the Irish delegate to the WMA objected to the proposed clause regarding therapeutic abortion in the Code, the committee formed to reconsider the offending paragraph recommended that the code be altered.

Whereas the original draft read, "A doctor must always bear in mind the importance of preserving human life from the time of conception. Therapeutic abortion may only be performed if the conscience of the doctor and the national laws permit", the revised version read "A doctor must always bear in mind the importance of preserving life from conception until death".[9]

In the early 1950s the WMA continued to revisit issues of medical ethics. The General Assembly passed in 1950 a resolution against euthanasia as contrary to the public interest and to medical ethical principles.[10] In 1951, at the request of the United Nations the WMA cooperated with the WHO to ascertain the "number, location and condition of the survivors of Concentration Camps, who, under the Nazi regime, were victims of so-called scientific experiments".[11] Noting that the victims of experiments were scattered in many countries, the WMA requested that member organisations ask these individuals about their willingness to have their names and addresses reported provided they were safeguarded from publicity and that they were assured of satisfactory compensation for their disabilities. The WMA asked member nations to collect the names and addresses of "Victims of Nazi Medical Experimentation" and to forward this information to the WHO in preparation for compensation.[12]

One pressing issue that confronted the WMA Council in the late 1940s was the rehabilitation of the German medical profession. In October 1949, council members of the WMA had arranged to meet privately with leading members of the Arbeitsgemeinschaft Westdeutscher Ärztekammern (AWA). Otto Leuch (Switzerland) and Dag Knutson (Sweden), representing the WMA, met with AWA doctors Hans Neuffer and Theodor Dobler in January 1950.[13] The four physicians agreed that no minutes of the meeting be recorded and together decided that nothing about the conference should be published in the medical press. The WMA delegates were charged with inviting the German representatives into closer relations with WMA doctors with an eye to electing the Germans to membership. One obstacle to this invitation for the WMA was the

8   Ummel (1991).
9   Minutes (1949), p. 9.
10   Resolutions (1950), p. 134.
11   Victims (1951), pp. 241-242.
12   Annual Report (1952).
13   Report on Conference in Stuttgart 21-22 January 1950.

AWA's employment of Karl Haedenkamp, a physician known to have connec-
tions to the Nazi party in the years between 1934 and 1939:

> "The employment of Dr. Haedenkamp has been deemed irreconcilable with the principles
> and views, expressed in the said declaration, which categorically disclaims all connections
> with Nazi ideology and condemns those members of the German medical profession, who
> took part in or tolerated acts against the noble tradition of medical men".

For their part, the German physicians argued that Haedenkamp's services were
indispensable to their professional organisation. They defended his moral
character by "repeatedly stressing" that even those with prominent positions in the
Nazi regime knew little about what was going on – the Nazi leaders, the two
German physicians claimed, were "past-masters in the art of drawing iron
curtains".[14] After extensive discussion and negotiation, the German medical
association prepared a statement acknowledging the numerous acts of cruelty and
oppression perpetrated by some German doctors during the Third Reich and
solemnly promising to do everything to prevent such a future betrayal of medicine
by German doctors.[15] The AWA noted, for example, how since 14 June 1947
every physician, who obtained his medical license, was required to take the
Hippocratic Oath as revised by the WMA (the Declaration of Geneva). In 1951,
when the Secretary General of the WMA canvassed member nations about
admitting West Germany and Japanese physicians, thirty of the thirty-one national
medical associations who responded voted in favour of admitting Japan; twenty-
eight voted in favour of admitting Germany. The General Assembly of the WMA
subsequently authorised the Council to accept the Japanese and West German
medical associations as members.[16]

These early difficulties with the Nazi affiliations of some prominent German
participants in the WMA continued to trouble the organisation. In 1993, German
physician and WMA president-elect, Hans Joachim Sewering, resigned his
position following revelations that he had sent a 14-year-old girl with epilepsy to
a "healing clinic" in 1943 where he knew she would be killed. A one-time
member of the Nazi party and the Nazi SS, Sewering first joined the WMA in
1959 and had served as treasurer of the organisation for twenty years. In the face
of calls from individual German physicians and from Canadian, American and
Israeli medical associations for Sewering to resign, the WMA, which owed much
of its financial backing to German medical interests, continued to defend
Sewering's selection as president.[17]

---

14   Ibid.
15   Report on the Statement about German Medical War Crimes (1949).
16   Memorandum (1951).
17   Seidelman (1996); White (1996).

III. The Problem of Human Experimentation

In 1953, the Royal Netherlands Medical Association asked the WMA to consider the use of human subjects in scientific experiments. L. A. Hulst, the Dutch medical delegate, proposed that the WMA request that editors of medical journals around the world consider the importance of protecting "test persons" and to develop guidelines to judge whether subject protection was adequate.[18] The issue of clinical research was already under review in France, where in 1952 the French National Academy of Medicine had reviewed some features of experiments on human beings.[19] In their deliberations, French doctors distinguished between the use of new methods intended to benefit an individual patient and experiments performed to benefit others. Whereas experiments on patients were regarded as "not only the right but the duty of the physician", the Academy ruled that experiments for science could only be performed on "informed volunteers free to accept or reject" the intervention.[20]

Paul Cibrie, a French physician-delegate to the WMA, chaired the WMA's committee on medical ethics, which was asked to evaluate issues regarding human experimentation. From the start, Cibrie sought to dissociate the WMA's considerations of human experimentation from the "scientific crimes" of Nazi medicine. The Nazi medical atrocities, he noted, could be eliminated as "true monstrosities, the commission of which ought always to result in merciless justice".[21] Under his guidance, the WMA committee on medical ethics formulated four regulations to serve as a framework for consideration in discussions of human experimentation. The four conditions for ethical human experimentation included: the scientific and ethical qualification of the experimenters; caution and discretion in the publication of early results; the distinction between experiments applied to sick and healthy subjects; and the requirement that subjects undergoing experimentation fully recognised the risks involved. Thus, under Ciprie's direction, the recommendations for ethical human experimentation reprised the French Academy's 1952 guidelines. In a supplemental report, Cibrie separated the requirements for experimentation on the sick and on the healthy to bring the number of regulations to five.[22]

Differences over the practice of human experimentation in different national settings became quickly apparent. When the Council of the WMA considered the report in October 1954, the American Austin Smith, one of Cibrie's fellow committee members (the other member of the committee on medical ethics was Spanish physician Lorenzo Garcia-Tornel), protested that the requirement that healthy human subjects be fully informed about an experiment would seriously undermine research in the United States. Smith had long been associated with the AMA. He served as secretary of its longstanding Council on Pharmacy and

18 Experiments on Human Beings (1953).
19 Human Experimentation (1952).
20 Frenkel (1978), pp. 131-132.
21 Report (1952).
22 Ibid.

Chemistry, and in 1949 he succeeded Morris Fishbein as editor of its influential journal, a position he held until 1958. Smith's reservations about informing healthy subjects stemmed from significant post-war changes in the organisation and performance of clinical trials. Placebos were becoming integral to the efforts on the part of elite researchers to impose rigorous criteria for the evaluation of new drugs and other therapies.[23] The introduction of new methodological constraints in the conduct of clinical trials directly conflicted with the attention in the post-Nuremberg period to insure that research subjects were fully informed.

Other representatives shared Smith's concerns. British physician Hugh Clegg and Danish physician Otto Rasmussen expressed similar reservations in light of the need for properly controlled (and blinded, although the word "blinded" was not used) scientific studies. Seeking to defuse the issue, the Dutch delegate L. A. Hulst observed that the difficulty was created by the language used. In the case of an experimental vaccine, he noted, it was important for the individual to know whether or not he had received the vaccine. It would not be appropriate to allow someone to think that he had been vaccinated when there existed a 50 per cent possibility that he had received a placebo injection. Because vaccination trials were rarely conducted in adults, however, Clegg moved that the example of vaccination be deleted from the document because children could not legally give their consent. Following the discussion about the need to inform healthy subjects and to have controlled and blinded studies, the WMA Council endorsed Smith's proposal that any mention of informing healthy subjects about their participation in a control group be deleted from the document sent to the General Assembly.

In October 1954, the eighth general assembly took up the Resolution on Human Experimentation and the Principles for Those in Research and Experimentation. Several delegates explored the regulation about the lay press and the danger of premature and sensational publication. Other delegates raised the issue of consent in the case of experimentation on mentally challenged persons and in children. The American delegate F. J. L. Blasingame requested that the requirement of written consent of the responsible individual or the written consent of the individual legally responsible for the subject be added. The General Assembly endorsed the resolution on human experimentation, including the requirement of written consent.

After the adoption of the Rome resolution, the issue of human experimentation continued to concern the WMA's committee on medical ethics and the Council. In 1959, when British physician Hugh Clegg was appointed chair of the committee on medical ethics, he found the Council seriously divided about the need for a revised code of regulations for human experimentation and the form such a code should take. To begin the work, the British physician (and editor of the *British Medical Journal* (*BMJ*)) solicited eleven member nations (including the US, Germany, France, Britain, Israel, Japan, India, Turkey, and Chile) for representative general guiding principles for the WMA to use in creating a code

---

23   Kaptchuk (1998); see also Davidovitch (2004).

on "this complicated subject".[24] To assist the medical societies in articulating their views about clinical research, Clegg identified five scenarios for which the Committee was interested in formulating regulations: the administration of drugs to medical students to test their effects; preventive inoculations using a control group not inoculated against whooping cough or tuberculosis; controlled therapeutic trials of a new drug; using inmates of prisons, penitentiaries, or mental institutions for controlled prophylactic or therapeutic trials, and investigations on hospital patients which had no relation to the condition which brought them to the hospital.[25] Several months later, at the request of French physician Marcel Poumailloux, Clegg's committee added a sixth situation for which guidance from member nations would be welcome: experiments undertaken on women in several countries in order to produce sterility either temporarily or permanently.[26]

Clegg's committee report to the WMA Council in April 1960 prompted considerable discussion. Council members offered a variety of observations and suggestions for revising and clarifying the recommendations for human experimentation. Some council members expressed concern about the use of "captive subjects". The Indian delegate A. P. Mittra noted that a prisoner offered remission in his sentence for submitting to an experiment could not exercise "judgment and conscience in the true sense of the word". The Philippines delegate urged Clegg and his committee to explore ethical aspects of sending humans into outer space. Otto Rasmussen, the physician representative from Denmark, advised that religious aspects should not be introduced in a code of ethics for human experimentation; instead the code should be based on a "common denominator" acceptable to all religious faiths. In a similar vein, Jean Maystre, the official liaison officer and a Swiss physician, requested Clegg and his committee to obtain additional information from other cultural and ethnic groups, especially Moslem and Buddhist countries. Several members expressed the need to consider experiments that altered or changed personality.[27]

The minutes of the 38th council session in Madrid illustrate how the Nuremberg Code of permissible human experimentation shaped WMA discussions about guidelines for clinical research. As some commentators have noted, the WMA's 1954 Rome Resolution and the drafts of what would become the Declaration of Helsinki did not explicitly mention the Nuremberg Code. In spite of this, nearly all commentators have concluded that the Declaration was greatly influenced by the Nuremberg Code – a conclusion which Sharon Perley and her colleagues have noted is "nowhere documented".[28] The minutes of WMA committee and council meetings offer documentary evidence for the salience of the Nuremberg Code for their deliberations. In their discussions over universally applicable guidelines for human experimentation, the WMA Committee on medical ethics debated, and rejected in some cases as too restrictive, specific

24 Special Reports (1960).
25 Report of the Medical Ethics Committee (1959).
26 Minutes (1959).
27 Minutes (1960).
28 Perley et al. (1992), p. 158.

principles in the Nuremberg Code. At the 1960 Council meeting, for example, members expressed concern that the requirement that all human experimentation be preceded by prior experimentation on animals would bar important research:

> "The third rule in the Nuremberg Code would seem to be too restrictive as it provides that no human experimentation should be undertaken without prior experiment on animals. Under certain condition it might provide impossible to try the experiment on animals".[29]

In his September 1960 report of the Committee on Medical Ethics in West Berlin, Clegg informed the Council members that he and his colleagues had briefly considered adopting the Nuremberg Code, published in the American periodical *Science* in February 1953, as a guide.[30] Clegg's committee quickly concluded that the Code was not a sufficient guide, and instead found it necessary to attempt "to draft a code which could serve at least as a guide to doctors working in different conditions and in different countries".[31] Even before this report, Clegg had suggested the inadequacies of the Nuremberg code for resolving the "doctor's dilemma". In a March 1960 article for the *World Medical Journal*, Clegg offered the story of BCG vaccination as a cautionary tale. Although the vaccination for tuberculosis had been introduced in 1922, it was not until 1956 that the efficacy of the vaccine in preventing tuberculosis was definitively established:

> "If only a properly controlled trial of B.C.G. had been conducted in 1923, then thirty-four years of doubt and controversy would have been avoided, and millions of lives would have been saved. And at the end of the thirty-four years one is left with the gnawing doubt about the justification of withholding a prophylactic for which there was reasonable evidence of its efficacy".[32]

Given the complexities of modern medical science, Clegg questioned the wisdom of laying down "hard and fast" rules to constrain investigators and their research subjects, but called on research workers to be saturated with the "Hippocratic ideal," the physician's commitment to provide "compassionate care for the sick person".[33]

Perhaps not surprising, by September 1960 Clegg acknowledged that preparing a code for human experimentation that would simultaneously protect research subjects and not constrain investigators would require considerable time. To speed up the discussion, Clegg personally drafted a provisional statement subject to modification and improvement by the Council and his fellow committee members (Italian physician A. Spinelli and Indian delegate A. P. Mittra joined Clegg on the medical ethics committee).

Clegg's draft code included several restrictions on experiments performed for acquiring knowledge. These included the stipulation that the subject of the experiment be in a mental, physical, and legal state to exercise fully the power of choice in decisions to participate. In addition, Clegg expressed disapproval for research

29   Minutes (1960), p. 22.
30   Report of Medical Ethics Committee (1960).
31   Report of Medical Ethics Committee (1960).
32   Clegg (1960), p. 77.
33   Ibid., p. 79.

in which the subject was in a dependent relationship to the investigator (including the medical student to his teacher, a patient to his doctor, and a technician to his laboratory supervisor). He insisted that prisoners of war should never be used as experimental subjects nor should the persons housed in prisons, penitentiaries, and reformatories – that is captive groups – be used as subjects. Clegg also identified the inmates of mental hospitals and hospitals for mental defectives as undesirable subjects for experimentation.[34]

The Committee on Medical Ethics continued to rework Clegg's draft code on human experimentation. The 1961 draft divided experiments into the sick and the healthy. In the case of experiments conducted solely for the acquisition of new knowledge, the draft code explicitly banned experiments on prisoners of war, on civilians detained as a result of military invasions or occupation, on persons retained in prisons, on those in mental hospitals, and on those incapable of giving consent because of age, mental incapacity, or being in a dependent position.

At the April 1961 Council meeting, the proposal received additional scrutiny from Council members. The use of children as research subjects generated much discussion among the physicians who debated the legal right of parents and guardians to consent to experimentation on their children. Although some rejected outright the idea that parents might benefit financially as a result of consenting to experimentation on their child, some insisted that children should categorically be excluded as subjects of experimentation. The issue of prisoners as subjects in research received similar scrutiny. Even though prisoners in some cases volunteered to participate in research, both Clegg and Spinelli insisted that these subjects be excluded as a captive group. The issues raised by children and prisoners in research were not the only sources of conflict. Council members disagreed about the need for defining what constituted a human experiment and about how input from member nations could be solicited to inform the deliberations.

In 1961, Spinelli succeeded Clegg as chair of the Committee on Medical Ethics, and continued to oversee the status of the draft code on human experimentation. In 1962 two American delegates to the WMA Council, Gerald Dorman and Austin Smith, raised several concerns about the legal and public relations status of the draft code. In May 1962, Dorman questioned the statements in the draft code about the use of prisoners in experimentation. He asked that the draft code of ethics on human experimentation be returned to the committee for further discussion in light of disagreements between the English and French texts, the divisions among the council on the regulations of experiments conducted for the advancement of medical knowledge, and the need to have public relations advice. Smith, who by 1962 had left his position as *JAMA* editor to become president of the Pharmaceutical Manufacturers Association, similarly warned that both legal experts and public relations experts should review the wording of the document in order to minimise misinterpretation on the part of laypersons.[35]

34   Supplementary Report (1960).
35   Minutes (1962); Campion (1984), p. 492.

In October 1962, the *BMJ* published the WMA's Draft Code of Ethics on Human Experimentation. A brief accompanying editorial note stressed that the code appeared as a service to British physicians and did not represent a final version: "some of the items in it will be re-ordered and modified, and that, in particular, it will eventually be prefaced by a general statement on the essential part played by research in medicine".[36] The draft code defined an experiment on a human being as "an act whereby the investigator deliberately changes the internal or external environment in order to observe the effects of such a change". The draft outlined conditions for acceptable human experiments and those that should not be undertaken, especially those involving "children in institutions and not under the care of relatives". The draft similarly excluded as subjects of experiments prisoners of war – military or civilian, political prisoners and persons retained in prisons, penitentiaries, or reformatories, mental hospitals and hospitals for mental defectives.[37]

Earlier that year, publication of an article by British physician Maurice H. Pappworth entitled "Human Guinea Pigs: A Warning" sparked widespread comment in the British national press. An editorial appearing in the same issue as the Draft Code provided another opportunity to advance Clegg's views that certain classes of human beings required special protections. Rules for human research became necessary when "general exhortation, letters in the press, and questions in Parliament seem to have little restraining effect on those who cannot always understand the difference between guinea-pigs and human beings, especially when they are collected together in penitentiaries, reformatories, and institutions for the mentally defective".[38]

In 1962, Clegg was the editor of the *British Medical Journal*.[39] The decision to publish the draft code as a service to British doctors simultaneously advanced his interests in publicising his version of the draft guidelines for human experimentation. American reservations about the draft code, especially the bans on using institutionalised children and prisoners as research subjects, may explain why the 1962 draft code did not appear in American medical or scientific journals. Even though Smith had resigned his position as *JAMA* editor, American physicians did not lack on-going access to the AMA's journals for publishing WMA news and documents. One American researcher, V. Knight, took the opportunity to criticise the Draft Code and its provision forbidding the use of "captive subjects" in a review of the use of volunteers in virological research. In 1964, he rejected the Draft Code's restriction on using prisoners as volunteers. "Prisoners in the present experiments," he explained, "were not unduly influenced by the modest privileges and comforts offered, and that there was no duress, stated or implied, with respect to their decision to participate".[40] Moreover, Knight, like other American defenders of prisoner research, identified the

---

36 Draft Code (1962), p. 1119.
37 Ibid.
38 Experimental Medicine (1962), p. 1108.
39 Bartrip (1990).
40 Knight (1964), pp. 18-19.

"positive rehabilitative benefits" that prisoners derived from their participation in medical research.[41]

IV. Resolving the Deadlock

Controversy over using children in institutions and the "captive-subjects" of mental hospitals, prisons, and reformatories continued to divide the WMA members. In 1963, the Committee on Medical Ethics (now composed of American Gerald Dorman, Spinelli, Jean Maystre, Ole Harlem of Norway, and U. Siirala from Finland) reported a deadlock. At Dorman's suggestion, the Committee agreed to insert a "frank statement" about the failure to reach consensus over the clauses governing both the participation of children in institutions and prisoners in clinical research.[42] The issue of using institutionalised children as research subjects pitted the Americans and Canadians against the French and British who argued that this population should not be used in research. American physicians similarly argued against restrictions on the use of prisoners, insisting that if a prisoner understood and consented to an experiment then he should be permitted to participate in clinical research. In 1963, the draft guidelines were sent to all member nations for study and comments. By 31 October, however, only Finland had registered its comments.

In 1964, the Chair of the Committee on Medical Ethics presented the Council with its final deliberations on the draft document "Ethical Principles Guiding Doctors in Clinical Research". The issue of using research subjects in a dependant relationship had not been determined. After lengthy debate, the Council agreed to resolve the issue by altering the name of the document to "Recommendations Guiding Doctors in Clinical Research".[43] When the document came to the General Assembly for a vote, no mention about using children in institutions or prisoners appeared in the text. In June, the General Assembly unanimously endorsed the recommendations for clinical research. To emphasise the importance of the document, the WMA decided to identify the recommendations as the "Declaration of Helsinki".[44]

The 1964 Declaration of Helsinki shared some features of the Nuremberg Code's requirements for permissible human experiments. The Helsinki Declaration followed the Nuremberg Code's insistence that animal and laboratory studies precede human studies and endorsed the requirement for scientifically qualified investigators. Both the Declaration and the Code stipulated the right of the subject to withdraw from research and the responsibility of the investigator to discontinue the trial if he or she foresaw injury to the research subject. Both called for the consent of the subject.

41   Ibid., p. 19.
42   Summary Minutes and Report (1963).
43   Minutes (1965).
44   XVIII World Medical Assembly (1964).

Unlike the Nuremberg Code, the Declaration of Helsinki distinguished clinical research combined with patient care and non-therapeutic human experimentation. In so doing, the Declaration echoed the conceptual framework adopted by the German Reich Health Council in 1931. On the heels of the "Lübeck tragedy" in which some seventy-five children died in trials of the BCG vaccine, the Reich Health Council issued its "Regulations on New Therapy and Human Experimentation", which distinguished "innovative therapy" and "scientific experimentation" undertaken for "research purposes without serving a therapeutic purpose in an individual case".[45] Although the distinction between therapeutic and non-therapeutic research did not appear in the Nuremberg Code, it was resurrected by the French in 1952 and endorsed by the WMA in the 1954 Rome Resolution. This distinction introduced different consent requirements for ethical human experimentation. The WMA document specified written consent from a healthy subject adequately informed of the aims, methods, anticipated benefits, and potential hazards of the study and the discomfort that it may entail. By contrast, physicians who combined clinical research with professional care were not advised to obtain patient consent in writing. "If at all possible, consistent with patient psychology, the doctor should obtain the patient's freely given consent after the patient had been given a full explanation".[46] In another striking departure from the Nuremberg Code, the Declaration permitted experimentation on individuals unable to exercise informed consent, including children, whose parents or legal guardians agreed to allow their participation in an experiment.

The Declaration of Helsinki was unanimously endorsed but not all participants were pleased by the outcome. Even before the formal ratification of the document, the *BMJ* recorded its dissatisfaction about the compromise of ethical principles necessary to achieve consensus. In 1963, an editorial in the *BMJ* had warned about the insidious "American influence" at work in the revisions of the code. "I am disturbed to learn that the WMA is now hedging on its clause about using – or not *using* – criminals as experimental material," noted the unsigned editorial. "The American influence has been at work on its suspension". Crediting the Americans for being the first to apply the terrible lessons of the Nuremberg Doctors Trial, the writer nonetheless rejected the American argument for a profound difference between experiments performed in American prisons and those conducted on the inmates at Auschwitz. "One of the nicest of the American medical scientists I know was heard to say 'Criminals in our penitentiaries are fine experimental material – and much cheaper than chimpanzees.' I hope the chimpanzees do not come to hear of this".[47] One month following the formal ratification of the Declaration of Helsinki, *BMJ* editorial sentiment remained skeptical about the changes wrought by American influences: "we welcome the

---

45   Grodin (1992), p. 130.
46   Human Experimentation (1964), p. 177.
47   Without Prejudice (1963), p. 1603.

revised code of the WMA, while regretting that its revision has to some extent weakened it".[48]

What was the nature and extent of this American influence on the Declaration of Helsinki? When asked nearly thirty years later about the "American influence" on the Declaration of Helsinki, Gerald Dorman, the sole American member of the WMA's committee on Medical Ethics in the critical years 1963-1964, confirmed that he made the case to his fellow committee members for the ethical use of prisoners in research. "At the time of the development of the Helsinki Declaration", he recalled in 1991, "the U.S. delegation did not wish to declare unethical such laws [permitting prison experimentation] per se. However, we did want to restrict and limit their usage by insuring that prisoners had full knowledge of the risks, mishaps or unforeseen immediate and longterm results of their decision to participate".[49]

George Annas, one of the most prominent contributors to the literature on research ethics, has suggested another American influence. The most important single event to push the final adoption of the 1964 Declaration of Helsinki, he has argued, was the United States Food and Drug Administration's (FDA's) proposal to streamline and standardise the process for granting approval for experimental drugs.[50] In the wake of the thalidomide tragedy, the large-scale trials of new drugs made it necessary, Annas claimed, to confront the issues of human experimentation in a context far removed from both the Nazi concentration camps and the Hippocratic doctor-patient relationship model. As Ruth Faden and Tom Beauchamp have argued, the Drug Amendments of 1962 enacted by the U. S. Congress called for fundamental and potentially far-reaching changes in governmental regulation of the drug industry, including the need to inform patients that they were receiving an experimental drug. The FDA responded with "poorly developed" consent provisions that "repeated the vague wording and broad exception in the law".[51] Confusion over the FDA regulations persisted, until the agency clarified its policy with a new set of regulations issued in August 1966. The new regulations – "Consent for Use of Investigational New Drugs on Humans: Statement of Policy" – drew extensively on both the Nuremberg Code and the Declaration of Helsinki.

Drug development and the large-scale trials of new drugs may have played an even more important and immediate role in the formulation of the Declaration of Helsinki. Funding for the WMA and its activities depended on dues from members and other sources. Although the Americans had initially declined to participate in the 1946 meeting that resulted in the WMA, American financial support played a crucial role in the organisation's early years. In September 1947, the AMA organised a luncheon for pharmaceutical manufacturers and their representatives. Already assured of interest on the part of drug makers about "the

48   Ethics of Human Experimentation (1964), p. 136.
49   Harkness (1996), p. 161.
50   Annas (1991).
51   Faden/Beauchamp (1986), p. 204.

desirability from many angles of the W.M.A.", those lunching at the Waldorf Astoria Hotel in New York City heard the president of Warner-Hudnut speak about the humanitarian aims of the WMA.[52] Elmer Bobst emphasised that the "pharmaceutical industries are part of medicine and their contributions to this project are really a business expense, since funds are an essential factor".[53] The American supporting committee, Canadian physician T. C. Routley, chair of the WMA council, acknowledged, "guaranteed to underwrite the cost of maintaining and operating the central office up to $50,000 a year for five years".[54]

In 1949, some 1200 American physicians each contributed $10 to the United States Committee.[55] In addition to these individual doctors, "interested business friends" comprised the leaders of major American pharmaceutical companies. Among the life members of the US Committee were Bobst, L. D. Barney, president of Hoffman-LaRoche, DeWitt Clough, chair of the board of directors of Abbott Laboratories, Adam Fiske, a vice-president at Eli Lilly, Howard Fonda, senior vice-president at Burroughs-Wellcome, Willard Greenwald, scientific consultant for Philip Morris, John McKeen, president of Charles Pfizer and Company, Robert Lincoln, founder of McNeil Laboratories, and Carleton Palmer, chairman of the board of the American pharmaceutical company, E.R. Squibb.[56]

The financial support of the United States Committee was critical to the survival of the new organisation. The US Committee played an important role in the daily life of the WMA. The Committee required that the WMA maintain its headquarters in America; the offices for the WMA were located at the New York Academy of Medicine in New York City until 1974, shortly after the AMA resigned in protest over funding and voting arrangements.[57] American physicians occupied prominent positions in the new organisation. Louis Bauer, who served as the WMA's Secretary General, chaired the Board of Trustees of the AMA. American surgeon Elmer Henderson, a member of the AMA's Board of Trustees, served on the WMA Council. Morris Fishbein, ousted in 1949 from his longtime position as editor of *JAMA*, served as the initial editor of the *WMA Bulletin*.[58] Austin Smith, who succeeded Fishbein as JAMA editor, also assumed the role of executive editor of the *World Medical Journal*. Smith's editorship at JAMA represented a peak period in the development of new pharmaceutical products, especially antibiotics. At the *Journal*, annual advertising revenues rose from $2.7 million in 1951 to more than $8 million in 1959.[59]

In 1958 Austin Smith left the AMA and WMA to become president of the Pharmaceutical Manufacturers of America, a trade group to promote the interests

---

52   Irons (1947), p. 3.
53   Ibid., p. 5.
54   Routley (1949), p. 18.
55   World Medical Association (1949).
56   Life Members (1951).
57   Richards (1994).
58   Fishbein (1969).
59   Campion (1984), p. 491.

of American drug-makers.[60] Even after his departure from the AMA and WMA, Smith's position as president of the US Committee gave him a voice in the affairs of the WMA. In the late 1950s and early 1960s the US Committee continued to finance "approximately one-third of WMA activities".[61] In 1959, following the WMA meeting in Montreal, Smith warned that he would be unable to recommend the continued participation of the US Committee in light of the administrative problems in the organisation and its troubled finances. To address the concerns of the Americans, the AMA Board of Trustees in 1963 appointed a committee on AMA–WMA relations; this committee was asked to advise the Trustees about the activities of the WMA and its relationship to the US Committee. Among the members of this committee was Gerald Dorman, the American delegate to the WMA Committee on Medical Ethics and the one who opposed any explicit restrictions on using prisoners and institutionalised children in experimentation. Shortly after the Declaration of Helsinki was adopted, in December 1965, the US Committee to the WMA was dissolved.[62]

Drug development in the United States relied extensively on the use of prisoners and reformatories. After the US Congress passed amendments to the Food, Drug and Cosmetic Act in 1963, prisoners became essential to the performance of the clinical trials of new drugs. By 1972, FDA officials estimated that more than 90 per cent of all investigational drugs were tested initially on the inmates of American prisons.[63] The AMA delegates to the WMA, especially physicians like Austin Smith who worked closely with pharmaceutical company executives, recognised a potential threat to American drug development by restrictions on the use of prison inmates. Even before the Draft Code of Ethics of Human Experimentation was published in 1962, the minutes of the WMA's committee on medical ethics and the council demonstrate that an American influence was already at work to forestall any restrictions on the use of inmates of prisons and reformatories from the document that became the Declaration of Helsinki.

American pharmaceutical companies were similarly invested in the development and testing of new vaccines. As physicians recognised, vaccine testing necessarily involved children, and American researchers and the pharmaceutical companies that supported their research had depended on institutionalised children as the initial recipients for many of the vaccines developed in the 1950s and 1960s. Jonas Salk's polio vaccine, for example, developed in cooperation with the Parke, Davis pharmaceutical company was initially tested in homes for retarded children.[64] Vaccines for measles were tested in women's prisons, which allowed young children to remain with their mothers,

---

60 He later became chair and chief executive officer of Parke, Davis & Company, and vice chairman of the board of Warner-Lambert Company, two of America's preeminent pharmaceutical houses.
61 WMA, AMA Archives.
62 Ibid., p. 20.
63 Harkness (1996), p. 158.
64 Smith (1990).

and in group homes for retarded and crippled children. At the Willowbrook State School, pediatric infectious disease researcher Saul Krugman hoped to develop a vaccine against hepatitis using the population of severely retarded infants and children in that institution.[65] It is hardly surprising that the American delegates to the WMA resisted restrictions on the use of these populations – institutionalised children – in the development of new drugs and vaccines.

American medical organisations quickly embraced the Declaration of Helsinki. Publication of the new recommendations produced almost immediate changes. By 1966, eight American biomedical organisations had endorsed the Declaration, including the AMA, the American College of Physicians, the American College of Surgeons, and the American Academy of Pediatrics.[66] Investigators who submitted abstracts for presentations at conventions for the American Federation of Clinical Research learned that they were now required to sign statements that their work had been conducted in accordance with the Helsinki Declaration. Authors who submitted articles to medical and scientific journals were similarly required to sign statements before publication.[67]

The Declaration of Helsinki has been hailed as one of the most successful efforts to redeem medical research from the shadow of the atrocities committed in the name of biomedical research in Nazi Germany. Struggling to reconcile protections for the human subjects of biomedical research with the needs and constraints of the emerging clinical sciences, physicians representing many nations found the process protracted and difficult. But the long and winding road to the Helsinki Declaration also suggests that the Declaration, like the Nuremberg Code that preceded it, reflected a strong American slant. In light of the professional commitments of American physicians and political and fiscal realities in the early years of the WMA, America was first among equals on the world stage and in world medicine.

65   Rothman (1991).
66   Human Experimentation (1966).
67   Levine (1996), pp. 242-243.

References

Annas, G. J. (1991): Mengele's Birthmark: The Nuremberg Code in United States Courts, Journal of Contemporary Health Law and Policy 7 (1991), pp. 17-45.

Annas, G. J./Grodin, M. (1992): The Nazi Doctors and the Nuremberg Code. Oxford: Oxford University Press.

Bartrip, P. W. J. (1990): Mirror of Medicine: A History of the British Medical Journal. Oxford: Oxford University Press.

Burrow, J. G. (1963): AMA: Voice of American Medicine. Baltimore: Johns Hopkins University Press.

Campion, F. D. (1984): The AMA and U.S. Health Policy Since 1940. Chicago: Chicago Review Press.

Carmi, A. (ed.) (1978): Medical Experimentation. Israel: Turtledove Publishing.

Clegg, H. (1960). Human Experimentation, World Medical Journal 7 (1960), pp. 77-79.

Cunningham, A./Andrews, B. (eds.) (1997): Western Medicine as Contested Knowledge. Manchester: Manchester University Press.

Davidovitch, N. (2004): From a "Humble Humbug" to the "Powerful Placebo". The Image of the Placebo in the Orthodox-Alternative Medicine Debate, in: Roelcke/Maio (2004), pp. 293-307.

Faden, R./Beauchamp, T. (1986): A History and Theory of Informed Consent. New York: Oxford University Press.

Fishbein, M. (1969): Morris Fishbein, M.D.: An Autobiography. New York: Doubleday & Co.

Frenkel, D. (1978.): Human Experimentation: Codes of Ethics, in: Carmi (1978), pp. 127-137.

Grodin, M. A. (1992): Historical Origins of the Nuremberg Code, in: Annas/Grodin (1992), pp. 121-144.

Harkness, J. (1996): Research Behind Bars: A History of Nontherapeutic Research on American Prisoners. Ph.D. dissertation, University of Wisconsin, Madison.

Howard-Jones, H. (1981): The World Health Organization in Historical Perspective, Perspectives in Biology and Medicine 24 (1981), pp. 467-482.

Howard-Jones, H. (1982): Human Experimentation in Historical and Ethical Perspectives, Social Science and Medicine 16 (1982), pp. 1429-1448.

Kaptchuk, T. J. (1998): Powerful Placebo: The Dark Side of the Randomised Controlled Trial, Lancet 351 (1998), pp. 1722-1725.

Knight, V. (1964): The Use of Volunteers in Medical Virology, Progress in Medical Virology 6 (1964), pp. 1-24.

Lee, S. (1997): WHO and the Developing World: The Contest for Ideology, in: Cunningham/Andrews (1997), pp. 24-45.

Levine, R. J. (1996): International Codes and Guidelines for Research Ethics: A Critical Appraisal, in: Vanderpool (1996), pp. 236-259.

McNeill, P.(1993): The Ethics and Politics of Human Experimentation. Cambridge: Cambridge University Press.

Perley, S./Fluss, S./Bankowski, Z./Simon, F. (1992). The Nuremberg Code: An International Overview, in: Annas/Grodin (1992), pp. 149-173).

Pridham, J. A. (1951): Founding of the World Medical Association, World Medical Associaiton Bulletin 3 (1951), pp. 207-209.

Richards, T. (1994): The World Medical Association: Can Hope Triumph Over Experience? British Medical Journal 308 (1994), pp. 262-266.

Roelcke, V./Maio, G. (eds.) (2004): Twentieth Century Ethics of Human Subject Research. Stuttgart: Steiner.

Rothman, D. J. (1991): Strangers at the Bedside. New York: Basic Books.

Routley, T. C. (1949): Aims and Objects of the World Medical Association, WMA Bulletin 1 (1949), p. 18.

Schmidt, U. (2004): Justice at Nuremberg. Leo Alexander and the Nazi Doctors' Trial. Basingstoke: Palgrave.

Seidelman, W. (1996): Nuremberg Lamentation: For the Forgotten Victims of Medical Science, British Medical Journal 313 (1996), pp. 1463-1466.

Smith, A./Benford, R. J. (eds.) (1963): Birth of A Drug: Research and Development in the Pharmaceutical Industry. Washington, D.C.: Pharmaceutical Manufacturers Association.

Smith, J. (1990): Patenting the Sun: Polio and the Salk Vaccine. New York: Anchor Books.

Sohl, P./Bassford, H.A. (1986): Codes of Medical Ethics: Traditional Foundations and Contemporary Practice, Social Science and Medicine 22 (1986), pp. 1175-1179.

Ummel, M. (1991): Genève, le temps d'un serment, Gesnerus 49 (1991), pp. 517-525.

Vanderpool, H. (ed.) (1996): The Ethics of Research Involving Human Subjects: Facing the 21st Century. Frederick, Maryland: University Publishing Group.

Weijer, C./Anderson, J. A. (2001): The Ethics Wars: Disputes over International Research, Hastings Center Report 31 (2001), pp. 18-20.

Weindling, P. (2001): The Origins of Informed Consent: The International Scientific Commission on Medical War Crimes, and the Nuremberg Code, Bulletin of the History of Medicine 75 (2001), pp. 37-71.

White, L. W. (1996): The Nazi Doctors and the Medical Community; Honor or Censure? The Case of Hans Sewering, Journal of Medical Humanities 17 (1996), pp. 119-135.

Winton, R. (1976): The Significance of the Declaration of Helsinki: An Interpretative Commentary, World Medical Journal 25 (1976), pp. 58-59.

Published Citations with No Authors:

Dedication of the Physician (1949), WMA Bulletin 1 (1949), p.4.

Draft Code of Ethics of Human Experimentation (1962), British Medical Journal 2 (1962), p. 1119.

Ethics of Human Experimentation (1964), British Medical Journal 2 (1964), pp. 135-136.

Experimental Medicine (1962), British Medical Journal 2 (1962), p. 1108.

Human Experimentation. Code of Ethics of the World Medical Association (1964), British Medical Journal 2 (1964), pp. 177-183.

Human Experimentation: Declaration of Helsinki (1966), Annals of Internal Medicine 65 (1966), pp. 367-368.

Human Experimentation in Medicine (1952). Foreign Letters - Paris, J.A.M.A. 150 (1952), pp. 426-427.

Life Members of the World Medical Association, United States Committee, Inc. (1951), WMA Bulletin 3 (1951), pp. 256-258.

Special Reports: Aspects of Human Experimentation (1960), World Medical Journal 7 (1960), pp. 84-86

Victims of So-Called Experimentation Under Nazi Regime (1951), WMA Bulletin 3 (1951), pp. 241-242.

War Crimes and Medicine (1949), WMA Bulletin 1 (1949), p. 4.

Without Prejudice (1963), British Medical Journal 1 (1963), p. 1603.

World Medical Association General Assembly in London (1949), British Medical Journal 2 (1949), p. 175.

XVIII World Medical Assembly (1964), World Medical Journal 11 (1964), p. 284.

Manuscript Citations from WMA Archives, Geneva, Switzerland

Experiments on Human Beings by L. A. Hulst, 10 April 1953. 38.3/53.

Memorandum from Secretary General to All Member National Medical Associations, 22 May 1951.

Minutes of the 37th Council Session, Montreal Canada, September 1959, 4 February 1960.

Minutes of the 44th Council Session, Chicago, Illinois, 4 March 1962.

Minutes of the 51st Council Session, Helsinki, Finland, 4 January 1965.

Report on Conference in Stuttgart 21-22 January 1950; Dr. Dag Knutson and Dr. Otto Leuch. C.16/50.

Report on the Statement about German Medical War Crimes, by Dr. O. Leuch, 9 September 1949. C. 41B/49.

Report of the Medical Ethics Committee at the 35th Council Session, 25 March to 3 April 1959. 17.1/59.

Report of the Medical Ethics Committee at the XIVth General Assembly, 15-22 September 1960. 17.2/60.

Summary Minutes and Report of the 47th Council Session. 4 March 1963, p. 4.

Supplementary Report of the Medical Ethics Committee, 17.2a/60.

Other Archival Sources

Irons, E. E. (1947). Notes on a Trip of Representatives of the A.M.A. for (1) Organization of the World Medical Association (2) An Informal Mission for the Surgeon General U.S. Army to Inquire into Possibilities for Improving Educational Conditions for Medical Officers in Europe. (Typescript, Countway Library, Harvard University.)
World Medical Association, American Medical Association Archives. Typescript, 35 pages.

Acknowledgements: I would like to thank Jon Harkness and Jay Katz for the archival materials relating to the World Medical Association. I am grateful to Volker Roelcke, Giovanni Maio and the editors for their thoughtful suggestions. Robert Levine generously gave comments on the paper.

Povl Riis

Forty Years of the Declaration of Helsinki: Progress in Medical Ethics?

I. Introduction

As one of the three authors[1] of the second Declaration of Helsinki, the Tokyo version, adopted in 1975, I am able to contribute to the history of the Declaration and its implications in the decades after 1976.[2] Medical ethics as well as research ethics have undergone similar developments and are part of a wider history of medicine, yet it was a history which was shaped in large parts by individual medical experts or influenced through national initiatives; the Declaration of Helsinki, on the other hand, has a global history which needs to be contextualised within the international, political and professional developments after the Second World War.

II. The Randomised Controlled Trial Paradigm
and the Need for a Medical Ethics Code

The history of post-war medical ethics codes, especially those concerned with research ethics, was greatly influenced by war crimes and crimes against humanity which German researchers had conducted on concentration camp inmates and other vulnerable populations during the Second World War. Those writing the first version of the Helsinki Declaration in 1964 were determined to condemn medical atrocities and ensure that medical scientists would "never again" conduct criminal experiments on man, not only prisoner populations in totalitarian regimes but also on patient-subjects in modern democratic societies.

One of the factors why the first version of the Helsinki Declaration did not appeal to modern medical research was the fact that controlled clinical trials only gradually became the dominating paradigm after Sir Arthur Bradford Hill's trial from 1948 into the effect of streptomycin in treating pulmonary tuberculosis.[3] By then, Johannes Fibiger's controlled trial from 1897-1898 on serum therapy of

---

1   The other two authors were Erik Enger, Norway, and Clarence Blomquist, Sweden.
2   World Medical Association (1976).
3   Medical Research Council (1948), pp. 597-609.

diphtheria had long been forgotten, given that the First World War had cast a shadow over research which had been performed in Europe in the years before 1914.[4]

The paradigm of the controlled clinical trial (also called randomised controlled trial, RCT) only gradually influenced international medical research, mainly
because of the human suffering which had engulfed the post-war world and the
necessary reconstruction of Europe which went along with it. In the late 1960s,
however, Europe regained its intellectual potential with a new generation of
medical scientists, who adopted the RCT as the gold standard in clinical research.
This development created a need for patients and healthy volunteers willing to
participate in clinical trials, and consequently tested the extent to which the first
Declaration of Helsinki controlled the ethics of this new paradigm. As a result, the
World Medical Association (WMA) appealed to the Nordic Medical Associations
which commissioned the above-mentioned three authors to revise the 1964-
version. Our task was to revise the Declaration in line with our own experience in
applying ethics standards in practice and in our training courses for young
researchers.

III. The Origins of the Declaration of Helsinki

Given that German doctors had been directly involved in medical atrocities during
the Second World War, the WMA took the lead in establishing an international
medical ethics code[5] rather than biomedical and scientific societies or academies.
The most obvious reason for the WMA's initiative was the lack of a strong
international network for medical research in general. With the arrival of RCT-
methodology, which was primarily related to the testing of drugs, the first
version(s) of the Helsinki Declaration closely reflected a clinical pharmacological
paradigm. Those drafting the first version of the Helsinki Declaration did not
anticipate that the Declaration might also have to be applied in the area of testing
diagnostics, preventive measures, surgery, and many other fields in the future.[6]

Given the experience of the Second World War *individual ethics*, i.e. the protection of, and respect for, the individual trial participant, became the central aim
of ethics codes (and still is). Yet the role of *collective ethics* neither played a part
in the Declaration of Helsinki nor in the discussions and educational initiatives
which accompanied its formulation. Although the autonomy of the research
subject has to be respected at all times, it is important to recognise the need for
clinical research in our global society in which patient groups and citizens depend
to a large extent on clinical research as a public good.

4   Fibiger (1898), pp. 309-325 and pp. 337-350.
5   World Medical Association (1964).
6   Riis (2003), pp. 15-25.

IV.   Scientific Quality as a Reason for Ethical Analysis

The ethics of clinical research is closely connected with the quality of the methodology which is applied in a research project or trial. If the methods which have been chosen or the overall methodology (= the architecture of the research protocol) are flawed or invalid, then even risk-free studies which involve human participants are judged to be unethical because the time spent by the participants is unlikely to lead to useful results. Given the interaction between medical ethics and the quality of research methodology, clinical researchers should be trained in both research ethics *and*, at the same time, in scientific methodology, including logics, statistics, diagnostic taxonomy and definitions, as well as sources of bias.

V. Establishing a Control System

The Tokyo version of the Helsinki Declaration from 1976 stressed the necessity of an ethical control system based on independent committees, whose assessment would be an integral part of the planning phase in research studies. However, at the time it seemed not possible, or perhaps not desirable by the WMA, to tackle some of the central issues and organisational questions of "ethics committees":

- Should "ethics committees" deal with the originality of the idea, methodo-lo-gical quality and ethical acceptability?
- Should "ethics committees" be established within an institutional context in order to be in the place where research is carried out (but where they also might loose some of their independence and impartiality) or should they be regionally based or centralised by national agencies in order to ensure independence (which involved the risk that they would remain at an administrative distance to research)?
- Should the membership of "ethics committees" include lay people and in what proportion?
- Can lay members of "ethics committees" serve as representatives of ethics standards in society in the same way as, for example, ethicists and theologians?

VI. Progress in Medical Ethics?

Compared to the situation some forty years ago, the role and quality of medical ethics in clinical research has undoubtedly improved. For countries which have a national research ethics control system, whether legally-based or official in other ways, *individual ethics* is now an accepted requirement for clinical scientists. Safety and the respect for informed consent are now established principles of biomedical research involving human subjects, not only in science-driven societies, but also as a part of the general knowledge of an existing ethical control system in society. People today understand that patient-oriented research is not just a way by which ambitious scientists improve their career options, but also a central element to improve diagnostics, treatments and preventive measures.

Given that science is by nature not static but dynamic, new ethical problems and dilemmas appear quite frequently. The same is true for a large number of biomedical scientists who join the research community. Although medical ethics standards and research practice may have improved in most places, there are no grounds for complacency. On the contrary, it is necessary to closely monitor the increasingly global biomedical research community, and, if necessary, continuously revise the existing international and national ethics codes.

VII. New Challenges for Ethics Codes and Control Systems

During the last forty years the international research community has had to face up to many new ethical challenges and ethical dilemmas. Whereas many of the problems have been resolved in a satisfactory fashion, others are still open to debate. In the following, I will briefly survey the areas in which ethical challenges have occurred and will occur in the future:

New research methods and fields have broadened the scope of the original approach of the first Declarations of Helsinki from 1964 which was oriented towards the individual.

Genetics has influenced both individual ethics and collective ethics through the establishment of new diagnostics, forensic methods and perspectives which take occupational issues into consideration. Research on stem cells has been, and still poses, a great challenge to research ethics, not only in relation to general research projects but also with regard to stem cells as agents to combat diseases. The ethics of research on family pedigrees cannot be carried out and assessed from the perspective of a single person, given that often the consent of three generations of family members is needed for this kind of genetic research.[7] Another aspect of genetic research which poses ethical problems relates to new methods of procreation which preserve the anonymity of sperm donors or which concern preimplantation diagnostics and "tailor-made babies" as potential donors for sick siblings.

Today's *Biobanks*, which were established as potential sources for research data or to provide information on clinical files, also create a number of ethical problems. These range, for example, from issues of ownership to informed consent and authorised access without time-limit.[8]

Epidemiology has obtained an increasing application and importance in modern research, for instance in relation to the influence of life-style on health and disease, or with regard to new genetic techniques. It can be a difficult undertaking for nation-wide or even multi-nation-wide projects to obtain informed

7   UNESCO (2000).
8   Riis et al. (1987).

consent from all participants involved, which can create subsequent ethical problems.

The *globalisation* of research, especially collaborative research projects between developing and developed countries, creates new ethical problems which relate to potential exploitation, consent in illiterate populations, inequality of genders, and capacity building.[9]

Throughout the last decades the *ethics of researchers* had been the focus of attention. Issues which cause concern often relate to false information which researchers provide to participants as part of the consenting procedure, as well as to the subsequent invalid research findings which represent another deception of the participant and his or her good will. Yet the prevention and exposure of scientific dishonesty is not an appropriate field of activity of research ethics committees, but its existence, forms and interactions must be known by committee members and scientists.

Finally, the change in terminology from *medical science* to *health science* reflects the large number of health professionals who have joined the biomedical research community during the latest decades: nurses, physiotherapists, ergotherapists, midwives, biochemists, psychologists, engineers, health economists, pharmacists and many more. Clinical methodology and research ethics in all of these professions ought to be identical with research conducted by medical scientists and controlled by the same ethics codes and supervisory control systems.

VIII. The Abundance of Research Ethics Codes

The large number of existing ethics codes creates problems of priority and hierarchy. Researchers often face great difficulties in identifying and selecting the appropriate ethics codes for their research projects, given that the codes are not concordant and do not have the same importance within a national and international context.[10]

In Europe, for example, researchers have to prioritise their national laws and regulations over the Directives of the European Union in the relevant member state.[11] This is followed by the conventions and explanatory reports of the Council of Europe, especially for those member states which have signed and ratified the conventions.[12] Finally, there are many advisory codes and regulations, published,

---

9   Nuffield Council on Bioethics (2002).
10   Council of Europe (1997a); Council of Europe (1997b); World Health Organisation (1999); World Medical Association (2000); European Union (2001); Council of Europe/Steering Committee on Bioethics (CDBI) (2002); World Health Organization (2002); Council of Europe/Working Party on Biomedical Research (CDBI-CO-GT2) (2003).
11   European Union (2001).
12   Council of Europe (1997a); Council of Europe (1997b); Council of Europe/Steering Committee on Bioethics (CDBI) (2002); Council of Europe/Working Party on Biomedical Research (CDBI-CO-GT2) (2003).

for example, by the WMA (The Fifth Helsinki Declaration),[13] the UNESCO,[14] the World Health Organisation (WHO)[15] and the Nuffield Foundation.[16]

In today's world, Europe has an important and even global influence on research practices through the ethics codes of the Council of Europe and European Union, because these codes are not written by professional organisations but are formulated in close cooperation with independent health scientists and researchers. Europe has thus a strong obligation to preserve and further develop its influence on global research ethics and control measures in the future.

13   World Medical Association (2000).
14   UNESCO (2000).
15   World Health Organization (2002).
16   Nuffield Council on Bioethics (2002).

References

Council of Europe (1997a): Convention for the Protection of Human Rights and Dignity of the Human Being with regard to the Application of Biology and Medicine: Convention on Human Rights and Biomedicine. Oviedo, Spain.

Council of Europe (1997b): Explanatory Report to the Convention on Human Rights and Biomedicine, Strasbourg.

Council of Europe/Steering Committee on Bioethics (CDBI) (2002): Draft Additional Protocol to the Convention on Human Rights and Biomedicine, on Biomedical Research, Strasbourg.

Council of Europe/Working Party on Biomedical Research (CDBI-CO-GT2) (2003): Draft Explanatory Report to the Draft Additional Protocol to the Convention on Human Rights and Biomedicine, on Biomedical Research, Strasbourg.

European Union (2001): Directive 2001/20/EC of the European Parliament and of the Council of 4. April 2001 on the Approximation of the Laws, Regulations and Administrative Provisions of the Member States, Relating to the Implementation of Good Clinical Practice in the Conduct of Clinical Trials on Medical Products for Human Use, Luxembourg.

Fibiger, J (1898): Om Serumbehandling af Difteri, Hospitalstid 6 (1898), pp. 309-325 and pp. 337-350.

Medical Research Council (1948): Streptomycin Treatment of Pulmonary Tuberculosis: a Report of the Streptomycin Tuberculosis Trials Committee, British Medical Journal 29 (1948), pp. 597-609.

Nuffield Council on Bioethics (2002): The Ethics of Research Related to Healthcare in Developing Countries. London: The Nuffield Foundation.

Riis, P./Nielsen, L./Strandberg Pedersen, N./Almind, G. (1987): Health Science Information Banks: Biobanks. Copenhagen: Danish Central Scientific Ethical Committee, Danish Council of Ethics, Danish Medical Research Council.

Riis, P. (2003): Thirty Years of Bioethics: The Helsinki Declaration 1964-2003, New Review Bioethics 1 (2003), pp. 15-25.

UNESCO (2000): The Universal Declaration on the Human Genome and Human Rights: From Theory to Practise, Geneva: UNESCO.

World Health Organisation (1999): International Guidelines on Bioethics, Geneva: WHO.

World Health Organization (2002): Council for International Organizations of Medical Sciences. International Guidelines for Biomedical Research involving Human Subjects, Geneva: WHO.

World Medical Association (1964): The Declaration of Helsinki, Helsinki: WMA.

World Medical Association (1976): The Second Declaration of Helsinki. Tokyo: WMA.

World Medical Association (2000): Fifth Declaration of Helsinki, Edinburgh: WMA.

Kati Myllymäki

Revising the Declaration of Helsinki:
An Insider's View

I.   Introduction

In 1953, the World Medical Association (WMA) first discussed the idea of a
position paper on research ethics. In 1961, the first draft of the Declaration of
Helsinki was tabled after several years of constructive discussion. Finally, in June
1964, following further revisions, the Declaration was approved by the general
assembly of the WMA in Helsinki.

The Declaration was drafted by the WMA but it has been adopted by the
larger research community. National and international patient and citizen organisations also refer to it as well as legislative bodies in many countries. The Declaration was formulated in order to complement the Declaration of Geneva (1948), a
form of modernised Hippocratic Oath, as well as the International Code of
Medical Ethics (1949). The decision to establish the WMA after the Second
World War and issue these documents happened in response to medical atrocities
which German scientists had conducted in Nazi concentration camps.

The Declaration of Helsinki has been revised five times. It is a "living document" which is continuously revised in order to take account of the changing
research culture and new biomedical technologies. Throughout the last forty years
medical research has undergone enormous changes; new technologies and fields
of scientific enquiry pose new and difficult challenges for the protection of
individuals, not only with regard to their physical and mental well-being but also
in relation to the protection of personal data in patient records, including genetic
information. Medical research is not only about randomised double-blind controlled pharmaceutical trials. Research is also about personal data, epidemiology,
human tissue material, embryos, surgery, and prophylactic measures like vaccinations and rehabilitation.

The major revision of the Declaration of Helsinki in 2000 in Edinburgh was
accompanied by a lengthy discussion process by several WMA working groups
and expert hearings. In addition, those tasked with the revision of the Declaration
also received comments from the various national medical associations. The final
working group was one of the so-called "three wise women" or "the three
witches", as we called ourselves: Nancy Dickey (the former president of the
American Medical Association), Judith Kazimirski (the former president of the
Canadian Medical Association) and myself, Kati Myllymäki, president of the
Finnish Medical Association. The assistant and secretary of our working group

was Delon Human, the General Secretary of the World Medical Association, South Africa. It is noteworthy, perhaps, that all three of us were general practitioners rather than medical scientists and researchers. Although we clearly understood the responsibility we had towards future research, our clinical expertise concentrated our minds on the patients' point of view and his or her protection.

Our working group was set-up in April 1999 during a meeting of the WMA Council in Santiago, Chile, and after a report from a working group led by Robert Levine (Yale, USA) had led to a heated debate. Levine made a forceful case that the Declaration needed to be revised and published his views in *The New England Journal of Medicine*:

> "The Declaration of Helsinki requires revision because it is defective in two important respects. First, it relies on a distinction between the therapeutic and nontherapeutic research; all documents that rely on this spurious distinction contain errors not intended by their authors. Second, it includes several provisions that are seriously out of touch with contemporary ethical thinking. As a consequence, many researchers routinely violate its requirements. Such routine violations and their associated attitudes rob the Declaration of its credibility". [1]

Levine singled out two specific issues which apparently were "out of touch" with contemporary research practice and therefore needed to be addressed. According to the Declaration, "placebo controls" were not permitted if there existed a "standard" therapy in the field. The other issue related to the fact that "every patient is entitled to receive the 'best proven therapy' which is available in industrialised nations even though such therapy is not available in the country in which the patient resides". [2]

Levine's report to the WMA Medical Ethics Committee caused a substantial amount of confusion among delegates, perhaps because of the way in which he had criticised the Declaration or perhaps because some delegates felt that he represented wider pharmaceutical and US financial interests. Levine's report had been thorough and had identified important issues in the Declaration which had raised concern among scientists, but the response to his presentation can only be described as "emotional". Some delegates responded particularly strongly, perhaps because they felt that his presentation had been aggressive and impolite towards the international community of medical associations. Given that the Declaration of Helsinki is seen as the corner stone of medical research ethics in the world, it was disconcerting to hear that somebody called it "meaningless" and "out of date". Some delegations even believed that Levine's report was little more than the voice of the multinational pharmaceutical industry and some thought that his views, and those of his followers, would open a Pandora's box by introducing double standards to research and research exploitation in the developing world.

1   Levine (1999); see also Briefing Notes from Professor Robert J. Levine to the Working Group on the the Revison of the Declaration of Helsinki and to the WMA Medical Ethics Committee meeting on 14 October 1998.
2   Briefing Notes from Professor Robert J. Levine to the Working Group on the Revison of the Declaration of Helsinki and to the WMA Medical Ethics Committee meeting on 14 October 1998.

As a result of the debate about Levine's report, the Council decided to proceed with a new working group in conjunction with the consultation of all national medical associations and other interested parties. During the lunch break delegates from the national medical associations were discussing ways of how to move forward. Disappointment and tensions were clearly noticeable. There had been a strong response to Levine's report and various delegations expressed their will to take part in the next phase. It became clear, however, that too many countries wanted to participate in the redrafting of the Declaration; a multi-national and multi-lingual working group would not only have been unwieldy and probably inefficient, but also expensive and impractical.

During our lunch break with Enrique Accorsi from Chile, Markku Äärimaa from Finland and Delon Human we discussed various possibilities on how to break the deadlock. I eventually made a joke, saying that if men are unable to produce an acceptable document maybe women could succeed in the job. To my surprise the gentlemen took up my suggestion and stated that if we had a female working group – given that only few women were present at the meeting – it would only have one working language and male colleagues would not insist on their participation. This solved the problem of a working group which would not be too large and unwieldy, given that all the major delegations would otherwise have wanted their own representative in the group. I was even more surprised when the Council of the WMA accepted the proposal for this working group. I do not remember who first coined the term "three wise women". It may well have been our General Secretary, Delon Human, but from the beginning we referred to ourselves as the "three witches".

Although the draft proposals of Levine's group were not adopted, his group had identified important issues which needed to be resolved; their notes were also very useful for our working group and for the subsequent public discussion.[3] Looking back at events at the time, I would say that our group carefully studied Levine's briefing notes and tried to work through all the problematic areas, including the role of the research subject, informed consent, financial concerns and publication issues. This paper is primarily based on my personal notes and recollections as well as on records of WMA meetings.

II.   The Process of Revising the Declaration of Helsinki

During the process of revising the Declaration it became clear that any changes to this document would be difficult. At times, emotions were running high. Several individuals and organisations argued that any changes to the Declaration would not only undermine the meaning of the document, but its heritage. Linguistic and cultural differences did not make the revision process any easier. Sometimes certain concepts, even when translated correctly, do have a slightly different con-notation and meaning in different parts of the world. Moreover, English, Spanish

---

3   WMA Medical Ethics Committee meeting, Levine briefing notes, 14 October 1998.

and French words seemed to have different meanings among native speakers, depending on the country and culture they came from. In some cases certain phrases apparently could not be changed because the phrase had been used in national legislations; even general concepts like national or federal, country or state raised problems of interpretation and led to sometimes passionate exchanges. Others, like Levine and his group, criticised the Declaration for being "out of touch with contemporary ethical thinking".[4]

The process of revising the Declaration was designed to be as transparent as possible. All the member associations of the WMA had the possibility of discussing ideas and suggestions on a national level in their own ethics committees, and consult with the research community and patient organisations. Individuals and non-medical organisations were invited to comment on specific web-pages which had been set up by the WMA. Representatives of the WMA also attended several international meetings to gather feedback from the international medical community. They attended, for example, the meeting of the Council for International Organisation of Medical Sciences (CIOMS), the European Forum for Good Clinical Practice (EFGCP) and the World Congress on Medical Law. Moreover, in 1999, the *Bulletin of Medical Ethics* organised an international workshop about the planned revisions of the Declaration and published the papers.[5] Juhana Idänpään-Heikkilä, General Secretary of CIOMS, provided us with good contacts to the World Health Organisation (WHO) and helped me in editing the language during the revision process. It was also important that CIOMS delayed any publication of the new guidelines until the WMA had finalised the revised Declaration. The CIOMS guidelines state:

> "The Declaration of Helsinki, issued by the World Medical Association in 1964, is the fundamental document in the field of ethics in biomedical research and has influenced the formulation of international, regional and national legislation and codes of conduct. The Declaration, amended several times, most recently in 2000 (Appendix 2), is a comprehensive international statement of the ethics of research involving human subjects. It sets out ethical guidelines for physicians engaged in both clinical and non-clinical biomedical research".[6]

Our working group communicated primarily by e-mail and met twice a year during the official WMA meetings. We also held an additional meeting at Miami Beach in the United States. A memorable day included a trip to the Everglades to see alligators and feed local mosquitoes with our own blood. Another meeting took place in Finland where we worked, for most of the time, at the headquarters of the Finnish Medical Association. I also invited the working group to my home in the countryside, where Nancy Dickey and Judith Kazimirski enjoyed a traditional Finnish sauna. All of these meetings were full of intense discussions and included the reading of comments from national medical associations and other feed-back which we received, including the comments from the WMA web-site. The atmosphere during these discussions was particularly friendly and construc-

4   Levine (1999).
5   Bulletin of Medical Ethics (1999).
6   http:/www.cioms.ch/frame_guidelines_nov_2002.htm.

tive and we shared many good laughs. All three of us had a similar sense of humour and I believe that we all enjoyed working together.

III. The Contentious Issues in the Declaration of Helsinki (1996 version)

By the end of 1990s the research community engaged in a debate about the future role of the Declaration. It became clear that new developments in medical research together with a process of revising one paragraph at a time, and adding explanatory details, had led to a somewhat incoherent document which had lost some of its integrity and responsiveness in protecting subjects as well as possible. From the start we identified the following problems which needed to be resolved:[7]

1. The concept *biomedical* was considered to be unclear and confusing. It also proved difficult to translate the term into other languages or apply it to different cultural contexts. Some felt that the term *biomedical* referred too much to biotechnology or biochemistry. The term *medical*, on the other hand, can be understood to refer only to pharmaceutical issues or to internal medicine, depending, of course, on language and culture. The majority of the national medical associations nonetheless supported the proposal to change the heading from *biomedical* to *medical*.

2. We also engaged in intensive discussions about the prospective *target group* of the Declaration. The document was understood to be used by different health and medical professionals as a general point of reference on research ethics. Whereas the 1996 version mentions the term *physicians* in the subtitle, the new version does not. The new subtitle is more general: "Ethical principles for Medical Research Involving Human Subjects". During the discussions, it became apparent that the WMA has no mandate to issue declarations on behalf of other professions, although it is obviously appreciated that other professional groups and legislative bodies have taken up some of the concepts of the WMA declarations. We discussed the possibility of cooperating with the official organisations of other health professionals, but we had to acknowledge that finding an acceptable compromise for the medical profession alone posed a considerable challenge in itself. Negotiations on a multi-national and multi-professional level would probably have taken years. In the first paragraph of the new Declaration we nonetheless included the following sentence: "guidance to physicians and other participants in medical research involving human subjects".

3. There was also some debate about the formal status of the Declaration. During our discussion it became clear that different people were reading the Declaration of Helsinki in different ways. Whereas some read the Declaration as a legal document which was binding and official, others interpreted it as a general state-

7   Bulletin of Medical Ethics (1999).

ment which could be applied within the specific national and cultural context. To solve this problem we changed the subtitles. Rather than speaking of "recommendations guiding physicians", the new Declaration speaks of "ethical principles". The term *guidance* is then mentioned in paragraph 1 of the Declaration.

4. Another issue which informed our discussion was the extent to which the scope of medical research had broadened over the last decades. Originally, the Declaration referred to medical experimentation involving human subjects. In 1964, human tissue could not be identified by means of gene technology, as it can today, and in vitro fertilisation or human embryo research were things of the future. Research and the ethics of research are therefore not only concerned with the well-being of individuals; this is why we included the issue of identifiable human material or identifiable data to the Declaration. The aim of the revised version of the Declaration is to demand respect and protection (integrity) in research. People need to know what their blood samples, pieces of tissue or egg cells and sperms are used for. For this kind of research the issue of consent is critically important but also quite challenging.

Epidemiological research on databases is another contentious issue, especially with regard to the question of consent; as a result we carried out further work in order to protect patient records and the integrity of individuals. The notorious case of the Icelandic database, which included the plan to link patient records and genetic data into a national database which was run and controlled by a private company, highlighted the problems in this area. We decided that epidemiological research would not be included in the Declaration of Helsinki; instead a separate document, called "The World Medical Association Declaration on Ethical Considerations Regarding Health Databases", was prepared and accepted by the General Assembly of the WMA in Washington in 2002. It was recognised, at the same time, that many countries have national cancer registries. Some of these databases have a legal status and are accepted by the public, which means that physicians are obliged to collect patient data and patients do not have the opportunity or the right to opt out. The importance and usefulness of these kinds of registries is widely accepted. Compared to the Declaration of Helsinki, the issue of consent is phrased somewhat differently. Paragraph 18 of the WMA Declaration on Databases states:

> "Under certain conditions, personal health information may be included on a database without consent, for example where this conforms with applicable national law that conforms to the requirements of this statement, or where ethical approval has been given by a specifically appointed ethical review committee. In these exceptional cases, patients should be informed about the potential uses of their information, even if they have no right to object".[8]

The issue of databases compiled in connection with epidemiological works was seen as sufficiently important to warrant a separate declaration, mainly because the risks for the patient are quite different compared to research on human

8   WMA (2002)

subjects. It was also believed to be important to ensure the consistency of the Declaration of Helsinki in which patients must be able to opt out and withdraw from the research if he or she so wishes. The above mentioned example of a national, legally binding cancer register generally does not allow individuals to opt out.

5. Another important aspect of the Declaration was the distinction between clinical and non-clinical research. The earlier versions of the Declaration were divided into three parts: basic principles, clinical and non-clinical research. The Declaration included the principle that extra precaution is necessary whenever research is conducted on healthy volunteers and all risks must be evaluated carefully because there is no benefit for the subject. On the other hand, extra precaution is needed when the subjects are patients, because of their vulnerable position. In other words, both groups need specific protection. Moreover, medical research has developed to such an extent that basic research (e.g. pathogenesis of a disease, which is not therapeutic research) is also performed on patients. Cases in point are basic research on diabetes mellitus, the taking of blood samples and/or research which explores the family history and living habits of diabetic patients. In this kind of basic research (which is not a therapeutic, diagnostic or prophylactic trial or intervention) one group is generally made up of patients who are suffering from the disease under investigation and the other group comprises healthy volunteers for comparison. Paragraph 2 of the 1996 version of the Declaration of Helsinki states: "The subjects should be volunteers – either healthy persons or patients for whom the experimental design is not related to the patient's illness". This formulation was not considered to be in line with contemporary research practice. Levine, for example, argued that the paragraph ruled out "all rational research on the causes of diseases or on the pathogenesis or pathophysiology".[9] That is why the structure of the Declaration was changed to take account of general principles which applied to all research, on the one hand, and specific principles which are related to the protection of patients, on the other: Basic principles for all medical research and additional principles for medical research combined with medical care.

6. The issue of prophylaxis was also high on the agenda. In recent years some of the major concerns in medical research ethics have been research programmes involving vaccination and other prophylactic measures. The issue of prophylaxis had already been mentioned in the 1975 Tokyo version of the Declaration, but we wanted to emphasise this point throughout the document. That is why the list "prophylactic, diagnostic and therapeutic" is repeated in several paragraphs. This also underlines the fact that medical research nowadays is a much broader field than only Randomised Controlled Trials (RCTs) or pharmaceutical experimentations.

9   Levine (1999), p. 531.

7. Another aspect of research concerned financial transparency. The Finnish Medical Association was especially active in raising financial issues. The fact that tobacco companies were funding and selecting research projects had raised major concerns around the world. For a patient, a nurse, a physician or a hospital it is important to know who funds a particular research project. The same applies to the editors and readers of medical journals. If research is funded by a tobacco or pharmaceutical company, by a national institute of health, university or public or private hospital or patient organisation, issues of impartiality and conflicts of interest may arise. That is why paragraph 13 states:

> "The researcher should also submit to the (ethical review) committee, for review, information regarding funding, sponsors, institutional affiliations, other potential conflicts of interest and incentives for subjects".[10]

8. The issue of the informed consent is and remains at the heart of the Declaration of Helsinki. One of the most profound violations of medical ethics standards was the fact that Nazi medical scientists had performed human experiments without the subjects' consent. We hoped to improve and better define the issue of consent as part of the revision process. International discussions on paediatric drugs have been important in this respect. It is recognised today that children are suffering because research is generally conducted on adults and the results are not easily applicable to minors. At the same time it is difficult to find the right balance between helping children, on the one hand, and protecting them as research subjects, on the other. The discussion about paediatric clinical trials continues both within the European Union and among the members of the United States Institute of Medicine (IOM).[11] Children today need more protection in clinical trials, certainly not less, but children also need evidence-based medical care. The issue of consent was also discussed in relation to different cultural contexts. In certain Moslem-dominated countries, for example, women are unable to give legally valid consent and it is the husband or father of the woman who consents on her behalf.

9. The role of the environment and of animals also had to be taken into consideration in revising the Declaration. Although the aim of medical research is to help and alleviate the suffering of human beings it is important not to overlook environmental aspects and animal protection. A new statement was therefore added to the Declaration: "Appropriate caution must be exercised in the conduct of research, which may affect the environment, and the welfare of animals used for the research must be respected".[12]

10. Another important aspect of the Declaration related to the publishing of research findings and the handling of negative results. For example, we discussed cases where published data was biased. Medical journals tend to publish positive

10   WMA Declaration of Helsinki (2000).
11   Ault (2004).
12   WMA Declaration of Helsinki (2000).

results instead of negative findings or so called "0-results". There have also been cases where a pharmaceutical company has prohibited a researcher from publishing his or her research findings because they might have a negative effect on the business. As a result, patients do not necessarily receive the best possible form of therapy. At the same time, new groups of people are exposed to unnecessary risk because the information of any experiments which failed or where the data was negative is not publicly available. That is why it is central to have the highest degree of transparency and be able to track ongoing research through an international register of research projects.

During the discussions it was noted that editors of medical journals have their own ethics rules as far as publishing is concerned. It was also noted that neither the WMA nor anyone else can or should interfere with the responsibilities of an editor or publisher to decide whether research data will be published or not. Instead, Internet and publicly available databases should be used to share information of clinical trials which have taken place. The large number of "abandoned molecules" is remarkable and it is important that humans are not unnecessarily exposed to repetitive experiments and risks to their health when the results are already known. As a counter-argument, some have suggested that the worldwide sharing of research data could jeopardise commercial interests and slow down the development of new drugs. The flip side of this argument, however, is that many national and federal drug administrations are in control of enormous databases which contain detailed information of clinical trials. In most cases the information is not open to the public and in the public domain, a situation which clearly needs to be addressed in the future.

It is a great piece of news that the WHO has signed up to an initiative which aims to keep the international community informed of clinical trials. The WHO plans to make information about RCT's available on the Internet free of charge. The International Standard Randomised Controlled Trial Number (ISRCTN) register is a good instrument to protect people for being unnecessarily exposed to repetitive trials and to help the scientific community to track and keep up to date with current research developments.[13] Paragraph 27 of the revised Declaration took account of these issues:

> "Both authors and publishers have ethical obligations. In publication of the results of research, the investigators are obliged to preserve the accuracy of the results. Negative as well as positive results should be published or otherwise publicly available. Sources of funding, institutional affiliations and any possible conflicts of interest should be declared in the publication. Reports of experimentation not in accordance with the principles laid down in this Declaration should not be accepted for publication".[14]

11. Obviously, we also had to address the role of placebos. The issue was one of the most contentious during the revision process. The 1996 version of the Declaration stated:

---

13   Zarocostas (2004).
14   WMA Declaration of Helsinki (2000).

"In any medical study, every patient – including those of the control group, if any – should be assured of the best proven diagnostic and therapeutic method. This does not exclude the use of inert placebo in studies where no proven diagnostic or therapeutic method exists".[15]

This wording was considered to conflict with the ethics of medical publishers, given that most medical journals and institutions were demanding placebo-controlled trials as a necessity and the golden standard of research. Trials without a control group were considered to be of a low quality and left unpublished.

The debate revolved around the conflict between the scientific quality of the research, on the one hand, and the protection of human subjects in clinical trials, on the other. Some argued that the formulation in the 1996 version of the Declaration was not realistic and, as a result, made the document irrelevant. Representatives of the pharmaceutical industry and the Federal Drug Administration in the United States were particularly forthcoming in making this argument. Others argued that a wording which allowed for greater discretion would open up a "Pandora's box" and undermine the aim to protect human subjects in the future. We also discussed at length the concept of "best proven method". Given that science is a dynamic process which is never complete or perfect or final, we needed to recognise that "best proven methods" change with time and with the discovery of new research data; they also depend on the health care system, culture and population in which medical care is provided.

Some of us drew attention to the problems which developing countries are facing in this respect. There is a risk that some scientists might find it easier to carry out their research with placebos in poor countries or on disadvantaged populations; in those cases local and national research ethics committees would not be powerful or competent enough to demand proper care for control groups, for example in AIDS research in sub-Saharan Africa. Dirceu Greco from Brazil was one of the strong advocates in defending poor populations against the extensive use of placebos with existing therapy, and he used Brazilian AIDS research as an example. Some African colleagues also argued that the Declaration of Helsinki is the only valid protection which exists for poor population against the exploitation by multi-national companies.

Although a compromise was found during the negotiations in Edinburgh in 2000, I was convinced that the issue with regard to placebos (paragraph 29) and post-trial-care (paragraph 30) were matters which would be soon back on the agenda. The new wording in the Declaration did not resolve the placebo issue. However, given that the revision process had already taken up an extensive amount of time it was agreed to approve the major structural change of the Declaration in 2000, and continue the work with that document for the time being. At the back of our minds was also the danger that the whole revision process, which at times had been arduous and difficult, might be undermined or terminated. The wording in paragraph 29 of the revised Declaration therefore reads as follows:

"The benefits, risks, burdens and effectiveness of a new method should be tested against those of the best current prophylactic, diagnostic and therapeutic methods. This does not

15   WMA Declaration of Helsinki (1996).

exclude the use of placebo, or no treatment, in studies where no proven prophylactic, diagnostic or therapeutic method exists".[16]

As I had foreseen, the discussion on placebos continued and new working groups tried to find a consensus. The issue of placebos was addressed with a note of clarification to paragraph 29 in Washington in 2002. It seems that some members of the medical profession and citizen groups think that the current formulation is too weak; equally, there are those who argue that the present wording in the Declaration prevents reasonable science. The note of clarification is as follows:

"The WMA hereby reaffirms its position that extreme care must be taken in making use of a placebo-controlled trial and that in general this methodology should only be used in the absence of existing proven therapy. However, a placebo-controlled trial may be ethically acceptable, even if proven therapy is available, under the following circumstances:

Where for compelling and scientifically sound methodological reasons its use is necessary to determine the efficacy or safety of a prophylactic, diagnostic or therapeutic method; or

Where a prophylactic, diagnostic or therapeutic method is being investigated for a minor condition and the patients who receive placebo will not be subject to any additional risk of serious or irreversible harm

All other provisions of the Declaration of Helsinki must be adhered to, especially the need for appropriate ethical and scientific view".

12. A closely related issue which needed to be addressed concerned post-trial access to health care. During the revision process it became clear that there was a danger that vulnerable or disadvantaged groups could be exploited if special attention was not given and additional safeguards were not provided. Certain interested parties, like, for example, pharmaceutical companies, might find it cheaper to organise a clinical trial in geographical areas which do not possess a proper health care system. The whole issue centres on distributive justice. In order to prevent instances where researchers from outside the community appear in a certain geographical location, run their trial, collect the information and then disappear, we tried to put the design of the study into the context of the community in which the trial takes place. The aim of this was to ensure that a disadvantaged population would benefit from the trial.

The major criticism against the proposal was the argument that it would be unfair to burden researchers with the financial responsibility for failing health care systems. It was also considered to be impractical and impossible to imagine that after a trial the tested drug would be commercially available as a legally registered pharmaceutical product. Others objected that medical practice in a certain country or location was unlikely to change after only one clinical trial. We also discussed the costs of post-trial care and whether this kind of obligation would put universities under financial strain. As a result of these interventions it was decided to give the responsibility to ethical review committees which are in a better position to assess the local circumstances and needs. It was also noted that post-trial access to care does not refer only to the developing countries but also to disadvantaged

16   Declaration of Helsinki (2000), paragraph 29.

groups in developed countries. Paragraph 30 of the revised Declaration therefore reads:

> "At the conclusion of the study, every patient entered into the study should be assured of access to the best proven prophylactic, diagnostic and therapeutic methods identified by the study".[17]

In 2004, the WMA added a note of clarification to Paragraph 30:

> "The WMA hereby reaffirms its position that it is necessary during the study planning process to identify post-trial access by study participants to prophylactic, diagnostic and therapeutic procedures identified as beneficial in the study or access to other appropriate care. Post-trial access arrangements or other care must be described in the study protocol so the ethical review committee may consider such arrangements during its review".

13. Almost all of the above issues relate to the general issue of research exploitation. The process of globalisation has placed the issue of distributive justice centre stage for medical research. The controversy over the use of placebos in trials of zidovudine-treatment in order to halt perinatal transmission of HIV infection in developing countries is a case in point. Researchers argued, however, that the standard of care in the rural areas was such that there was essentially no treatment and that the study enrolees would therefore be receiving care which met with the local standard.[18] This obviously raised the question whether the local standard of care could be judged as sufficient or acceptable?

The lack of collaboration between academia and public health systems in developing countries has created an environment in which inappropriate and unethical research is commissioned and carried out. For developing countries unethical research encompasses scientifically unsound research, duplicate studies and research which does not relate to the health priorities of the population under investigation.[19]

14. Finally, we dealt with the issue of compassionate care. The 1996 version of the Declaration included the following paragraph: "In the treatment of the sick person, the physician must be free to use a new diagnostic and therapeutic measure, if in his or her judgement it offers hope of saving life, re-establishing health or alleviating suffering". We discussed whether compassionate care has anything to do with research at all or whether it is part of general medical ethics. We acknowledged that in some cases compassionate care can produce new ideas for further research and untraditional, creative or even "revolutionary" thinking which can break barriers. We decided therefore that these cases should be published so that the research community can learn from the results. Paragraph 32 reads:

> "In the treatment of a patient, where proven prophylactic, diagnostic and therapeutic methods do not exist or have been ineffective, the physician, with informed consent from the patient, must be free to use unproven or new prophylactic, diagnostic and therapeutic measures, if in

---

17 WMA Declaration of Helsinki (2000).
18 Brennan (1999).
19 Clark/Smith (2003).

the physician's judgement it offers hope of saving life, re-establishing health or alleviating suffering. Where possible, these measures should be made the object of research, designed to evaluate their safety and efficacy. In all cases, new information should be recorded and, where appropriate, published. The other relevant guidelines of this Declaration should be followed".[20]

Most of the suggested revisions in the Declaration were welcome, like, for example, broadening the concept of medical research, clarifying the issue of informed consent, addressing financial transparency and raising the problem that certain information of clinical trials was not published. The process of revising the Declaration of Helsinki was multi-faceted, transparent and truly international. It has been an interesting and rewarding process for those involved; I myself feel that it has been a great honour to be part of the WMA process. The discussions about research ethics will surely continue, given that the Declaration is far from perfect and probably never will be. In today's world and research community, which is highly complex, the Declaration is not meant to be a legal document but a text which expresses the ideals, values and aspirations of the medical profession in protecting human subjects.

At the centre of current and future medical research stand the high ethical principles as expressed in the Declaration, in particularly those standards which aim to ensure the protection of human subjects in experimental research. In 2003, Solomon Benatar expressed this sentiment during the WMA General Assembly when he said: "Scientific progress must be coupled to moral progress, and in particular in relation to social justice. The Helsinki Declaration has the potential to stimulate moral progress in research. Such progress, if made, will be reflected in reductions in health inequity, and in improvements in population health".[21] I could not agree more.

---

20   WMA Declaration of Helsinki (2000).
21   Benatar (2004).

References

Ault, A. (2004): Children Need more Protection in Clinical Trials, says IOM, Lancet 363 (2004), p. 1119.

Benatar, S. (2004): Linking Moral Progress to Medical Progress: New Opportunities for the Declaration of Helsinki, World Medical Journal 50 (2004), pp. 11-13.

Brennan, T. A. (1999): Proposed Revisions to the Declaration of Helsinki – Will they Weaken the Ethical Principles Underlying Human Research? New England Journal of Medicine 341 (1999), pp. 527-530.

Bulletin of Medical Ethics (1999): Revising the Declaration of Helsinki: A Fresh Start, Bulletin of Medical Ethics 150 (1999), pp. 3-44.

Clark, J./Smith, R. (2003): Practising Just Medicine in an Unjust World, British Medical Journal 237 (2003), pp. 1000-1001.

Levine, R. (1999): The Need to Revise the Declaration of Helsinki, New England Journal of Medicine 341 (1999), pp. 531-534.

WMA Declarations of Helsinki (1964), (1974), (1996), (2000).

WMA (2002): The World Medical Association Declaration on Ethical Considerations Regarding Health Databases, adopted by the WMA General Assembly, Washington D.C. 2002 (see http://www.wma.net/e/policy/d1.htm)

Zarocostas, J. (2004): WHO Boosts Internet Access to Clinical Trials, Lancet 363 (2004), p. 1206.

Websites

http://www.wma.org
http://www.controlled-trials.com
http://www.cioms.ch/frame_guidelines_nov_2002.htm

Acknowledgements: I would like to thank my colleagues Judy Kazimirski and Nancy Dickey for a wonderful time during the process of revising the Declaration of Helsinki. I also would like to thank Delon Human for all his help and expertise and, of course, all the colleagues around the world for their trust and support.

Robert Carlson, Kenneth Boyd, David Webb

The Interpretation of Codes of Medical Ethics:
Some Lessons from the Fifth Revision of the Declaration of Helsinki

I.   Introduction

In this chapter we seek to summarise how the text of the Declaration of Helsinki (DoH) came into its current form. We will briefly describe the changes with the first four revisions from the original 1964 version and then consider in more detail the discussions leading up to the fifth and current revision of the Declaration of Helsinki. This revision has given rise to considerable controversy and we will focus on what are the three most controversial paragraphs (paragraphs 19, 29 and 30) in the current version. We make use of archival material made available by the World Medical Association (WMA) to trace in detail how these particular paragraphs evolved. By undertaking this analysis, we have the twofold aim of exploring in further detail the apparent ethical intentions behind these paragraphs and to consider what lessons this process may provide when the DoH, at some point in the future, is further revised.

II.   The Evolution of Previous Versions of the Declaration of Helsinki

We have published elsewhere a detailed analysis of how the text of the DoH changed with each of the revisions and only a brief outline is provided here.[1]

II.1. The Original (1964) Declaration of Helsinki

In September 1964, the WMA officially published in its quarterly journal, the World Medical Journal, the text of the original DoH.[2] As with all Declarations of the WMA, the DoH was published in the three official languages of the organisation: English, French and Spanish. Although not officially published until September, the contents of the DoH were already widely available. For example, the British Medical Journal (BMJ), on 18 July 1964 contained the following very brief statement:

---

1   Carlson et al. (2004), pp. 695-713.
2   World Medical Association (1964).

"A draft code of ethics on human experimentation was published in the British Medical
Journal (BMJ) of 27 October 1962. [...] A revised version was accepted as the final draft at
the meeting of the World Medical Association in Helsinki in June 1964. [...] It is to be
known as the Declaration of Helsinki".[3]

This modest "birth announcement" in the BMJ belied just how important this
document would become over the ensuing four decades.

Sev Fluss has undertaken a detailed comparison of the DoH with the Nuremberg Code of 1947 and notes the extensive influence of Nuremberg on the DoH.[4]
In a detailed analysis, Herranz identifies within the Nuremberg Code's ten paragraphs, twelve statements that serve as markers to determine whether a particular
medical experiment conformed to appropriate ethical standards. He noted that ten
of these twelve markers from Nuremberg are retained in the DoH.[5] The original
DoH, at just over 700 words in length, was a very brief document when compared
with future (and the current) revision(s). Each of the subsequent revisions has
added material and very little has been removed.[6] We now turn to a brief review
of each of the earlier revisions.

II.2. The First Revision: Tokyo (1975)

In proportionate terms, this was the most substantial of all the revisions (including
the present revision) of the DoH. The length of the document nearly doubled. This
revision was the work of three Scandinavian professors of medicine[7], one of
whom, Professor Povl Riis, remains very active in academic commentary on
codes of ethics pertaining to medical research[8] and has contributed one of the
chapters to this volume.

Given the very minor nature of the second, third and fourth revisions (see
below), it is reasonable to assert that it is this – the 1975 version – that became the
form of the DoH that rose to prominence in the medical research community over
the next quarter-century.

Since the focus of this chapter is the fifth (Edinburgh, 2000) revision we only
briefly review the changes in 1975. Arguably the most far-reaching practical
development in the 1975 revision was the introduction of a paragraph outlining
the requirement that research protocols be submitted to an independent committee
for review prior to the conduct of the research (paragraph I.2 under the heading
"Basic Principles"). Also new in the 1975 version was the important statement of
the principle that the well-being of the participants in research must outweigh
considerations of the benefit that the knowledge gained through the research may
provide for "science and society". This is stated initially in a "positive" grammati-

3   Anonymous (1964), p. 177.
4   Fluss (1999), pp. 18-21.
5   Herranz (1998), pp. 127-139.
6   Carlson, Boyd and Webb (2004), pp. 695-713; see Figure 1.
7   Flanagan (1997), p. 926.
8   Riis (2000), pp. 3045-3046.

cal format in the "Basic Principles" section: "Concern for the interests of the subject must always prevail over the interest of science and society". It is restated (in its opposite grammatical format) in the section pertaining to "Non-therapeutic biomedical research involving human subjects (Non-clinical research)": "In research on man, the interest of science and society should never take precedence over considerations related to the well-being of the subject".

II.3. The Second Revision: Venice (1983)

This was a minor revision in comparison to the extensive remodelling of the DoH undertaken in 1975. Apart from the essentially cosmetic changes (the word "doctor" was replaced by the word "physician" and the Latin phrase "a fortiori" was replaced by "especially"), a paragraph was added regarding the issue of research on minors. Where a minor was capable of giving a degree of consent, then that consent for research participation was to be obtained in addition to the consent of the legal guardian.

II.4. The Third Revision: Hong Kong (1989)

This, along with the fourth revision, is one of the most minor of all the revisions. Although the actual number of words added was greater in this revision than in the fourth revision (29 words versus. 19 words in the fourth revision), the fact that the fourth revision changed a paragraph that was at the heart of one of the most controversial aspects of the DoH leads me to this assertion.

In the third revision, additional detail was added to the paragraph stating the requirement for independent review. The paragraph now specifies further the nature of the independence of the committee reviewing the research protocol and makes explicit the requirement that the committee must conform to the laws of the country in which the review takes place. The WMA does not publish any formal commentary to accompany the paragraphs or revisions and in this case it is perhaps regrettable because it would be interesting to know why this amendment was deemed necessary. This paragraph (now paragraph 13 in the Declaration of Helsinki) has been retained in the current version and is by far the longest and most detailed of the paragraphs. Arguably there is much redundancy. Given that the alternative is that a review committee might operate *outside* the law of the country, perhaps this should go without saying. Additionally, it could be argued that there is contradiction with the new paragraph 9 of the fifth revision whereby the requirements of the DoH are now stated to supersede any legal instruments that might have the effect of reducing the protections offered by the DoH. Up to the fifth revision, the DoH simply indicated a requirement that researchers be aware of and compliant with relevant legislation in addition to the ethical requirements of the DoH. By mentioning the fifth revision, we realise that we risk confusing the chronological structure of this chapter. However, we mention this potentially very controversial issue here as some of the roots of it are highlighted by the 1983 revision. A detailed debate about this is beyond the scope of this chapter, but we will take the subject somewhat further in the later discussion of whether documents such as the DoH should be aspirational or prescriptive in nature.

II.5. The Fourth Revision: Somerset West, South Africa (1996)

As with the revision in 1989, the actual changes to the text in the fourth revision were minimal. Regarding the fourth revision, Williams observed: "Before 1996 there was no mention of placebos in the DoH. A strict reading [...] from the version in force in 1995 would seem to prohibit placebos altogether".[9] The only change in 1996 was to add the sentence shown below in italics to paragraph 3 in the section pertaining to "Medical Research Combined with Professional Care (Clinical Research)":

> "In any medical study, every patient – including those of a control group, if any – should be assured of the best proven diagnostic and therapeutic method. *This does not exclude the use of inert placebo in studies where no proven diagnostic or therapeutic method exists*".

No change was made to the preceding paragraph II.2 which also relates to the standard of control to be used in research studies and which reads "The potential benefits, hazards and discomfort of a new method should be weighed against the advantages of the best current diagnostic and therapeutic methods". Williams goes on to observe,

> "Throughout the recent revision process this [i.e. use of placebo] was one of the most contentious issues. It was exacerbated by revelations of placebo-controlled trials in developing countries where a standard treatment exists but is not widely available in those countries".[10]

This sets the stage well for a detailed consideration of the controversial paragraphs that emerged in the fifth (Edinburgh, 2000) revision of the DoH.

III. The Fifth Revision of the Declaration of Helsinki, Edinburgh, 2000.

The process for the fifth revision of the Declaration of Helsinki lasted from September 1997 to October 2000. It began with a submission by the American Medical Association (AMA) to the WMA Council and finally ended with the near unanimous adoption of the revised form of the Declaration of Helsinki at the WMA Assembly in Edinburgh, Scotland, in October 2000. The process essentially went through three major phases, the first two of which proved largely to be "false starts". It was decided in 1998 not to proceed with the version

9   Williams (2004), pp. 31-42.
10   Ibid.

proposed by the AMA but rather to convene a Working Group, chaired by Robert Levine of Yale University, to consider the proposed revision of the DoH. Once again, in 1999, the WMA decided against accepting the revision proposed and assembled a new working group in April 1999. This group comprised Nancy Dickey of the United States, Kati Myllymäki of Finland, and Judith Kazimirski of Canada.[11]

These three became colloquially known as the "three wise women" and it was their committee's deliberations that eventually provided the basis for the 2000 revision of the DoH. This Working Group reported to the Medical Ethics Committee of the WMA Council. The central focus of the analysis in the remainder of this chapter will be to consider the evolution of the text of what eventually became the three controversial paragraphs (paragraphs 19, 29 and 30) as the Working Group deliberated, reported to the Medical Ethics Committee (MEC), and received modifications based on the outcome of MEC and WMA Council meetings. To understand more fully the process, it is necessary to describe in further detail the operating procedures of the WMA and it is to this description that we now turn.

III.1. An Aside: World Medical Association Procedures for Drafting and Adopting Ethical Declarations

The process by which the WMA adopts Declarations has been described by Lurie and Greco as "quasi-democratic".[12] This is in contrast to a fully democratic, "one person-one vote" procedure. In this section, we aim to describe more fully the WMA's "quasi-democratic" process.[13] It is through this process that the text of the Declaration of Helsinki passed to take on its current form. To understand the process requires some understanding of the structure of the WMA.

To finally become a Declaration of the World Medical Association, a Declaration must be approved at the WMA's annual assembly. Annual assemblies are usually held in October of each year. The delegates to the annual assemblies are representatives of the constituent National Medical Associations (NMAs) that form the membership of the WMA.

Within the WMA there are six WMA regions: Africa, Asia, Europe, Latin America, North America and the Pacific. It is intended that the venue for the

---

11   Ibid.
12   Lurie/Greco (2005), pp. 1117-1119.
13   The WMA kindly invited one of us (Robert Carlson) to observe its medical ethics committee meetings, council meetings and annual assemblies throughout 2003 and 2004 while a note of clarification to paragraph 30 of the Declaration of Helsinki was under consideration. This description is based both on observations of these meetings and extensive discussions with WMA delegates and staff. We are grateful to John Williams, currently Director of Ethics at the WMA and formerly a Canadian Medical Association delegate to the WMA, for his helpful comments. These comments clarified many misperceptions on our part. The responsibility for any remaining inaccuracies rests with us.

annual assembly rotate through the six regions although for a variety of reasons, a strict order of rotations is not always followed. (For example, in 2001, the events of September 11 and the subsequent disruption to travel necessitated the cancellation of the planned annual assembly in New Delhi though the WMA Council did manage to meet at WMA Headquarters in Ferney-Voltaire, France.)

As mentioned above, regular members of the WMA are not individuals but the NMAs of the various member countries. It is possible for individual physicians to join the WMA as associate members. The associate members meet just prior to the Assembly and at this meeting they elect two representatives to the General Assembly. These representatives have the right to speak but not to vote.

There are eighty-one national medical association members (NMAs) currently listed at the WMA's website.[14] However, that does not mean that there are potentially eighty-one votes cast on any resolution at the annual assembly. Voting strength is weighted according to the "declared" number of members that each national medical association has. An individual national medical association can "declare" any number of members up to its actual number of members. The reason why an NMA would choose to declare fewer than its actual number of members is that the dues paid for WMA membership are linked to the number of declared members. Such an arrangement permits countries whose NMA has a relatively large membership (because of the large population of the country even taking into consideration the higher population: doctor ratio often observed in resource-poor countries) but has limited financial resources to "declare" fewer members. This allows some NMAs to participate in the WMA that would otherwise be unable to do so.

Individual NMAs must weigh the advantage of lower membership dues against the advantage of declaring the full number of members and receiving its full voting strength (and perhaps a place on the WMA Council – see below).

III.1.1. WMA Council

The WMA Council meets three times a year: usually in May at a venue near the WMA headquarters and in September or October, immediately prior to and immediately after the Annual Assembly. Although individual NMA members could, in theory, table a motion or resolution on the floor of the Assembly, the chances are very small that it would be accepted if it had not already been discussed and endorsed at a Council meeting (and the Committee stages – see below). Council meetings are both more frequent and longer, allowing much more scope for detailed debate than at the Annual Assembly.

Each of the six WMA regions must always have at least one representative from at least one of the six NMA regions. These regional representatives are elected for a period of two years at a time. Additionally, any NMA with 50,000 or more "declared" members (see above) is also entitled to a seat on the Council.

14   http://www.wma.net/e/members/list.htm.

Therefore, the Council tends to have more representation from countries with relatively large populations, whose NMAs are financially relatively well off.

III.1.2. The Medical Ethics Committee

There are three standing committees of the WMA: the Finance and Planning Committee, the Socio-medical Affairs Committee, and the Medical Ethics Committee. Membership of these three standing committees is drawn from the membership of the Council. Each of the three committees meets during Council sessions. With respect to the text of its Declarations, it is the job of the latter two committees to undertake the detailed "word-smithing" required and to bring to the full Council the recommended text of Declarations pertaining to socio-medical issues, or to medical ethics issues respectively. Where the Council cannot agree on the wording of a document, it will usually refer the document back to the relevant committee. In cases where there are deep divisions over the wording of a Declaration, or where a very important Declaration is put forward for major revision, an ad hoc Working Group may be formed that will draw up the text of a document for discussion, first at the Standing Committee stage and, subsequently at the Council stage. Such Working Groups will always canvass individual NMAs for their opinions. In some cases, including the revision of the Declaration of Helsinki, and the note of clarification to paragraph 30, the WMA will canvass opinion more broadly and invite comment from a wide range of experts whose interests impinge upon or are impinged upon by the text of the Declaration.

III.1.3. Voting Procedures

In both Council meetings and in the Standing Committees, each NMA member has one vote and a simple majority is required for resolutions to be passed. This situation changes completely at the Annual Assembly. Prior to the Assembly there is always a "credentialing" meeting. At this meeting, those NMAs who have paid the appropriate dues for the number of "declared" members are allocated their number of votes. Every NMA has at least one vote. For those with more than 10,000 "declared" members, an additional vote is allocated for each 10,000 "declared" members. Thus, for example, an NMA with 50,000 declared members would have six votes (assuming they had paid the appropriate membership dues by the time of the Assembly).

For resolutions at Assembly that do not relate to medical ethics a simple majority of these allocated votes suffices for the resolution to pass. A resolution to adopt or amend any of the WMA's ethics documents requires 75 per cent or more of these votes.

To be revised in October 2000, the Declaration of Helsinki had to pass through all of the procedures described above. Voting at Council is done by a show of hands. At the Assembly it is done by a show of cards, each one printed with the number corresponding to that delegation's voting strength. The particular voting decisions of NMAs are not officially recorded by the WMA. All we can be certain of is that the text of any revision of the Declaration of Helsinki received at least 75 per cent voting support although the decision to adopt the text of the Declaration has been described as "near unanimous".[15]

III.2.   The Evolution of the "Controversial Paragraphs"

Most of the contention that arose out of the fifth (Edinburgh, 2000) revision surrounded three paragraphs – paragraphs 19, 29 and 30.[16] That paragraphs 29 and 30 raised a storm of controversy is evidenced by the WMA's unprecedented step of issuing notes of clarification to these paragraphs. Paragraph 19 was considered for a note of clarification but the final decision was that such a step was unnecessary. The final versions of these three paragraphs are as follows:

> "Paragraph 19: Medical research is only justified if there is a reasonable likelihood that the populations in which the research is carried out stand to benefit from the results of the research.
>
> Paragraph 29: The benefits, risks, burdens and effectiveness of a new method should be tested against those of the best current prophylactic, diagnostic, and therapeutic methods. This does not exclude the use of placebo, or no treatment, in studies where no proven prophylactic, diagnostic or therapeutic method exists.
>
> Paragraph 30: At the conclusion of the study, every patient entered into the study should be assured of access to the best proven prophylactic, diagnostic and therapeutic methods identified by the study".

It is our aim at this point to consider, based on the material that was available in the WMA archives, how these three paragraphs evolved through the process of drafting the text. This analysis is based on unpublished documents made available to me by the WMA. The WMA kindly allowed me free search of their archives. However, because of limited space, limited staff numbers and a recent relocation of the headquarters, the archives were not systematically filed. Some relevant documents appear to be no longer extant – at least in the WMA archives.

The series of documents available that tracked the evolution of the text are all entitled "Proposed Revision of the Declaration of Helsinki" and are serially numbered as follows: 17.C/WW1/2000, 17.C/WW2/2000, 17.C/WW3/2000, 17.C/WW4/2000 and 17.C/WW5/2000. From the minutes of the WMA General Assembly in Edinburgh, 2000 it became apparent that the version presented to the Assembly was 17.C/WW8/2000. This was unchanged in the Assembly so the text of 'WW8' corresponds to the actual text of the fifth revision of the Declaration of Helsinki. Documents 17.C/WW6/2000 and 17.C/WW7/2000 are not extant in the WMA archives and the possible reason for this is discussed below. Although the deliberations of the Working Group began in 1999, documentation of these

---

15   Williams (2004), pp. 31-42.
16   Ibid.

deliberations is unavailable. We begin therefore with the text of the proposed revision (17.C/WW1/2000) that was presented by the Working group to the Medical Ethics Committee at the WMA Council meeting in May 2000.

III.2.1. May 2000 – 17.C/WW1/2000

Paragraph 19: This paragraph was not yet in the proposed text.

> Paragraph 29: "24. In any medical study, every patient – including those of a control group, if any – should be assured of proven diagnostic and therapeutic methods. This does not exclude the use of inert placebo in studies where no proven diagnostic or therapeutic method exists.
>
> 23. The potential benefits, hazards and discomfort of a new method should be weighed against the advantages of the best current diagnostic and therapeutic methods".

Comment: This document had what eventually became paragraph 29 numbered as paragraphs 24 and 23. The order of occurrence of what were previously paragraphs II.2 and II.3 in the 1996 version has been reversed (and this accounts for the numbering 24. and 23. in this document). With respect to the wording, what is labelled here as paragraph 24 is very similar to the 1996 version that reads: "In any medical study, every patient – including those of a control group, if any – should be assured of the best proven diagnostic and therapeutic method. This does not exclude the use of inert placebo in studies where no proven diagnostic or therapeutic method exists". The wording of what is labelled here as paragraph 23 is unchanged.

The only proposed change therefore at this stage was to require assurance of "proven ... methods" rather than the "best proven" method.

Paragraph 30: This paragraph was not yet in the proposed text.

This document was considered by the Medical Ethics Committee and changes were made. The next version (17.C/WW2/2000) was presented by the MEC to the WMA Council. This Council meeting was held shortly after the MEC during the series of meetings on 4-5 May 2000.

III.2.2. May 2000 – 17.C/WW2/2000

The text as proposed by the MEC to WMA Council was as follows:

> Paragraph 19: "Medical research is only justified if there is a reasonable likelihood that the populations in which the research is carried out stand to benefit from the results of the research".

Comment: What eventually became paragraph 19 is now included in the proposed text. The documentation indicates that the text initially proposed by the MEC was "Medical research is only appropriate..." and the word appropriate was changed to "justified" during the MEC meeting.

In this document this paragraph is numbered paragraph 24a. Apparently it had originally been included as a preamble to the statement about placebo controls. It was subsequently separated from this statement and moved forward in the DoH to be in the section entitled "Basic Principles (for All Medical Research)".

> Paragraph 29: "24b. In any medical study, every patient – including those of a control group, if any – should be assured of proven effective prophylactic, diagnostic, and therapeutic methods.
>
> 24c. This does not exclude the use of inert placebo in studies where no proven diagnostic or therapeutic method exists
>
> 23. The potential benefits, risks and discomfort of a new method should be weighed against the advantages of the best current prophylactic, diagnostic and therapeutic methods".

Comment: It can be seen that what entered these deliberations as paragraph 24 has emerged in three pieces, i.e., 24a, 24b and 24c. Paragraph 24a, as mentioned, was moved to a place earlier in the proposed text. 24b and 24c are still consecutive. The only change to the wording of 24b or 24c is the addition of the two words "effective prophylactic". The previous version therefore required assurance of "proven diagnostic and therapeutic methods". It was now proposed to require assurance of "proven effective prophylactic, diagnostic and therapeutic methods".

In what is labelled here as paragraph 23, the word "hazards" has now been changed to "risks" and the word "prophylactic" added so that the phraseology matches that of paragraph 24b.

Paragraph 30: This paragraph was not yet proposed in the text.

The above changes were then deliberated by the WMA Council and the ensuing text (17.C/WW3/2000) was approved for distribution by the Council to the various NMAs.

III.2.3. May-October 2000: 17.C/WW3/2000

Some minor changes were made to other portions of the proposed text but no changes were made to any of the texts described above under 17.C/WW2/2000. Thus, with respect to what eventually became paragraphs 19, 29 and 30,:there is no difference between WW2 and WW3 in the series of documents under consideration. It was the text of 17.C/WW3/2000 that was then released to the various NMAs and further comment invited. The Working Group along with the then Secretary General of the WMA, Delon Human, then met in August 2000 to consider the proposed revision in the light of these further comments. They presented the updated proposed text (17.C/WW4/2000) based on these deliberations and this text was to be considered by the MEC in early October prior to the pre-Assembly Council meetings.

III.2.4. October, 2000: 17.C/WW4/2000

> Paragraph 19: "24a. Medical research is only justified if there is a reasonable likelihood that the populations in which the research is carried out stand to benefit from the results of the research. The protocol presented to the review committee must include a realistic plan to deliver those treatments identified through such research to the populations from which the subjects have been drawn".

Commentary: This proposed paragraph now contains a newly drafted second sentence.

> Paragraph 29: "24b. In medical research, every patient – including those of a control group, if any – should be assured of the best proven prophylactic, diagnostic and therapeutic methods. This does not exclude the use of inert placebo in studies where no proven prophylactic, diagnostic or therapeutic method exists.
>
> 23. The potential benefits, risks and discomfort of a new method should be weighed against those of the best current prophylactic, diagnostic and therapeutic methods".

Commentary: What were previously paragraphs 24b. and 24c. have now been combined into one paragraph 24b. The word "effective" has been replaced by "the best" so that patients are now to be assured of "the best proven prophylactic, diagnostic and therapeutic methods". This in fact restores the wording (with the exception of the addition of "prophylactic") of the adjectival portion of the sentence to what it was in the 1996 version of the DoH.

In paragraph 23 the indicative pronoun "those" has replaced "the advantages". "Those" makes reference to "benefits, risks and discomfort". Interestingly, the logic of the previous form of the sentence would have required that the "potential benefits, risks and discomfort" of a new method were weighed only against "the advantages" of the existing method. This potential inconsistency had been present in the DoH since 1975.

Paragraph 30: There remains no mention of the issue that would eventually appear as paragraph 30 in the revised Declaration of Helsinki. We can see that it did not emerge completely de novo but rather appears to be a re-interpretation of the implications of the former 24b., i.e. "In medical research, every patient – including those of a control group, if any – should be assured of the best proven prophylactic, diagnostic and therapeutic methods". This is the version that was considered by the Medical Ethics Committee (MEC) in its deliberations just prior to the General Assembly in Edinburgh in October 2000.

III.2.5. October 2000: 17.C/WW5/2000

As mentioned above there is no trace of documents 17.C/WW6/2000, 17.C/WW7/2000 and 17.C/WW8/2000 in the WMA archives. However, as the minutes of the Assembly indicate 17.C/WW8/2000 was the version adopted by the WMA Council and recommended to the WMA General Assembly. Since no changes were made at the Assembly, we can conclude that WW8 was identical to the adopted text of the revised Declaration of Helsinki.

The MEC met for long hours in the days leading up to the General Assembly in an attempt to finalise the wording of the revision of the Declaration of Helsinki. Working documents were created very quickly at various points in the deliberations and changes were ongoing. The following indicates the status of the text of the three paragraphs under consideration according to the working document 17.C/WW5/2000.

> Paragraph 19: "24a. Medical research is only justified if there is a reasonable likelihood that the populations in which the research is carried out stand to benefit from the results of the research".

Comment: The proposed second sentence requiring a "realistic plan to deliver" treatments identified as beneficial to the population has been removed. This sentence has now reverted to exactly the same wording as proposed by the MEC to the Council in May (see WW2 above). This is also the exact wording of what became paragraph 19 in the revised DoH. Therefore we can conclude that even if the non-extant WW6 and WW7 contained any differences, they were restored to this text by WW8.

> Paragraph 29: "23. The potential benefits, risks and discomfort of a new method should be weighed against those of the best current prophylactic, diagnostic and therapeutic methods. This does not exclude the use of placebo, or no treatment, in studies where no proven prophylactic, diagnostic or therapeutic method exists".

Comment: This paragraph has been extensively restructured from the previous version. The entire sentence relating to "assurance of access" has been removed (and the issue of assurance of access now appears in what was to become paragraph 30 – see below). The sentence beginning "The potential benefits…" is unchanged from its earlier version but it has now been placed before the sentence beginning "This does not exclude…".

> Paragraph 30: "24b. At the conclusion of the study, every patient in the study should be assured of access to the best proven prophylactic, diagnostic or therapeutic methods identified by the study".

Comment: This is the first appearance, at this late stage, of what became the controversial paragraph 30. It was initially a re-wording of the sentence formerly seen as paragraph 24b (see above).

III.2.6. October 2000 – the Fifth Revision of the Declaration of Helsinki, Edinburgh, 2000.

Paragraph 19: Apart from the re-numbering of the paragraph from its interim number 24a to its final position at 19 – a task that could only be finalised when the wording of the Declaration was finalised – there was no change to this paragraph. Paragraph 29:

> "The benefits, risks, burdens and effectiveness of a new method should be tested against those of the best current prophylactic, diagnostic, and therapeutic methods. This does not

exclude the use of placebo, or no treatment, in studies where no proven prophylactic, diagnostic or therapeutic method exists".

Comment: Between the working document 17.C/WW5/2000 and the final version of the revised Declaration of Helsinki the phrase "the potential benefits, risks and discomfort should be weighed against ..." was changed to "The benefits, risks, burdens and effectiveness of a new method should be tested against ...". This represents three changes: (i) the word "potential" is removed; (ii) the more metaphorical verb "weighed" (medical research does not usually involve actually determining the weight of the new treatment under investigation) is changed to the more literal "tested"; (iii) the word "effectiveness" has been added to the list of attributes of the new method that need to be tested against the existing method.

Paragraph 30: "At the conclusion of the study, every patient in the study should be assured of access to the best proven prophylactic, diagnostic or therapeutic methods identified by the study".

Comment: Apart from finalising the paragraph number (see comment above), no changes were made from 17.C/WW5/2000.

IV. Lessons from the Fifth Revision of the Declaration of Helsinki

We have now traced in detail the evolution of the text of the three controversial paragraphs of the Declaration of Helsinki. It is time to reflect on some of the lessons that can be learned from this analysis?

1. How important is the original intent of the authors of the DoH? We have already observed the structure of the WMA. It is the largest global grouping of doctors. The efforts of the WMA represent a much sought-after international consensus as to what is and what is not ethically acceptable in the conduct of medical research. As such, ethical proclamations by this organisation must be taken seriously. Through this analysis, we can take steps to get closer to understanding the intent of the authors of this Declaration.

2. It must be remembered, however, that once the deliberations of the WMA become fixed in the text of the Declaration of Helsinki then the text can take on a proverbial "life of its own". Although the WMA have been very open and generous in allowing access to their meetings and archives, for the most part those who will read, interpret and apply the Declaration of Helsinki will not be party to these deliberations. Therefore, it is also important that the text can stand alone and be interpreted by its readers in such a way that there is an understanding of what the ethical guidelines established by the Declaration of Helsinki mean in actual research practice. The notion of whether the meaning of a text lies in its author's intent, in its reader's interpretation or, indeed, somewhere else, remains a complex and vexed philosophical problem. It is reasonable to assert that, despite this, it is certainly disingenuous to deliberately misinterpret the author's intent. For example, an overly literal interpretation of paragraph 19, requiring a reasonable likelihood of benefit to populations from which research subjects are drawn, could

lead to the conclusion that research on populations of "healthy volunteers" was ruled out. It seems, however, that the explicit mention of research in "healthy volunteers" (paragraphs 16 and 18) and "those who will not directly benefit" (paragraph 8) would mean that such an interpretation requires a deliberate decontextualisation and misinterpretation of the intent of the paragraph.

3. There are hazards involved in drafting a document "by committee". The sudden appearance of paragraph 30 seemed to have taken the medical research community by surprise. The great difficulty involved in developing a Note of Clarification (the process took 4 years compared with 1 year for paragraph 29) may be a reflection of the fact that the implications of this paragraph were not subject to the same process of consultation with NMAs and others that was the case for paragraphs 19 and 29. That being said, it should also be noted that even though paragraph 29 was deliberated in this way, it also gave rise to considerable controversy following the October 2000 revision of the Declaration of Helsinki. Certainly the introduction of a longer time period between the finalisation of a proposed form of its most important declarations and the final vote on these declarations in its General Assembly may avoid the turbulent and somewhat controversial process of adding a Note of Clarification.

4. There needs to be further thought given to whether the Declaration of Helsinki is essentially an aspirational document or whether it is a prescriptive document. Ruth Macklin raises this question without answering it:

> "Beyond these debates lies a deeper question about the nature of ethical guidelines. Should they be 'pragmatic' or 'aspirational'? Adherents of the view that statements such as the Declaration of Helsinki ... must be 'pragmatic' are likely to rely on current and past practices as a guide to what is possible. The pragmatists dismiss 'aspirational' guidelines as too lofty and, therefore, unrealistic. For their part, the 'aspirationists' tend to be reformers who judge past or current practices to be ethically insufficient to ensure that the highest standards for research apply everywhere ...".[17]

Philosopher Dorothy Emmet has considered in detail from several philosophical perspectives the value of what she terms a "regulative ideal": "To say that something is unrealisable is to speak with reference to a goal or standard which may be approached but which cannot be attained. Nevertheless, practice may be oriented towards it".[18] Essentially Emmet sees considerable value in the notion of setting out aspirational standards as giving a direction or orientation to practice.

With respect to the Declaration of Helsinki, the WMA seems not to have finally settled upon whether the guidelines are prescriptive or aspirational. The detail in paragraph 13 (pertaining to the function of independent review committees and, as mentioned above, the longest and most complex paragraph in the DoH) suggests a prescriptiveness. On the other hand, the far-reaching implications of paragraphs such as 19 and 30 have a more aspirational character.

At the same time the possibility that there is value in the ambiguity cannot be ruled out. The suggestion of prescription negates the aspirational nature of the

17   Macklin (2004), p.27.
18   Emmet (1994), pp. 2-3.

guidelines being used as a convenient excuse for not fully meeting the apparent requirements. On the other hand, ascendance of aspiration over prescription means that research that is correctly oriented and moving in the "right direction", but not fully "there yet", will not be excluded.

V. Summary

In summary, we have traced very briefly the first to the fourth revisions of the Declaration of Helsinki. This set the stage for a detailed consideration of the process by which three of the most debated paragraphs of the fifth (Edinburgh, 2000) revision of the Declaration of Helsinki were formulated. In doing so, we described the relevant operating procedures of the WMA and then tracked the relevant portions of the proposed revision through these procedures. The aim of this exercise has been to illuminate further the process of "authorship" of the Declaration of Helsinki. To the extent that understanding the intent of the author is necessary in understanding the meaning of a text, it is hoped that this exercise provides additional insight into the potential ethical implications of the fifth revision of the Declaration of Helsinki.

References

Anonymous (1964): Human Experimentation: Code of Ethics of the World Medical Association, British Medical Journal 2 (1964), p. 177.

Carlson, R. V./Boyd, K. M./Webb, D. J. (2004): The Revision of the Declaration of Helsinki: Past, Present and Future, British Journal of Clinical Pharmacology 57 (2004), pp. 695-713.

Emmet, D. (1994): The Role of the Unrealisable: A Study in Regulative Ideals. New York: St. Martin's Press.

Flanagan, A. (1997): Who Wrote the Declaration of Helsinki?, Journal of the American Medical Association 277 (1997), p. 926.

Fluss, S. (1999): How the Declaration of Helsinki Developed, Good Clinical Practice Journal 6 (1999), pp. 18-21.

Herranz, G. (1998): The Inclusion of the 10 Principles of Nuremberg in Professional Codes of Ethics: an International Comparison, in: Tröhler/Reiter-Theil (1998), pp. 127-139.

Lurie P./Greco, D. B. (2005): US Exceptionalism Comes To Research Ethics, Lancet 365 (2005), pp. 1117-1119.

Riis, P. (2000): Perspectives on the 5th Revision of the Declaration of Helsinki, Journal of the American Medical Association (2000), pp. 3045-3046.

Macklin, R. (2004): Double Standards in Medical Research in Developing Countries. Cambridge: Cambridge University Press.

Tröhler, U./Reiter-Theil, S (eds.) (1998): Ethics Codes in Medicine: Foundations and Achievements of Codification since 1947. Aldershot, Brookfield, Singapore, Syndney: Ashgate.

Williams, J. R. (2004): The Promise and Limits of International Bioethics: Lessons from the Recent Revision of the Declaration of Helsinki, Journal International De Bioethique 15 (2004), pp. 31-42.

World Medical Association (1964): Declaration of Helsinki, World Medical Journal 11 (1964), p. 259 (Spanish), p. 281 (English), p. 301 (French).

Acknowledgements: Robert Carlson's post was funded by an unrestricted educational grant from Johnson & Johnson Ltd. The assistance of the World Medical Association secretariat in making their archives available, and in particular the invaluable advice given by the WMA's Director of Ethics (John Williams) is also gratefully acknowledged.

David R. Willcox

Medical Ethics and Public Perception:
The Declaration of Helsinki and Its Revision in 2000

I.   Introduction

The debate surrounding the 2000 revisions of the World Medical Association's
(WMA) Declaration of Helsinki is notable for the controversy it generated. It was
not the first time the document had been revised by the WMA, but infighting
within the interested parties on ethical research was rife in professional medical
literature. The decisions being made would affect the rights of research subjects
and the obligations of researchers worldwide. The debate involved issues of
exploitation, profiteering, informed consent and the future of the Declaration and
medical ethics. With such public interest at stake the public perception of the
medical research community, the Declaration and nations' adherence to sound
medical ethics was open for examination.

This article will examine how the debate over the revisions found its public
voice. It will analyse medical literature, namely publicly-available journals and
articles that carried the debate in Britain and to a lesser extent in the United States.
It will ask how the debate was reflected in the wider public domain, through
parliamentary debate and the mass media. Was the public perception of the
Declaration altered by such coverage? Did the 2000 revisions alter the way in
which medical ethics was perceived? On the basis of published material, the
article will argue that despite raising issues of public importance the debate
surrounding the 2000 revisions of the Declaration of Helsinki did little to alter the
public perception of medical ethics.

II. The History behind the Fifth Revision

The Declaration of Helsinki constitutes an important guidance document relating
to ethical research involving human subjects. The necessity for such a framework
was brought into sharp focus following the Nuremberg Doctors' Trial in 1947 and
a proposal was first discussed by the WMA in 1953.[1] The changes made in 2000
were the fifth alterations since the document's inception in 1964.[2] The 52nd

---

1   World Medical Association (no date), p. 1.
2   The other revisions are as follows: Tokyo, Japan, October 1975; Venice, Italy, October 1983;
     Hong Kong, September 1989 and Somerset West, Republic of South Africa, October 1996. A

General Meeting of the WMA, held in Edinburgh in October 2000, sought to resolve a number of problematic issues. Clarifications were made throughout the document, but the public and professional debate centred on two key aspects.[3] These related to the use of placebos during trials and the post-trial access to medication for research subjects. The changes being discussed will be briefly outlined in order to understand the context of the debate.

The first issue, relating to the debate over the ethical use of placebos during trials, was addressed by the WMA in paragraph 29:

> "The benefits, risks, burdens and effectiveness of a new method should be tested against those of the best current prophylactic, diagnostic, and therapeutic methods. This does not exclude the use of placebo, or no treatment, in studies where no proven prophylactic, diagnostic or therapeutic method exists".[4]

This principle sought to address the question when the use of placebo could be ethically justified. The issue figured predominantly in the debate up to, and beyond, the 2000 revision. In case the WMA had hoped to encapsulate a clear-cut and long-standing definition they were to be disappointed. Further public discussion about the revision led to the WMA issuing a note of clarification in 2002:

> "The WMA hereby reaffirms its position that extreme care must be taken in making use of a placebo-controlled trial and that in general this methodology should only be used in the absence of existing proven therapy. However, a placebo-controlled trial may be ethically acceptable, even if proven therapy is available, under the following circumstances:
>
> – Where for compelling and scientifically sound methodological reasons its use is necessary to determine the efficacy or safety of a prophylactic, diagnostic or therapeutic method; or
>
> – Where a prophylactic, diagnostic or therapeutic method is being investigated for a minor condition and the patients who receive placebo will not be subject to any additional risk of serious or irreversible harm.
>
> All other provisions of the Declaration of Helsinki must be adhered to, especially the need for appropriate ethical and scientific review".[5]

The clarification reflected the difficulty in creating an all-encompassing set of ethical guidelines to govern research. The final sentence alone drew attention to the fact that such ethical decisions overlap and impact upon all levels of research planning. The difficulty in planning ethical research extends beyond the trial itself and the second contentious issue of the 2000 revisions, addressed in paragraph 30, dealt with post-trial care:

> Note of Clarification on Paragraph 29 was added in 2002 and a Note of Clarification on Paragraph 30 in 2004.

3   Further examples of alterations include the sub-heading for the Declaration which was altered from "Recommendations Guiding Physicians in Biomedical Research involving Human Sub-jects" (the 1996 version) to "Ethical Principles for Medical Research involving Human Sub-jects". Furthermore, specific attention was drawn to the need to protect vulnerable research populations in paragraphs 8 and 9 to ensure that national regulations should in no way "reduce or eliminate any of the protections for human subject set forth" in the Declaration.

4   World Medical Association (2004).

5   Ibid.

"At the conclusion of the study, every patient entered into the study should be assured of access to the best proven prophylactic, diagnostic and therapeutic methods identified by the study".[6]

The ethical legitimacy of medical research involving humans was deemed dependent upon continuing medical support for participants. The concerns expressed about this issue revolved around the prohibitive cost which would be incurred and the threat to funding for future research trials. Thus, the WMA added a further note of clarification in 2004:

"The WMA hereby reaffirms its position that it is necessary during the study planning process to identify post-trial access by study participants to prophylactic, diagnostic and therapeutic procedures identified as beneficial in the study or access to other appropriate care. Post-trial access arrangements or other care must be described in the study protocol so the ethical review committee may consider such arrangements during its review".[7]

The emphasis focused on review committees' requirement to judge proposals based not only on the merits of the experiment but also to ensure that the research subjects would not be abandoned after the trial's completion. Both of these revisions stimulated a debate which transcended the domains of official policy makers, and extended from the professional media of medical publications to the popular press.

Previous revisions met with less controversy despite arguably altering the document on a grander scale. In the 1975 Tokyo revision eight new paragraphs were added to the Declaration, in 1983 obtaining consent from a minor was added, while in 1989 the appointment of committees overseeing the protocol was the subject of an amendment. However, the 2000 revisions were particularly controversial, sparking international discussion which had the potential to influence the public perception of the Declaration and the processes involved in constructing it.

III. The Moral High Road to Edinburgh. The Debate in the Medical Literature

The period before the meeting in Edinburgh saw medical journals and publications awash with contrasting views.[8] The discussions formed a component of the overall debate about the role of the Declaration, but the debate itself was also a factor in how the document was perceived. This was particularly true on the subject of placebo use in medical research. In April 1997, Peter Lurie and Sidney Wolfe and others from the American group "Public Citizen" wrote to Donna Shalala, the Secretary of the US Health and Human Services, complaining about the nature of research into the transmission of AIDS from mother to child in developing nations.[9] The argument propounded was that studies which used a

6   Ibid.
7   Ibid.
8   See, for example, Josefson (1997), pp. 763-766.
9   Lurie et al. (1997).

placebo were denying that arm of the study group treatment and increasing the risk of a child being born with HIV. Instead the drug on trial, Zidovudine, should be compared with existing drugs.[10] The letter warned of a "dangerous double standard" as similar trials funded by the same group in developed nations did provide alternative treatments.[11] The trials were said to be both a breach of the Declaration of Helsinki in not providing the best proven method, and of four articles of the Nuremberg Code.[12] Herein lay the heart of the concerns over placebo use.

At around the same time, the *British Medical Journal* (*BMJ*) voiced concern on another aspect of research in developing nations, namely the provision of post-trial care. One article asked if poor people in developing countries were being exploited with trials conducted differently in South America and Africa than would be in Great Britain.[13] The criticism proposed that the existing ethical position perpetuated the testing of drugs in the developing world, which could only ever be afforded in developed states.

These two issues formed the basis of the debate and prompted the American Medical Association in 1997 to call for revisions. On the one hand, commentators such as Robert Levine, director at the Centre for Interdisciplinary Research on AIDS at Yale University, favoured the abolition of the distinction between therapeutic and non-therapeutic trials.[14] At a London workshop on ethics, he argued that one had to recognise that developing countries could not afford the same drugs as those in the developed world. This position was referred to in a *BMJ* article, somewhat misleadingly, as the "US position".[15]

In the other camp, the *BMJ*-article quoted Dirceu Greco from the Federal University, Brazil, as being against the "best attainable" approach.[16] Confirmation of a movement towards diametrically opposed groups was then surmised with the assertion: "Dr Vivienne Nathanson, head of science and ethics at the British Medical Association, said that the proposed revisions had led to increasing polarisation".[17] On the basis of this evidence one could be forgiven for concluding that the dividing line over the issues was between the "US position" and the developing world.

The disagreement over the proposed revisions was more complex and layered than divisions on a national or supra-national level. The assertion that the issue was divided between a "US position" and the rest of the world is not generally applicable. In Britain, one journal published a "for and against debate" on whether

---

10 Ibid.
11 Ibid.
12 The authors alleged that principle 2, 4, 5 and 7 of the Nuremberg Code had been violated; for the history and role of the Nuremberg Code in modern research ethics, see Schmidt (2004).
13 Wilmshurst (1997), p. 840.
14 Levine (1999), p. 531.
15 Woodman (1999), p. 660.
16 Ibid.
17 Ibid.

the Declaration needed strengthening.[18] Kenneth Rothman and Karin Michels of the Boston University School of Public Health and Harvard Medical School Obstetrics and Gynaecology Epidemiology Centre, respectively, championed the desire for a strengthened document. The pair argued that the United States Food and Drug Administration (FDA) was pressuring the WMA into making changes and that FDA mandates required placebo trials even if approved treatments existed, in contravention to the Declaration of Helsinki.[19] The authors proposed that the Declaration should assert that "no investigator or regulatory official has the right to decide how much sacrifice in terms of risk or discomfort a patient should endure in the name of science".[20] On the issue of consent the authors stressed that informed consent should not in itself be enough and the rest of the Declaration remained applicable. Furthermore, such consent should be gained through the use of understandable language.[21] In essence, the article called for a global as opposed to local or national ethics standards. Although critical of American organisations, specifically the FDA, the position was forwarded by two employees of American institutions. Therefore, a distinction should be made between, for example, the British or US position and the position of a British or US funding organisation; to do otherwise would overlook the diversity of opinions in different countries.

Contrary to Rothman and Michels' position stood that of Michael Baum from the Department of Surgery at University College London. His response was forth-right: "Rothman and Michels spit out the epithet 'in the name of science' as if science was a neo-Nazi movement rather than a disciplined search for an objective reality in the service of mankind".[22] Such association would not have been mis-placed in a tabloid newspaper attempting to provoke the reader's interest; conside-ring the origins of the Declaration and its intention, Baum's comment is parti-cularly stimulating. The retort of the original authors was to accuse Baum of being "historically off-key" by pointing out the historical roots of the Declaration.[23]

Such exchanges highlighted strong opinion generated by the issues in question. The historical foundations are never far from any discussion about the document and act as a constant reminder of "the alternative" – the image of Nazi atrocities and the Nuremberg Trials. The problem with this is the effect it has on the document's perception by the public. In the same way as the Second World War is introduced into media coverage, especially during conflict when it serves a propagandistic value, the Nazi image is thrust upon the Declaration. In doing so it threatens to divert the genuine debate away from the issues in hand.[24]

The revisions struck to the core of ethical issues about the relationship bet-ween scientists and research subjects. Those against any perceived weakening

18   Michels et al. (2000), pp. 442-445.
19   Ibid, p. 442.
20   Ibid, p. 443.
21   Ibid.
22   Ibid, p. 444.
23   Ibid, p. 445.
24   See also Willcox (2006) on issues of propaganda in conflict.

wanted to retain the central premise of the well-being of the research subject. Troyen Brennan of Harvard Medical School, writing in *The New England Journal of Medicine*, encapsulated this approach to the debate, fearing that the revisions would instigate

> "a shift to an efficiency-based standard for research involving human subjects and weaken the principles of the investigator's moral commitment to the research subject and the just allocation of the benefits and burdens of research, which have heretofore been the hallmarks of ethical research".[25]

In this context the debate is focused on the rights of the subject and herald back to the Nuremberg roots of the Declaration. The juxtaposed position can all too easily be viewed as promoting the opposite to this, placing the needs of society at a higher priority. However, the threat to the positive portrayal of the research profession arises when clouded by the issue of for-profit pharmaceutical companies. Such organisations, if arguing for a more efficient system, could be seen to be acting not from principle but for profit.

Thus it was in the context of the arguments in professional publications above that the revisions of 2000 were discussed. The subject in issue was immense, a fact not missed by commentators. After the WMA meeting in Santiago, Chile, in April 1999, *The Lancet* stated that the undertaking was "extremely ambitious" but that the proposals provided "little or no help to those who are charged with the practical application of agreed ethical principles".[26] A later editorial criticised the WMA's process of arriving at the revisions, arguing it had not been transparent enough.[27] The mechanics of both arriving at agreeable revisions and introducing them in the work-place added to the problems. At the root of the debate, however, were the issues of placebo and post-trial drug access. Concern about the revisions also had ramifications for politicians and the public perception of the profession as reflected in mass media.

IV. The Wider Audience: Members of Parliament and the Media

The deliberations over the proposed revisions were not restricted purely to the pages of medical literature, though it formed a substantial body of public material on the issue. In the period preceding the WMA meeting in Edinburgh the proposed revisions also received some attention in the deliberations of British politicians and the popular media. The coverage was obviously different in nature, but it is interesting to compare how the debate was treated in the wider public domain. In a specialist area such as health and science the medical literature can stimulate discussion in popular formats where editors then seek to distil the

---

25 Brennan (1999), p. 527. Incidentally, in keeping with the for and against format, Brennan's article featured in the same edition as Levine's; see Levine (1999).
26 Lancet (1999), p. 1285.
27 Lancet (2000), p. 1123.

discussion in terms that are accessible to lay-persons.[28] Perhaps most importantly for the issue of a public debate and the public perception of that debate is that the discussions become less about professional opinions about medical ethics but more about humanising the consequences of ethical decisions. Theoretical ethical discussions are connected by contextualisation through real medical scenarios proposed by the media to the human beings whose lives would ultimately be influenced by the guidelines.

The Declaration of Helsinki was approached in similar ways by both the media and politicians. Inference to the Declaration was often made by way of a reference to support the statement being made, rather than as the focus of the discussion. This is not surprising and could be said of numerous rules and guidelines. However, it is interesting insomuch as the Declaration became synonymous with the guiding principles of medical ethics. For example, when Nicholas Soames, Secretary of State for Defence, was questioned about the exposure of veterans to radio-labelled tracer materials at Porton Down, he responded:

"All studies involving volunteers at Porton Down are governed by the principles for ethical control of human experiments as stated in the Nuremburg code, the Helsinki declaration and the guidelines of the Royal College of Physicians. My Department does not issue guidelines to the independent ethics committee of experts who oversee the volunteer programme at Porton Down".[29]

Soames invoked the Declaration as one of the main guiding principles by which ethical research was being conducted. This had the benefit of acting as a higher authority than the department in question for regulating work at a government institution. The Declaration was widely utilised in this way and demonstrated its international role as a policy document on medical ethics. Lord Donoughue, the Parliamentary Secretary, Ministry of Agriculture, Fisheries and Food, used the Declaration in a similar manner:

"The Ministry of Agriculture, Fisheries and Food and other relevant departments have made further inquiries into the research reported in the press last summer and have been assured that it was conducted in accordance with the international guidelines which govern human volunteer studies. Through the operation of the Health and Safety at Work Act, the COSHH Regulations and the national and international protocols (such as the Declaration of Helsinki and the guidelines issued by the Royal College of Physicians) which apply in this area, there is a control system in place which aims to ensure that the safety of the volunteers is protected in the same way as anyone else who may be exposed to chemicals in the course of their work. Doctors involved in such research who do not comply with the Royal College's guidelines would be liable to a charge of serious professional misconduct".[30]

It is worth reproducing the text at length to understand the context in which the Declaration is invoked. There is little or no expansion upon the content of the

28   Boseley (2006).
29   Soames (1997), Col. 125-6. Porton Down is the British government's research establishment in Wiltshire. For more information about the subject of human experimentation at Porton Down see Schmidt (2006); see also the article by Ulf Schmidt on Porton Down in this volume.
30   Donoughue (1999), Col. WA141-2.

document but its relevance to the subject and its importance as a guideline to ethical research is unchallenged. The Declaration was depicted as being above departmental and even political control and bedded within the remit of the medical profession. For a lay-person, even one interested enough in politics to follow debates in Parliament, the exact nature of the Declaration would not be revealed here, only its importance. As mentioned above, this in itself is not surprising. It would be difficult for commentators to expand upon every reference, but the public image of deference to the Declaration is different here than to informed readers of medical literature. This in turn affected the consideration which the popular media gave the Declaration. If the Declaration was seen as above political influence and discussion, its existence, content and any changes made to it may seem clouded in secrecy yet inherently relevant to the public at large. Concerns about the perception of the process were evident in one letter to a medical journal by a paediatrician on the issue of informed consent:

> "I would think that of all the professions, only in medicine would there be any sort of debate about whether people need to be told that they, their bodies, their body fluids, their emotions, or whatever were to be subjects of research. This is arrogance on the part of doctors. Has anyone thought of asking these 'patients' what their opinions are?"[31]

Independent of whether one agrees with this conclusion, the fact is that the revisions and debates about what is best for research subjects can be perceived differently in different circumstances. While political commentators state their subservience to the Declaration and the professional debate, the public image created by the discussion is one of deference rather than inclusion.

The top-down perception of the WMA's revision process, which may be an unfair criticism, takes on greater ramifications when an issue directly related to the guidelines becomes a newsworthy story. There was scant discussion of the revision process in the popular media and the Houses of Parliament between 1997 and early 2000. However, the Declaration did become a matter of deliberation when combined with a provocative human interest story. During a debate on human stem cell research in 1999, Lord Ashbourne cited the Declaration in defence of his position. He went further than merely mentioning the name, but remarked: "In research on man, the interest of science and society should never take precedence over considerations related to the well-being of the subject". It continued:

> "The doctor can combine medical research with professional care, the objective being the acquisition of new medical knowledge, only to the extent that medical research is justified by its potential diagnostic and therapeutic value for the patient".[32]

Once again the Declaration was invoked as a benchmark for ethical considerations in human experimentation. Here, the commentator elaborates on a specific aspect of the document on a contemporary issue. Significantly, Lord Ashbourne referred to the 1975 Declaration of Helsinki, overlooking the later revised versions of

31   Bratt (1997), p. 1477.
32   Ashbourne (1999), Col. 340.

October 1983, September 1989 and October 1996.[33] The relevance to contemporary issues was nonetheless clear.

Little consideration was given to the debate surrounding the revisions of the Declaration up until 2000 outside of the medical literature. In the media, the Declaration was cited in reference to other news stories, such as human versus animal testing or as a component of another debate.[34] However, as the Edinburgh meeting drew closer, some discussion began in the mass media while political dialogue in public forums continued. The argument in the media began to reflect the discussion in the medical literature of the previous three years, albeit on a smaller scale. The British Broadcasting Corporation (BBC) referred to the "Public Citizen" condemnation of trials, where the participants had been denied treatment.[35] The BBC also made reference to an unspecified *New England Journal of Medicine* article questioning the trials.[36] While this initial BBC web-site article emphasised the concern that the current guidelines were to be relaxed, another one emphasised the likelihood that the Declaration might be strengthened to ensure ethical standards were met by researchers, a month later.[37] The switch to a more positive perception of the proposed changes was primarily the result of Anders Milton, Chairman of the WMA, talking to the BBC. His words set the tone for a more positive approach to the proposed revisions:

> "It is very important that medical research is carried out ethically and does not adversely affect the subject. Pharmaceutical companies should not use non-industrial countries to test drugs which will be used in the industrial world. It is very important that medical associations throughout the world speak with one voice on the issue of experimentation".[38]

The BBC covered both sides in the debate, yet the tendency was towards a more positive tone of addressing relevant issues as opposed to reacting against change that may weaken the status quo. On this occasion the BBC also informed readers that a decision would be made in Edinburgh in October. The story began to resemble the discussion in the medical literature, although a nuance between them was the mentioning of pharmaceutical companies in developed nations exploiting individuals in developing countries, rather than the juxtaposition of the stance between developed and developing nations.

On the whole, the media coverage of the proposed revisions in the period leading up to the Edinburgh meeting was limited. One media outlet which gave the story some coverage was *The Guardian* newspaper. Traditionally a liberal broadsheet, *The Guardian* did not develop an editorial policy on the subject, but did cover the debate unlike other press publications.[39] The paper highlighted the

---

33   Ibid.
34   Nixon (1998).
35   BBC (2000a).
36   Ibid.
37   BBC (2000b).
38   Ibid.
39   Although the newspaper did not develop an explicit editorial stance over the issue, the most likely position, according to the newspaper's Health Editor S. Boseley, would have been to

split within the scientific and medical communities, so readily apparent in the medical literature, using the views of Robert Levine to balance the views of "Public Citizen".[40] While *The Guardian* may have had no editorial policy, one piece on the eve of the Edinburgh meeting condemned the perceived attempt to "water down severely the Helsinki Declaration, removing what are seen in some quarters as undue 'restriction' on research".[41] Margaret Wertheim's article, which first appeared in *The Age* in Australia and was reproduced in *The Guardian*, set out how the issues could affect not only individuals but referred to the overall processes in which decisions were made:

> "The WMA is not the only body considering these issues. Moves are also afoot to amend the guidelines of the Council for International Organisations of Medical Sciences (CIOMS), which set out how the Helsinki Declaration should be implemented. CIOMS deliberations are being conducted in near secrecy, which is outrageous for a body charged with upholding an important ethical charter.
>
> It is bad enough that the vulnerable slave in sweat shops so that we might have cheap trainers. There can be no excuse for exploiting them medically so that we might have better drugs. When it comes to human health, justice must be our guiding principle".[42]

The article addressed the issue in line with discussions in the medical literature. The debate raging between medical professionals was largely absent from the mass media and seemingly represented an elite making decisions on behalf of individuals across the world. Within the context of the debate concerning exploitation and informed consent the issue was of far-reaching importance and a human interest story, but the process itself went largely unnoticed, despite its public relevance.

V. Ethics after Edinburgh: Reaction to the Revisions in the Medical Literature

Days after the Edinburgh meeting concluded, the research community was pondering the results. According to Anders Milton, the WMA had achieved its task of protecting people of developing nations, although, as we have seen, the public had not always been convinced that the aim was to strengthen rather than to weaken the protection of research subjects:

> "We have strengthened the position of participants in research, where we have made it much clearer than before that the population involved should benefit, studies should be done against the best proven method, and there should be access to the therapy at the end of the study".[43]

---

favour treatment on a par with that which would have been provided in the UK after research had ended; Boseley (2006).

40   Boseley (2006).
41   Wertheim (2000).
42   Ibid.
43   Christie (2000), p. 913.

The belief that greater clarity had been achieved in the Declaration was echoed by the author of the article, describing it as producing "much clearer terms than ever before the duty that doctors owe to participants in medical research".[44] However, unsurprisingly in the context of the prior debate, the outcome was less than universally welcomed as addressing all the problems of the Declaration.

Over a year after the Edinburgh meeting the *BMJ* asked four groups for their opinions about the fifth revisions to the Declaration of Helsinki, from "researchers working in the developing world, the developed world, and the pharmaceutical industry, as well as a patient representative".[45] The results of this microcosm of interested parties revealed an ongoing scepticism of the Declaration's universality. Furthermore, the views demonstrated the kaleidoscope of attitudes and colours of opinion which existed. A representative of the developing world cautioned that the poor standard of health provision in much of the world and in particular sub-Saharan Africa was "extraordinarily weak".[46] The intention to provide research communities in such regions with the best-proven method of treatment after a trial was potentially beyond the capabilities of that region. Other responses were likewise sceptical that much progress had been achieved. Hilda Bastian from the Cochrane Collaboration Consumer Network, Australia, seemingly representing patients, was not convinced by the new revisions. Bastian argued that the WMA document was inherently skewed against the interests of the individual patient:

> "When it was first created, and for many years subsequently, the declaration was a vital pioneer in setting and raising ethical standards in research. Nevertheless, the World Medical Association is a political organisation, representing some of the 'doers' of research only (and with no mandate to speak on behalf of the 'researched')".[47]

Without a direct mandate to speak on behalf of patients, Bastian argued, the WMA Declaration was inherently biased towards the interests of researchers. Even if this is not the case, the organisation might still lose credibility because of the public perception that it is. The contributors chosen by the *BMJ* concluded that the revised Declaration was unlikely to strengthen the rights of individuals:

> "Perhaps it is simply too much to hope for – that an organisation that does not share decision making with the community should be able to lead ethical development in a more democratised world. Yet, a meaningful role for the community in determining in what is essential to enhance people's health and their ability to exercise their rights is long overdue, both at a global and local level".[48]

This opinion reverberates with the previous suggestions of arrogance and a closed policy-making protocol. It is also reflected, to some extent, in the public media coverage and political debate on the issue. If the medical research community wanted to dispel this type of accusation, more work needed to be done to inform the public and raise the profile of deliberations in the eyes of politicians and

44   Ibid.
45   Anonymous (2001), p. 1417.
46   Tollman (2001), pp. 1417-1419.
47   Bastian (2001), p. 1419.
48   Ibid, p. 1421.

journalists. The public debate in the medical literature shines with democratic deliberations, yet this glow fades the closer it gets to the larger public domain and ultimately the individual. While many people may continue to place their trust in the medical research community, the failure to extend the message of the Declaration can harm its image and leave it open to criticism.

The other two groups approached for their opinion also had reservations. Sir Richard Doll of the Clinical Trial Service Unit and Epidemiological Studies Unit, Radcliff Infirmary, Oxford, bemoaned the fact that the revisions had been established without due consideration to the nature of the circumstances they were intended to apply to.[49] Laurence Hirsch and Harry Guess of Merck Research Laboratories held moderate reservations, especially regarding paragraphs 29 and 30, but were encouraged by the note of clarification of the former.[50] The support for clarification, however, demonstrated that the initial revisions were not particularly suited to this group. In another publication Robert Temple, Director of Medical Policy at the US Food and Drug Administration, reportedly referred to the ethics of the document as "bizarre".[51]

There was some support for the revisions in the public domain. The Association of Research Ethics Committees (AREC) appeared to embrace the changes and set about outlining how best to implement them.[52] The revisions were seen by Richard Nicholson, Chairman of Council, AREC, within the context of redressing the ethical imbalance in the pharmaceutical industry and making profit and power subordinate to the patient and ethical principles.[53] To this end the revised document was a welcome addition to combating the dominance of the drug companies over the industry as a whole. One letter to the *BMJ* initially echoed this positive reception, expressing delight for the new paragraph 29, but like many of the references cited thus far the drawbacks were quick to surface.[54] Concern about the modification turned away from the revisions themselves and focused upon potential further alterations induced by continued pressure from pharmaceutical companies to dilute the changes.[55] Attempting to reconcile the conflicted interests of the multitude of interested parties on a global scale was as problematic as the public debate prior to 2000 had intimated.

The influence of the FDA in pressuring the WMA into altering the Declaration of Helsinki had prompted Karin Michels and Kenneth Rothman in 2000 to write their piece on strengthening the guidelines.[56] In 2003, the two authors returned to the subject in the aftermath of the revisions.[57] Despite assertions from the WMA that the guidelines had been improved, the changes meant

---

49   Doll (2001), pp. 1421-1422.
50   Hirsch (2001), pp. 1422-1423.
51   American Society for Experimental Neuro Therapeutics (2001).
52   Nicholson (2001), pp. 5-7.
53   Ibid.
54   Bland (2002), p. 975.
55   Ibid.
56   Michels et al. (2000).
57   Michels/Rothman (2003), pp. 188-204.

little if they were not introduced. The FDA was, according to Michels and Rothman, still demanding placebo-controlled research evidence in violation of the Declaration of Helsinki.[58] In 2006, at the time of writing this article, the FDA position on accepting foreign clinical studies was clear:

> "In October 2000, the World Medical Association revised the Declaration. FDA has not taken action to incorporate those revisions into its regulations. FDA is making available this guidance document to clarify that the action of the World Medical Association did not change FDA regulations".[59]

As of 2006, the FDA still did not require such trials to conform to the 2000 edition of the Declaration and its guidance for Institutional Review Boards, Clinical Investigators and Sponsors, referred to the 1983 and 1989 versions.[60] Michels and Rothman's concerns over the FDA therefore continued. They also argued that the note of clarification added to the Declaration in October 2001 regarding paragraph 29 had clouded the issue of placebo trials and represented a backward step on the part of the WMA.[61] Thus, even after the debate and the revisions of the document, the 2000 version of the Declaration had still been unable to convince a disparate range of interested parties, a factor that diminishes the perception of the document as an international cornerstone of ethical research practice.

VI. Generating Public Interest with Human Interest

The clarifications added to the Declaration of Helsinki, paragraphs 29 and 30, had sought to deal with two of the major concerns of the public and those involved in research. As we have seen, this had not been entirely successful in resolving the discussions which preceded the revisions. After the 2000 meeting of the WMA the political discussion and media coverage of the revisions reflected the preceding discussion and is generally noticeable by its absence.

Media coverage was only stirred by the proposed clarification of paragraph 30 which was introduced in 2004, and then only on a small scale. *The Guardian* reported the proposed changes and allied it to the human interest element of the potential impact for developing nations and the distinction with current practice in the UK and US.[62] The footnotes to the Declaration were seen as tools for the pharmaceutical companies to weaken the brevity and strength of the document itself.

58 Ibid, p. 188.
59 Center for Drug Evaluation and Research. Guidance for Industry. Acceptance of Foreign Clinical Studies. www.fda.gov/cder/guidance/fstud.htm (accessed 4 August 2006).
60 FDA, Information Sheet Guidances. Guidance for Institutional Review Boards, Clinical Investigators, and Sponsors, http://www.fda.gov/oc/ohrt/irbs/default.htm (accessed 4 August 2006).
61 Michels/Rothman (2003), p. 190.
62 Boseley (2003).

The opposite side of the debate was reported by *The Daily Telegraph,* a newspaper editorially to the political right of *The Guardian.* The focus was the abundance of red tape that threatened to bind the hands of researchers from conducting their work and leading inevitably to the detriment of patient welfare.[63] However, the overall coverage of the Declaration itself and the ongoing debate hardly registered on the public interest barometer.

While the public exposure to, and perception of, the ongoing debate about the revisions did not transpose into the public domain, the Declaration of Helsinki had not been forgotten. The Declaration is ubiquitous in human-interest stories where medical ethics is called into question and whereby one part of society potentially suffers. In stories concerning "sham surgery" with patients' heads being drilled into, the Declaration is summoned and the breach by US organisations condemned by British experts.[64] The issue of protecting patient data is also discussed in relation to the ethical security of information in line with the Declaration's commitments to protect dignity and privacy.[65] Israel was said to have routinely flouted the Helsinki principles in a scandal over the use of vulnerable people as guinea pigs for medical research without the obligatory corresponding informed consent.[66] Throughout the media, the Helsinki Declaration continued to provide a reference point for medical ethics guidelines when discussing ethical issues in predominantly human-interest stories. While the discussions in the medical literature revealed the fissures in the debate about the revisions, the media presented a more solidified picture.

On the political front there was some debate about the implementation of the 2000 revisions. In an echo of the FDA position, commentators questioned why some legislation referred only to earlier versions of the Declaration. In one instance, during a standing committee on medicines for human use, it was alleged the 1996 version was cited so that placebo trials would be permissible.[67] This occurrence led one member of the committee to suggest as a consequence questions were being raised in the patient community.[68] Thus the inference here was that the public would be concerned that the government and medical researchers were choosing to ignore the 2000 revisions in order to relax the regulations surrounding it. This perception undermines the validity of the Declaration and questions the political determination to adhere to the most recent revisions. However, in general, the Declaration continues to be used as the reference point for medical ethics standards. In contrast to the ongoing discussions in the medical literature, the debate about the 2000 revisions made little impact in the wider public domain.

---

63   Highfield (2004).
64   Laurance (2000); see also Laurance (1999).
65   BBC (2001).
66   Butcher (2005).
67   Murrison (2004).
68   Harris (2004).

VII. Conclusion

The analysis of the coverage of the 2000 revision of the Declaration of Helsinki reveals a vibrant and at times heated discussion of the future of medical ethics and research. However, the debate never shaped the perception of the wider public despite the fact that the Declaration potentially influences the lives of humans across the globe. In this respect the public perception of medical ethics, as depicted through the media and parliament, cannot be said to have shifted significantly as a result of the revisions in 2000. The public voice of the discussion was heard within the professional literature but stayed largely within that sphere. Its impact on the wider world was minimal. However, in one respect, the result appears advantageous. Although the infighting and turmoil prior to the revisions has remained, it has largely evaded the wider public discourse. In this respect the solidity and uniformity of the Declaration remains intact. The focus of much media coverage on issues of the medical profession emphasises the human-interest elements of stories and utilises the Declaration as a reference. This usage demonstrates a level of trust in the validity of the document and ultimately the profession that conceived it. Indeed, trust is a key component of the relationship between the public and the medical profession and something that media coverage does reflect. In a YouGov poll for *The Daily Telegraph*, it was reported that two-thirds of respondents supported medical researchers using "spare" early embryos.[69] The poll was presented as demonstrating public backing for medical researchers to develop treatments for life-threatening diseases.[70] Furthermore, a study commissioned by The Royal Society in 2002 saw just 39 per cent of respondents agreeing that the media presented science in a "responsible" way, compared with 47 per cent disagreeing.[71] The MORI poll was possibly reflecting a public uncertainty about the capability of the national media to accurately reflect complex scientific issues. Unlike the media, the medical profession enjoys a relatively high level of public trust, with a 2001 poll revealing 89 per cent of those surveyed were convinced that their doctors were telling the truth.[72] The validity of opinion polls is debateable and these figures provide only a snapshot of opinion. However, a connection can be made between a willingness to defer to professional opinion and the regular invocation of the Declaration of Helsinki as a coherent and authoritative benchmark for global ethical practices.

The Declaration of Helsinki continues to be used as a cornerstone of medical ethics. Its ubiquitous presence in political and media discussions on all aspects of medical ethics requires a coherence and solidity to fulfil its function as a reassuring benchmark for ethics standards. Without this cohesion the Declaration might not have the same impact. This should not hide the ongoing difficulties in reconciling drug companies with researchers in developed and developing nations, but it

---

69   King (2005).
70   Ibid.
71   Royal Society (2002).
72   MORI (2001).

does mean that the public perception of the document is of a coherent and universal nature. Whether this is desirable remains open to debate.

References

American Society for Experimental Neuro Therapeutics (2001): Declaration of Helsinki Revised, NeuroRx Newsletter (March 2001).

Annonymous (2001): What are the Effects of the Fifth Revision of the Declaration of Helsinki?, British Medical Journal 323 (2001), 7326, pp. 1417-1423.

Ashbourne, E. (1999): House of Lords Hansard Text, 28 April 1999.

Bastian, H. (2001): Gains and Losses for Rights of Consumer and Research Participants, British Medical Journal 323 (2001), 7326, pp. 1419-1421.

BBC (2000a): Row over Medical Tests on Humans, BBC News Online, 4 May 2000.

BBC (2000b): Moves to Outlaw 'Unethical' Drug Trials, BBC News Online, 24 June 2000.

BBC (2001): Doctors Try to Guard Data, BBC News Online, 7 October 2001.

Bland, J. (2002): Clause 29 Forbids Trials from using Placebos when Effective Treatment Exists, British Medical Journal 324 (2002), 7343, p. 975.

Boseley, S. (2006): Correspondence with the Author, 4 July 2006.

Boseley, S. (2003): Unease at Plan to Alter Doctor's Ethical Code, The Guardian, 3 September 2003.

Boseley, S. (2000): Row over Drug Tests on Poor that Leave Some to Die, The Guardian, 4 May 2000.

Bratt, D. (1997): Doctors are Arrogant to Think that They Need to Debate Issue of Patient Consent, British Medical Journal 314 (1997), 7092, p. 1477.

Brennan, T. (1999): Proposed Revisions to the Declaration of Helsinki – Will they Weaken the Ethical Principles Underlying Human Research?, The New England Journal of Medicine 341 (1999), 7, pp. 527-531.

Butcher, T. (2005): Israeli Hospitals used Old and Mentally Infirm as Human Guinea Pigs, The Daily Telegraph, 10 May 2005.

Center for Drug Evaluation and Research: Guidance for Industry. Acceptance of Foreign Clinical Studies', http://www.fda.gov/cder/guidance/fstud.htm.

Christie, B. (2000): Doctors Revise Declaration of Helsinki, British Medical Journal 321 (2000), 7266, p. 913.

Doll, R. (2001): Research will be Impeded, British Medical Journal 323 (2001), 7326, pp. 1421-1422.

Donoughue, B. (1999): House of Lords Hansard Text, 26 January 1999.

Harris, E. (2004): Medicines for Human Use (Clinical Trials) Regulations 2004. House of Commons Standing Committee on Delegated Legislation Pt 3, Hansard, 25 May 2004.

Highfield, R. (2004): Rules 'Threaten Medical Research', The Daily Telegraph, 26 February 2004.

Hirsch, L./Guess, H. (2001): Some Clauses will Hinder Development of New Drugs and Vaccines, British Medical Journal 323 (2001), 7326, pp. 1422-1423.

Josefson, D. (1997): US Journal Attacks Unethical HIV Trials, British Medical Journal 315 (1997), 7111, pp. 763-766.

King, A. (2005): Most Britons back Embryo Research – but Draw the Line at Cloning Babies, The Daily Telegraph, 29 August 2006.

Lancet (1999): Declaration of Helsinki – Nothing to Declare? Lancet 353 (1999), 9161, p. 1285.

Lancet (2000): A Fifth Amendment for the Declaration of Helsinki, Lancet 356 (2000), 9236, p. 1123.

Laurance, J. (2000): Doctors seek Volunteers Who don't Mind being Given a Hole in the Head, The Independent, 8 February 2000.

Laurance, J. (1999): Doctors Drill into Patients' Heads in Placebo, The Independent, 29 September 1999.

Levine, R. (1999): The Need to Revise the Declaration of Helsinki, New England Journal of Medicine 341 (1999), 7, pp. 531-534.

Lurie, P. et al. (1997): Letter to the Department of HHS Concerning their Funding of Unethical Trials which Administer Placebos to HIV-Infected Pregnant Women through NIH and the Centers for Disease Control, Public Citizen, HRG Publication (1997), no. 1415. www.citizen.org/publications/release. cfm?ID=6612.

Michels, K./Rothman, K. (2003): Update on Unethical use of Placebos in Randomised Trials, Bioethics 17 (2003), 2, pp. 188-204.

Michels, K./Rothman, K./Baum, M. (2000): Declaration of Helsinki Should be Strengthened, British Medical Journal 321 (2000), 7258, pp. 442-445.

MORI (2001): Doctors Win Overwhelming Vote of Confidence from Public, 22 March 2001. www.mori.com/polls/2001/bma2001.shtml.

Murrison, A. (2004): Medicines for Human Use (Clinical Trials) Regulations 2004. House of Commons Standing Committee on Delegated Legislation Pt 1, Hansard, 25 May 2004.

Nicholson, R. (2001): Concerns and Frustrations of Research Ethics Committees, The Association of Research Ethics Committees Newsletter, 5 April 2001.

Nixon, R. (1998): Rabbits Give way to Human Guinea Pigs, BBC News Online, 16 November 1998.

Royal Society (2002): Full Results of the Royal Society's Survey for its National Forum on Science. www.royalsoc.ac.uk/page.asp?id=2014.

Schmidt, U. (2004): Justice at Nuremberg. Leo Alexander and the Nazi Doctors' Trial. Basingstoke: Palgrave.

Schmidt, U. (2006): Cold War at Porton Down: Informed Consent in Britain's Biological and Chemical Warfare Experiments during the Cold War, Cambridge Quarterly for Healthcare Ethics 15 (2006), 4, pp. 366-380.

Soames, N. (1997): House of Commons Hansard Written Answers, 13 January 1997.

Tollman, S. (2001): Fair Partnerships Support Ethical Research, British Medical Journal 323 (2001), 7326, pp. 1417-1419.

Wertheim, M. (2000): Medical Sweatshops: The Third World is Providing a Cheap Source of Subjects for Research into Aids and other Conditions, The Guardian Science Pages, 5 October 2000.

Willcox, D. (2006): Propaganda, the Press and Conflict. The Gulf War and Kosovo. London: Routledge.

Wilmshurst, P. (1997): Scientific Imperialism, British Medical Journal 314 (1997), 7084, p. 840.

Woodman, R. (1999): Storm Rages over Revisions, British Medical Journal 319 (1999), 7211, p. 660.

World Medical Association (2004): Declaration of Helsinki: Ethical Principles for Medical Research Involving Human Subjects. WMA.

World Medical Association (no date): Summary History of the World Medical Association Declaration of Helsinki. Recommendations Guiding Physicians in Biomedical Research involving Human Subjects. WMA.

Acknowledgements: I am grateful to Dr Ulf Schmidt, University of Kent, for his advice on the article. I am also grateful to Sarah Boseley, Health Editor of *The Guardian*, for responding to my questions on this subject.

Dominique Sprumont, Sara Girardin, Trudo Lemmens

The Helsinki Declaration and the Law:
An International and Comparative Analysis

I.   Introduction

The Declaration of Helsinki constitutes one of the cornerstones of medical research ethics. It remains the most referred to, if not revered, "code of ethics" at an international level. Indeed, it is a major achievement of the World Medical Association (WMA) to have provided the scientific and medical communities with a set of fundamental rules that have guided them in the conduct of research with human beings for over four decades.

The uniqueness and success of the Declaration of Helsinki is particularly striking in view of the fact that it is far from being the only document of reference at an international level in the field of biomedical research.[1] For instance, there are legal instruments of public international law such as the Nuremberg Code (1947), which largely inspired the authors of the Declaration of Helsinki, the 1966 United Nations Covenant on Civil and Political Rights (art. 7), and the Geneva Conventions (1949), which prohibit any type of human experimentation in time of war. In international law, there are also regional regulations such as the European Union directives on drug trials (directives 2001/20 and 2005/28), the 1997 Council of Europe Convention on Human Rights and Biomedicine, and its 2005 additional protocol on biomedical research. There are other guidance documents with a general scope at the international level. For example, the Council of International Organisations of Medical Sciences (CIOMS) issued its International Ethical Guidelines for Biomedical Research Involving Human Subjects in 1982, which were later revised in 1993 and 2002. There are also a variety of guidelines and other directives in the field of biomedical research that focus on a particular type of research. For instance, the International Conference on Harmonisation of Technical Requirements for Registration of Pharmaceuticals for Human Use (ICH) established rules with respect to clinical trials for pharmaceutical products. The 1996 ICH Good Clinical Practice: Consolidated Guideline (ICH-GCP) was later introduced in the regulations of the European Medicine Evaluation Agency (now called the European Medicines Agency or EMEA), the US Food and Drug Administration (FDA), and the Ministry of Health, Labour and Welfare in Japan. Health Canada gave it also the status of a "guidance document" in its regulatory

---

1   See Knoppers/Sprumont (2000), pp. 566-576.

framework surrounding drug approval. The CIOMS also has a directive on epidemiological studies, namely the 1991 International Guidelines for Ethical Review of Epidemiological Studies, currently under revision. Finally, there are specific guidelines in specific areas of medical practice, such as the World Psychiatric Association's 1996 Madrid Declaration on Ethical Standards for Psychiatric Practice, revised in 2002, or the International Federation of Sports Medicine's 1997 Code of Ethics. Again, these are only a few examples of the numerous guidelines that have been drafted since the second half the 20th century. In 1969, Jay Katz was among the first to question this situation:

> "Taking as a point of departure the ten "basic principles" set forth by the Nuremberg judges, numerous attempts have been made to propose "improved" codes of ethics to guide medical research. The proliferation of such codes testifies to the difficulty of promulgating a set of rules that does not immediately raise more questions than it answers. At this stage of our confusion, it is unlikely that codes will resolve many of the problems, though they may serve a useful function later. Even the much endorsed Declaration of Helsinki – praised, perhaps, because it is the newest and therefore the least examined – will create problems for those who wish to implement it".[2]

This comment appears particularly premonitory today, knowing that the Declaration has since been revised five times (1975, 1983, 1989, 1996, 2000), or even seven times – if one includes the two recently adopted notes of clarification (2002, 2004). The Declaration of Helsinki is therefore not only one among many international guidelines and research ethics documents, but there are also many versions of it. This raises a significant problem, because not everyone refers to the same version. This issue is recognised by the WMA itself, as reflected by this statement on the WMA website:

> "The current (2004) version [of the declaration of Helsinki] is the only official one; all previous versions have been replaced and should not be used or cited except for historical purposes".[3]

Yet, despite the explicit warning, few documents refer specifically to the most recent, 2004 version. In fact, as we will show, and contrary to our initial expectations, there are very few explicit references to the Declaration in the statutes and regulations of biomedical research at the national and international levels.

It would be beyond the scope of this chapter to cover all international law documents and regulations concerning research with human subjects, or to analyse in detail the national legislations.[4] We also do not intend to study all aspects of the reception of the Declaration of Helsinki in national law. We will not address, for instance, the role of the Declaration of Helsinki in case-law and other courts' or administrative bodies' decisions, even though this is an important issue for a better understanding of its legal value. The goal of this chapter is to present

---

2   Katz (1970), p. 295.
3   See www.wma.net/e/ethicsunit/helsinki.htm
4   For an overview see Human/Fluss (2001); see also Herranz (1998), pp. 127-139.

different procedures by which the Declaration of Helsinki is explicitly referred to in legislation. We will limit our presentation to statutes that are exemplary of the way in which the Declaration of Helsinki is introduced or included in different legal systems. We will focus our analysis on the EU and US drug regulation, as well as on the legislation dealing with human subjects research from Switzerland, Germany, France, the United Kingdom and Canada. Our main focus will be to identify how and to what extent the Declaration of Helsinki is embodied in those regulatory regimes, and what impact this may have on its legal nature. Prior to this international and comparative law analysis, we will propose a theoretical framework of the procedures by which the law can refer to codes of conduct or professional norms such as the Declaration of Helsinki.

II.   Delegation of Regulatory Power

II.1.   Rule of Law

II.1.1. Nature and Scope

Most States are governed today by the rule of law, at least in the civil law and common law systems. This fundamental legal principle has a double characteristic: the principle of legality (or legal certainty) and the principle of separation of powers. First, it requires official authority to act only in accordance with laws adopted through procedures laid down in the constitution and, second and corollary to the former principle, it imposes the separation of powers between the legislative, executive and judiciary branches of government. The rule of law, as noted by John Adams' famous statement in the constitution of the Commonwealth of Massachusetts, is "to the end it may be a government of laws and not of men".[5] Respect for the rule of law means the end of privileges and of the arbitrary exercise of governmental powers. It safeguards legal equality between all individuals, regardless of their origin, race, gender, age, social status, or their political or religious opinions.

The rule of law also draws the line between the legal order and other normative systems. Law helps to establish a crucial framework for society and strong means of enforcement are therefore at its disposal. John Rawls distinguishes the legal order from private relations in the following way:

> "What distinguishes a legal system is its comprehensive scope and its regulative powers with respect to other associations. The constitutional agencies that it defines generally have the exclusive legal right to at least the more extreme forms of coercion. The kind of duress that private associations can employ are strictly limited. Moereover, the legal order exercises a final authority over a certain well-defined territory. It is also marked by the wide range of the activities it regulates and the fundamental nature of the interests it is designed to secure.

5   Massachusetts Constitution, Part The First, art. XXX (1780).

These features simply reflect the fact that the law defines the basic structure within which the pursuit of all other activities takes place".[6]

In short, the rule of law dictates the primacy of the law in prescribing acceptable human behaviours in a given society over other, private rules such as social, professional, ethical, etc. It is the precondition for safeguarding equal liberty to all, preventing a group of individuals from imposing their will upon others outside the scope of the law. In that sense, the rule of law is often mentioned as the basic foundation of democracy and human rights even if, *per se*, it does not define the "justness" or "fairness" of the law or, in other words, to what extent the law respects the principle of justice.

II.1.2. Principle of Legality According to the European Court of Human Rights

The principle of legality implies that an individual right can be restricted or limited by the State only "in accordance with the law" or "to the extent prescribed by the law".[7] Such expressions are mentioned *expressis verbis* in the 1950 Council of Europe Convention for the Protection of Human Rights and Fundamental Freedoms. For instance, article 8 paragraph 2 of this convention concerning the "right to respect for private and family life" reads as follows:

> "There shall be no interference by a public authority with the exercise of this right except such as is *in accordance with the law* and is necessary in a democratic society in the interests of national security, public safety or the economic well-being of the country, for the prevention of disorder or crime, for the protection of health or morals, or for the protection of the rights and freedoms of others".[8]

For the European Court of Human Rights in Strasbourg, the term "law" "comprises statutory law as well as case-law and implies qualitative requirements, notably those of accessibility and foreseeability".[9] In Cantoni v. France, the Court expressed the opinion that "the scope of the concepts of foreseeability and accessibility depends to a considerable degree on the content of the instrument in issue, the field it is designed to cover and the number and status of those to whom it is addressed".[10] Thus, the impugned measures should have a basis in domestic

---

6   Rawls (1971), p. 236.
7   The word "law" can be interpreted in a formal sense – legal norms adopted by the legislature according to the rules set by the Constitution, or in a material sense as a synonym for the entire body of law. See, for instance, Inter-American Court of Human Rights, Advisory Opinion OC-6/86 of 9 May 1986, The Word "Laws" in Article 30 of the American Convention on Human Rights.
8   http://conventions.coe.int/Treaty/en/Treaties/Html/005.htm. [our emphasis].
9   Cantoni v. France, Judgment of 15 November 1996 of the European Court of Human Rights, in: Reports 1996-V, § 29.
10   Groppera Radio AG and Others v. Switzerland, Judgment of 28 March 1990 of the European Court of Human Rights, in: Series A n 173, § 68.

law. In particular, the accessibility of the law to the persons concerned requires, according to the Court, that the law is

> "formulated with sufficient precision to enable them – if need be, with appropriate legal advice – to foresee, to a degree that is reasonable in the circumstances, the consequences a given action may entail. A law which confers a discretion is not in itself inconsistent with this requirement, provided that the scope of the discretion and the manner of its exercise are indicated with sufficient clarity, having regard to the legitimate aim in question, to give the individual adequate protection against arbitrary interference".[11]

These requirements of foreseeability and preciseness define the regulatory power of the State when individual rights and liberties are at stake. Yet, the European Court of Human Rights admitted that, under certain circumstances, the law may refer to other sets of rules, for instance professional guidelines reflecting state-of-the-art practices, in particular when the field being regulated is technical in nature.[12] In the Groppera v. Switzerland judgment, the Court recognised that a Swiss Federal Council Ordinance relating to the Act governing correspondence by telegraph and telephone referred to provisions of the International Telecommunication Convention of 25 October 1973, that were published in the Official Collection of the Federal Statutes, and to the international Radio Regulations, as well to those international conventions and agreements concluded within the International Telecommunication Union that were not reproduced in the Official Collection. The applicants contested the validity of the references made in the Ordinance to those latest regulations that were not published in the Official Collection of the Federal Statutes. They argued that those documents were not readily available and that therefore reference to them was contrary to the principle of legality which required accessibility to the law by the persons concerned. Yet, the court pointed out that in this case

> "the relevant provisions of international telecommunications law were highly technical and complex; furthermore, they were primarily intended for specialists, who knew, from the information given in the Official Collection, how they could be obtained ... In short, the rules in issue were such as to enable the applicants and their advisers to regulate their conduct in the matter".[13]

The relevance of this case in assessing the possibility of referring to the declaration of Helsinki in a statute is that it recognises the competency of the legislature to leave some aspects of the legislation to be covered by rules that are not directly linked to the law in question, that were adopted in a different setting, and that may not need to be reproduced in extenso in that law. Such reference corresponds in legal terms to a delegation of regulatory power to a third party, generally a professional body or a public or private institution recognised for its technical or scientific expertise in a given field.

---

11 Tolstoy Miloslavsky v. the United Kingdom, Judgment of 13 July 1995 of the European Court of Human Rights, in: Series A n 316-B, § 37.

12 ATF 123 I 112, 129.

13 Groppera Radio AG and Others v. Switzerland, Judgment of 28 March 1990 of the European Court of Human Rights, in: Series A n 173, § 68.

II.1.3. Principle of Legal Certainty According to the Court of Justice of the European Communities

The Court of Justice of the European Communities, in exercising its jurisdiction under the Treaties, is strongly influenced by the general principles of community law[14], including that of legal certainty, which "expresses the fundamental premise that those subject to the law must know what the law is so as to be able to plan their actions accordingly".[15] The principle of legal certainty requires that "legal rules be clear and precise, and aims to ensure that the situations and legal relationships governed by community law remain foreseeable".[16] This concept is close to that of the principle of legality recognised by the European Court of Justice as developed above in Section II.1.2. It includes both the requirements of accessibility and foreseeability.

The principle of legal certainty has to be respected not only by the institutions of the Community, but also by the member states.[17] In Commission v. Italy, the Court pointed out that

> "the principles of legal certainty and the protection of individuals require, in areas covered by community law, that the Member States' legal rules should be worded unequivocally so as to give the persons concerned a clear and precise understanding of their rights and obligations and enable the national courts to ensure that those rights and obligations are observed".[18]

The court often recalled that when member states implement the directives into the internal juridical order, they must implement them "in a way which fully meets the requirements of clarity and certainty in legal situations which directives seek [...]".[19] Moreover, member states cannot put forward the jurisdiction of regional authorities in a particular area to defend themselves against the claim that the national legislation does not respect the prohibitions that a directive foresees.[20]

---

14   Arnull (1999), p. 190.
15   Takis (1999), p. 163.
16   Duff and Others v. Minister for Agriculture and Food and the Attorney General (Ireland), Judgment of 15 February 1996 of the Court of Justice of the European Communities, case C-63/93, in: European Court Reports 1996, p. 569, para. 20.
17   Papadopoulou (1996), p. 204.
18   Commission of the European Communities v. Italian Republic, Judgment of 21 June 1988 of the Court of Justice of the European Communities, Case 257/86, in: European Court Reports 1988, p. 3249, para. 12.
19   Commission of the European Communities v. Kingdom of Belgium, Judgement of 8 May 1980 of the Court of Justice of the European Communities, Case 102/79, in: European Court Reports 1980, p. 1473.
20   Commission of the European Communities v. Italian Republic, Judgment of 17 January 1991 of the Court of Justice of the European Communities, Case C 157/89, in: European Court Reports 1991, p. 57.

Nevertheless, in a judgment of 18 May 1989[21], the Court of Justice of the European Communities recognised the normative character of deontological rules, characterising them as "measures".[22] Even if measures cannot be considered as legislation or regulation *stricto sensu*, they are rules created by the public authorities or by professional bodies which, in this case, subordinate the marketing of products to specific technical requirements[23] and have a binding effect. Answering the questions submitted to it by the Court of Appeal of England and Wales, the Court said:

> "Measures adopted by a professional body for pharmacy, in whose register all pharmacists must be enrolled in order to carry on their business, which lays down rules of ethics applicable to the members of the profession and which has a committee upon which national legislation has conferred disciplinary powers that could involve the removal from the said register, may, if they are capable of affecting trade between the Member States, constitute "measures" within the meaning of Article 30[24] of the EEC Treaty".[25]

Again, this is an issue of delegation of regulatory and even disciplinary power to a professional body, as opposed to an official authority directly dependent on or part of the government. The legislature is thus authorised to delegate some of its power to a third party.

II.2.   Theoretical Models in the Legislation

As discussed, the rule of law allows for some flexibility, perhaps even some exceptions. The legislature may under specific circumstances delegate some regulatory power to professional bodies or a group of experts, especially when the field to be regulated is technical in nature or presents a high level of complexity. It would be practically impossible, both in terms of resources and expertise, for the government to adopt detailed legislation in every domain, taking into account all the interests at stake and keeping abreast of all the latest technological innovations. This is true, as we have just shown, in the area of telecommunication. This is arguably also the case in the field of biomedicine and biotechnology. For the State to impose detailed legislation could prove to be a barrier to medical progress without necessarily improving the protection of the human dignity and rights of the human subjects involved. Thus, the delegation of regulatory power

---

21   The Queen v. Royal Pharmaceutical Society of Great Britain, ex parte Association of Pharmaceutical Importers and others, Judgment of 18 May 1989 of the Court of Justice of the European Communities, joined cases 266 and 267/87, in: European Court Reports 1989, p. 1295.
22   Gérard (1992), p. 763.
23   Louis (1989), n. 306.
24   Ex art. 30 EEC Treaty = new art. 28 EC Treaty.
25   The Queen v. Royal Pharmaceutical Society of Great Britain, ex parte Association of Pharmaceutical Importers and others, Judgment of 18 May 1989 of the Court of Justice of the European Communities, joined cases 266 and 267/87, in: European Court Reports 1989, p. 1295.

appears as a compromise between, on one hand, the protection of the interests and fundamental rights and liberties at stake, and, on the other hand, the practicability of the law, its efficiency to respond to the needs of the various actors involved in the regulated activity or domain.

The procedure of delegation of powers depends primarily on national legislation, in particular constitutional law. It would be beyond the scope of this chapter to present in detail how this procedure is applied in national law. At this stage, our objective is only to propose a theoretical framework on which we will base our international and comparative law analysis. This short presentation is largely based on the Swiss legal system, but we are confident that our conclusion can be generalised to other legal systems such that of the Council of Europe or the European Union mentioned in Section II.1 as well as to legal systems outside Europe.

A reference to the declaration of Helsinki can take several forms. We should first distinguish *direct* from *indirect references*. We will speak about a direct reference only when the law explicitly mentions the Declaration of Helsinki. By contrast, an indirect reference would apply to cases where the law only mentions the guidelines of the WMA on research without specifying which one, or refers in general to the fundamental principles of research ethics as recognised by the medical profession. As we have seen, there are numerous relevant documents concerning biomedical research at the international level. An indirect reference to them is only an indication that such documents exist. This has no other legal impact but to invite the investigators to respect the general rules of medical research ethics and to act with due care according to the state-of-the-art. It is a reminder of their professional obligations.

Concerning direct references, an important distinction should be drawn between the static ones and the dynamic ones. One speaks of a *static reference* when the law mentions, for instance, the 1996 or the 2000 version of the Declaration of Helsinki, while a *dynamic reference* designates cases where the legislature refers to the Declaration without specifying which version, or refers to the latest version of the Declaration. This model of dynamic reference to the Declaration raises a question of delegation of power in connection with the rule of law.

A hypothetical example could help to illustrate this concern. The forthcoming Swiss federal law on research involving human subjects could refer to "the latest version of the Declaration of Helsinki for all questions not directly dealt with in the law". In principle, this would mean that the Swiss parliament recognises the authority of the WMA to revise the Declaration and that such revision will automatically be introduced in the law. After the law is adopted and enters into force, the WMA could, for instance, decide to modify paragraph 22 of the declaration concerning the subject's right of information by removing the following sentence:

> "The subject should be informed of the right to abstain from participation in the study or to withdraw consent to participate at any time without reprisal".

If the law does not explicitly address the issue of the information to be provided to potential volunteers concerning their freedom not to participate in research or to withdraw from it, the amendment of the declaration could mean that the investigator would no longer be bound to provide the subject with this essential information. Yet such an amendment, in order to be valid within the Swiss legal system, would need to respect the rule of law and, in particular, the principle of legality.

Two main legal arguments could be raised in this case to reject the notion of dynamic reference to the Declaration of Helsinki. First, the freedom of the research subject not to participate in a project or to withdraw from it is a fundamental right. As such, it can be restricted only in accordance with the law, namely statutory law or case-law. The more severe the restriction of the individual right or liberty at stake, the more restrictively this requirement should be interpreted. The hypothetical amendment of the Declaration of Helsinki would not meet the formal criteria of the principle of legality as it would not be adopted according to the rules established in constitutional law. Second, there is an issue of foreseeability of the law and of legal certainty. If the rights of the research subjects could be altered by future amendments of the Declaration, it would deprive the concerned persons of a clear and precise understanding of their rights and obligations under Swiss law. It would also be a violation of the principle of legality. Either way, the degree of protection of the rights and welfare of the research subjects would be reduced.

Another approach would be to argue that the right to refuse participating in a research project or to withdraw from it is indeed a fundamental right rooted in the constitution in general and in the personality rights of every individual. The mere fact that the Declaration of Helsinki does not make an explicit reference to that right is not *per se* relevant for the recognition of that right. In that sense, it means that the Declaration does not in itself provide a broader and wider protection to the human subjects compared to the level of protection granted by the legal system in general. This brings us back to Jay Katz's opinion on the limits of the Declaration of Helsinki.[26] The Declaration appears indeed as nothing more than a guidance document without direct legal impact on the responsibilities of the investigator and the rights of the human research subjects.

To conclude our discussion of the legal validity of how legislators refer to the Declaration of Helsinki in the law, it is important to point out that we have not yet found a single instance where the procedure of dynamic reference has been used at the legislative level. There are also only few examples of indirect reference to the Declaration in legislation or regulation, particularly those instances where the ICH-GCP has been incorporated into the drug regulation of specific countries. This finding is not surprising in view of the above-mentioned requirements concerning the delegation of regulatory power as imposed by the rule of law. It is certainly an important element to be taken into account by the WMA when

26   See Katz (1970), p. 295.

revising the Declaration. Such amendments are unlikely to be implemented, at least at the legislative level, prior to a careful assessment of their potential legal consequences. This is directly linked to the rule of law and the corollary need to respect the principles of legality and legal equality. A systematic implementation of the latest version of the Declaration would mean a delegation of regulatory power to the WMA that is not only outside the authority of the legislature itself, but may not even be in the best interests of the WMA itself.

III.   International and Comparative Law Analysis

In this Section, we will review the regulations of different jurisdictions, more specifically the EU and US drug regulations as well as the legislative and regulatory provisions regarding research subjects in Switzerland, Germany, France, the United Kingdom and Canada. In each case, we have looked for direct references to the Declaration in relevant regulations, statutes or guiding documents on research ethics. We focused our overview in the first place on more formal sources of law, namely the acts adopted by the legislature as well as regulations emanating from the regulatory authorities that received a legal mandate to deal with issues of human subjects research. When we did not find any such reference in the official register or collection of the legislation, we looked in the professional rules to the extent that they are included in the legislation under a delegation of power, such as in France, Germany and the UK. In such cases, we also assessed how professional bodies are entitled to regulatory or disciplinary powers. Finally, in one country, Canada, the most important sources of rule-making in the context of human subjects research are neither statute-based, nor based on professional regulations. The research ethics rules are primarily emanating from funding agencies or are based on guidance documents adopted by the drug regulatory agencies. In that case, we looked into these documents for references to the Declaration of Helsinki.

We will first analyse the EU and US drug regulations, together with the ICH-GCP, as they play an important role in the overall regulation of biomedical research worldwide. By fixing the standards for clinical trials of medical products for human use, this regulation has a direct influence on all other research regulation, not only due to the globalisation of drug trials, but also because of its industrialisation. Any investigator doing research in the world must at least pay attention to this regulation if their research concerns a product likely to be marketed in the EU or the US, which are the biggest markets in the world. This creates a clear incentive to act accordingly. As we will also see, the legislation of biomedical research at the national level is usually associated with the regulations related to clinical drug trials.

III.1.   EU and US drug regulation

III.1.1. EU Directive 2001/20 and 2005/28

On 4 April 2000, the European Parliament and the Council adopted the directive 2001/20/EC on the approximation of the laws, regulations and administrative provisions of the Member States relating to the implementation of good clinical practice in the conduct of clinical trials on medicinal products for human use.[27] The scope of this directive covers all clinical trials of medicinal products for human use carried out in one or several member states of the European Union. It is meant to harmonise the implementation of Good Clinical Practice in the conduct of drug trials within the European Union. Directive 2001/20/EC has recently been completed by the new Commission Directive 2005/28/EC of 8 April 2005, laying down principles and detailed guidelines for good clinical practice as regards investigational medicinal products for human use, as well as the requirements for authorisation of the manufacturing or importation of such products.[28]

Paragraph 2 of the directive 2001/20 preamble explicitly refers to the Declaration of Helsinki. It reads as follow:

> "The accepted basis for the conduct of clinical trials in humans is founded in the protection of human rights and the dignity of the human being with regard to the application of biology and medicine, as for instance reflected in the 1996 version of the Helsinki Declaration".[29]

The preamble of a directive does not have a normative or binding power as such. It does not fall under the definition of a "legal provision". This reference to the Declaration remains more a political statement, a reminder of the fact that the Commission did not intend to deviate from the Declaration of Helsinki in its regulation on drug trials. Directive 2005/28 contains a more effective reference to the Declaration. In fact, article 3 paragraph 2 of that directive states clearly that:

> "Clinical trials shall be conducted in accordance with the Declaration of Helsinki on Ethical Principles for Medical Research Involving Human Subjects, adopted by the General Assembly of the World Medical Association (1996)".

This constitutes a direct static reference to the Declaration.[30] There is no doubt that it is valid according to the case-law of the Court of Justice of the European Communities[31] and to the general requirements of the rule of law as developed in Section II.1 above. Yet, it remains rather a symbolic gesture of the Commission, since both directives appear to be more detailed, and sometimes more stringent concerning the protection of human subjects, the responsibilities of the investigator and the sponsor, the authority of the Research Ethics Committee

---

27 OJ L 121, 1.5.2001, p. 34.
28 OJ L 91, 9.4.2005, p. 13.
29 OJ L 121, 1.5.2001, p. 34.
30 See chapter II.2.
31 See chapter II.1.3.

reviewing all research protocols, etc., than the Declaration of Helsinki. The references made here tend rather to confirm that the Declaration of Helsinki is a minimum standard. This is substantiated in Annex 1 of the Commission's Directive 2003/63/EC of 25 June 2003, amending Directive 2001/83/EC of the European Parliament and of the Council on the Community code relating to medicinal products for human use.[32] Paragraph 8 of Annex 1 of this directive recalls first that "all clinical trials, conducted within the European Community, must comply with the requirements of Directive 2001/20". Concerning "clinical trials, conducted outside the European Community, which relate to medicinal products intended to be used in the European Community", the Commission adds that they "shall be designed, implemented and reported on what good clinical practice and ethical principles are concerned, on the basis of principles, *which are equivalent to the provisions of Directive 2001/20/EC*. They shall be carried out in accordance with the ethical principles that are reflected, for example, in the Declaration of Helsinki".[33] This is an indirect reference to the Declaration of Helsinki, as the text emphasises the ethical principles of research ethics rather than the Declaration itself, which is cited as only an example of a document that reflects core ethical principles. The Declaration appears as a minimum standard, the main standard remaining Directive 2001/20.

Concerning the references in Directives 2001/20 and 2005/28, one cannot help noticing that they mention explicitly the 1996 version of the Declaration even though those two directives were adopted after the major 2000 revision. Most likely, this can be explained in view of the ICH-GCP having been finalised in July 1996. Paragraph 2.1 of its introductory chapter, entitled "The principles of ICH-GCP", states that:

> "Clinical trials should be conducted in accordance with the ethical principles that have their origin in the Declaration of Helsinki, and that are consistent with GCP and the applicable regulatory requirement(s)".

This reference to the Declaration of Helsinki is completed in appendix G of the ICH-GCP which reproduces *in extenso* its 1996 version. This is of particular importance, as the ICH-GCP has been formally incorporated into the drug regulations of the EU, the US FDA and the Ministry of Health, Labour and Welfare in Japan.[34] For the European Union to refer to the latest or simply a more recent version of the Declaration, for instance the 2000 version, would mean to depart from the ICH-GCP and thus create legal uncertainty, contrary to the very aim of the ICH-GCP. Indeed, the ICH-GCP's goal was to provide a harmonised standard for drug trials at the international level.

---

32   O.J. L. 159, 27.06.2003, p. 46.
33   O.J. L. 159, 27.06.2003, p. 46.
34   See Sprumont (1999), pp. 25-43.

III.1.2. US Drug Regulation

As we have already mentioned, the US FDA has formally included the ICH-GCP in its regulation by publishing it in the Federal Register.[35] Thus, the ICH-GCP gained some legal authority under American law. Concerning the Declaration of Helsinki, the situation is close to that in the EU drug regulation. There is a direct static reference to the 1996 version. Yet, this is not the only reference that can be found in the US regulations.

In the USA, the existing standards for the ethical treatment of human research have been embodied in federal regulations known officially as the "Federal Policy for the Protection of Human Subjects of Research" but generally referred to as the "Common Rule" adopted on 18 June 1991.[36] The Common Rule has been promulgated in regulations by fifteen federal departments and agencies and applies to all research funded by these departments and agencies and all research conducted in institutions that accept funding from these agencies. Even the Central Intelligence Agency must comply with all subparts of 45 CFR part 46 under Executive Order 12333. The Common Rule establishes a comprehensive framework for the review and conduct of proposed human research to ensure that it will be performed ethically. Like the EU directive 2003/63, the US Common Rule includes provisions concerning research conducted in foreign countries, namely outside the USA. According to 45 CFR 46.101:

> "(h) When research covered by this policy takes place in foreign countries, procedures normally followed in the foreign countries to protect human subjects may differ from those set forth in this policy. [An example is a foreign institution which complies with guidelines consistent with the World Medical Assembly Declaration (Declaration of Helsinki amended 1989) issued either by sovereign states or by an organisation whose function for the protection of human research subjects is internationally recognised.] In these circumstances, if a department or agency head determines that the procedures prescribed by the institution afford protections that *are at least equivalent to those provided in this policy*, the department or agency head may approve the substitution of the foreign procedures in lieu of the procedural requirements provided in this policy". [our emphasis]

As in the EU directive, the focal point remains the "Common Rule", not the Declaration. The requirement is to evaluate the foreign guidelines followed by the investigator compared to the Common Rule, the Declaration of Helsinki being only mentioned as a minimum standard. Such a provision has also been integrated into the FDA regulation. Title 21 (Food and Drugs) includes a Part 312 (Investigational New Drug Application) which prescribes that:

> "1) Foreign clinical research is required to have been conducted in accordance with the ethical principles stated in the 'Declaration of Helsinki" (see paragraph (c) (4) of this section)

---

35 International Conference on Harmonisation; Good Clinical Practice: Consolidated Guideline; Availability. Food and Drug Administration, Department of Health and Human Services. Federal Register, vol. 62, no. 90, Friday, 9 May 1997, pp. 25691-25709.

36 See i.e. 45 CFR 46 Protection of Human Subjects: Subpart A, Basic HHS Policy for Protection of Human Research Subjects.

or the laws and regulations of the country in which the research was conducted, *whichever represents the greater protection of the individual*".[37]

The full text of the 1989 version of the Declaration of Helsinki is reproduced in the paragraph (c) (4) mentioned in the provision.

What is interesting is that the Common Rule refers to the 1989 version, while the ICH-GCP, which is also part of the FDA regulation, but applies in the context of clinical trials conducted in the context of drug approval, mentions the 1996 version. This could create a legal uncertainty if the regulation does not provide guidance to solve potential conflict between the two versions. As we emphasised in the quotation of 21 CFR 312.120, the applicable rules should be the ones that represent "the greater protection of the individual". This can only be assessed case by case, not only in light of the diverging versions of the Declaration of Helsinki but also of the laws and regulations of the country in which the research is conducted. Paradoxically, this could lead to the application of the latest version of the Declaration, if it is the rule of reference in the country in question and it proves to provide more protection to human subjects.

III.2.　Switzerland

There is presently no direct reference to the Declaration of Helsinki in the federal and cantonal laws of Switzerland, with only one exception: the Federal Law on Therapeutic Products (LTP) of 15 December 2000. According to article 53, paragraph 2 LTP:

> "The Federal Council shall specify the recognised principles of good clinical practice. In particular, it shall lay down the obligations to which the investigator and the sponsor are subject and shall adopt provisions concerning the control procedure. *In doing so, it shall take account of internationally recognised guidelines and standards*".[38]

The Federal Council, in other words, the government, did so by adopting the Ordinance on clinical trials of therapeutic products (OClin) of 17 October 2001. Concerning the international directives to follow, article 4 OClin specifies that:

> "Clinical trials for medicines must conform with the ICH (International Conference on Harmonisation) Guideline for Good Clinical Practice, version of 1 May 1996".[39]

Indirectly, this static reference to the ICH-GCP should be understood as a reference to the 1996 version of the Helsinki Declaration. In that sense, the situation in the Swiss law is similar to the one in the EU and the US concerning drug trials.

37　21 CFR 312.120 (Foreign clinical studies not conducted under an IND) [our emphasis].
38　RS 812.21 [our emphasis]. An English version of this law is available on the website of Swissmedic (the Swiss Agency for Therapeutic Products): www.swissmedic.ch/files/pdf/ HMG_English_New_version. pdf.
39　RS 812.214.2. An English version of this law is available on the website of Swissmedic (the Swiss Drug Agency): www.swissmedic.ch/files/pdf/VKlin%20_e_%202005-03-14.pdf.

There is a direct reference to the Declaration of Helsinki in the code of ethics of the Swiss Medical Association (FMH), a private association defending the interests of the physicians at the national level. Contrary to the situation i.e. in Germany, France or the United Kingdom, but similar to Canada, the FMH does not have regulatory or disciplinary powers over the medical profession. Its rules apply exclusively to its members, and a Swiss physician remains free to join or not to join this private association. In particular, the affiliation to the FMH is not a requirement for the practice of medicine, as professional law is a competency of the cantonal authorities, not the FMH. Nevertheless, it is interesting to point out that concerning biomedical research, article 18 of the code of ethics of the FMH, last revised on 30 April 2003, makes a direct reference to the 2000 version of the Declaration of Helsinki, which is reproduced in annex 1 of the code. This is of particular importance since, in other domains that raise serious ethical dilemmas – such as organ transplants, sterilisation of mentally impaired persons, medically assisted reproduction, genetics, end-of-life decisions, etc. – article 18 of the FMH code of ethics refers systematically to relevant guidelines adopted by the Swiss Academy of Medical Science. Yet, even though the Swiss Academy of Medical Sciences has also adopted in 1997 a guideline on biomedical research, the FMH chooses explicitly not to refer to this research ethics guideline, but instead requires its members to act according to the 2000 version of the Declaration of Helsinki. This example shows diverging opinions within the medical profession in relation to what should be regarded as the standards for the protection of research subjects. This situation is not unique. In fact, it is unavoidable in view of the numerous versions of the Declaration, but also in light of the existence of so many other guidance documents in the field of biomedical research at the national and international level.

Yet, concerning Swiss law, the fact that the FMH code of ethics refers to the 2000 version is not only an issue of controversy within the medical profession. It also raises a problem of conflict of norms. On the one hand, a physician should follow the 2000 version according to his professional rules, while, on the other hand, he is obliged to comply with the 1996 version as required by the drug regulation. This may prove problematic if the two versions differ radically on specific issues.

III.3. Germany

The situation in Germany with respect to the impact of the Declaration of Helsinki is rather similar to that in Switzerland. There is no explicit reference to the Declaration of Helsinki in the law. Yet, since Germany is member of the European Union, it should comply with EU legislation. This includes the EU directives on clinical trials which we analysed in Section III.1.1. There is therefore an indirect reference to the 1996 version of the Declaration of Helsinki in article 40 of the Federal Law on Therapeutic Products (*Arzneimittelgesetz*, AMG)[40] as it mentions the EU directive 2001/20.

There are also references to the Declaration of Helsinki in the codes of ethics of some Medical Associations of Federal States (*Länder*), or "Medical Chambers" (*Ärztekammern*). The Federal States' Medical Associations are public-law corporations. Every doctor has to be a member of their regional association as a requirement to practice their profession.[41] Among other tasks, the *Länder*'s Medical Associations have the power – delegated by the laws of the medical profession of the *Länder* – to adopt regulations (*Satzungen*) on specific topics, such as the code of deontology and the code of continuing education.[42] The code of deontology defines what the doctor must respect in the exercise of his profession and what he must refrain from doing to prevent disciplinary sanctions.[43] Those codes need approval from the professional regulatory authorities to become legally binding. This authorisation procedure permits the *Länder* to ensure their sovereignty in controlling which medical professional duties are established by the Chambers.[44] For the Constitutional Court,[45] the regulatory power of the *Länder*'s Medical Associations is limited by the Constitutional order. The legislature cannot completely abandon its legislative power, especially in controlling the rules enacted by the Medical Associations. Fundamentally, only rules that are internal to the medical profession can have their source in the regulatory power of the Chambers.[46]

Besides the Federal States Medical Associations, the German Medical Association (*Bundesärztekammer*) is the central body of the self-regulatory system of the German medical profession. This private law association includes the seventeen Medical Associations of the *Länder*. It plays an active role in the opinion-forming process in relation to health policy in society, and in legislative procedures.[47] Among other tasks, it adopts model regulations (such as the model professional code, and model post-graduate training regulations) that are then introduced (without or with small modifications) in the legal framework of the *Länder*. Some federal laws also give explicitly a regulatory power to the German Medical Association to draft binding medical guidelines. Such delegation of regulatory authority is, for instance, mentioned in the Act regulating transfusion practice (*Transfusionsgesetz*, TFG) (§ 18) and in the Act on donation, removal and transmission of organs (*Transplantationsgesetz*, TPG) (§ 16). Finally the German Medical Association has promulgated several medical ethics guidelines on its own initiative, guidelines that complete the codes of deontology of the

40   www.bundesrecht.juris.de/amg_1976/BJNR024480976.html.
41   Hamann/Fenger (2004), p. 171.
42   Laufs/Uhlenbruck (1999), p. 52.
43   Ibid.
44   Vesting (1998), p. 169.
45   Beschluss des Bundesverfassungsgerichts (1972), p. 1506.
46   Vesting (1998), p.170; Laufs/Uhlenbruck (1999), pp. 52-53.
47   See the website of the German Medical Association: www.bundesaerztekammer.de

Federal States Medical Associations.[48] Those guidelines have an important role in practice,[49] but their legal force is controversial.

As a private-law association, the German Medical Association does not have a regulatory power. As we have seen, however, some federal laws delegate to the German Medical Association the duty to enact guidelines that can become binding based on this delegation. In other cases, the guidelines can be included in the Federal States Medical Associations' regulations. For some authors[50], the fact that a guideline of the German Medical Association is embedded into a local guideline gives it binding legal force. The guidelines can also be attached as annex to the code of deontology (*Satzung*).[51] Through the approval mechanism by the regulatory authority, the guidelines adopted by the Chamber become binding documents. By contrast, Laufs argues that[52], even if a code of deontology of a Chamber refers to a guideline, this guideline does not acquire the status of regulation (*Satzung*), because the Chamber may not have explicitly taken a position on the document and, in fact, may even ignore its existence. In other words, Laufs rejects in principle the possibility of an explicit dynamic reference to a guideline of the German Medical Association. Fuchs[53] considers that, in any case, the guidelines of the Federal States Medical Associations should be legally binding for the physicians. In his view, this is the only way to show society that the medical profession is entitled to identify ethical issues in medical practice and to elaborate the necessary framework to deal with them. The guidelines of the German Medical Association can, in any case, be considered as standards of good medical practice, whether they are later adopted by the regional Medical Associations or not.

The code of deontology (*Musterberufsordnung*) of the German Medical Association used to make a direct reference to the Declaration of Helsinki in article 15, paragraph 2. For a long time, this was not problematic until the Helsinki Declaration was revised in 2000. This revision of the Declaration created heated debate and controversy in the medical profession. While the reference to the Declaration in the code of deontology was usually to the latest version, the introduction of the 2000 revision was rejected during the 105th session of the German medical assembly (*Ärztetag*), which is composed of 250 delegates from the seventeen Federal States Medical Associations and acts as the parliament of the association. At the time, the *Ärztetag* decided to make no reference to the Declaration of Helsinki any longer. One year later, the decision was partially

---

48 Christoph Fuchs and Thomas Gerst, Medizinethik in der Berufsordnung, in: www.bundes aerztekammer.de/30/Berufsordnung/15Ethik/index.html.
49 Laufs/Uhlenbruck (1999), p. 54.
50 Vesting (1998), p. 169; Bachmann/Heerklotz (1994), p. A587.
51 For example in the code of deontology of the Baden-Württemberger Ärztekammer: www. aerztekammer-bw.de/20/arztrecht/05kammerrecht/bo.pdf.
52 Laufs/Uhlenbruck (1999), p. 54.
53 Christoph Fuchs and Thomas Gerst, Medizinethik in der Berufsordnung, in: www.bundes aerztekammer.de/30/Berufsordnung/15Ethik/index.html.

reversed. The solution, which was finally accepted in 2003, and which remains in place today, was to adopt a new paragraph 4 of article 15 which reads as follows:

> "Physicians observe in the conduct of research involving human subjects the ethical principles of research with human being laid down in the Helsinki Declaration of the World Medical Association".[54] (translated by the authors)

On the website of the German Medical Association, there is a translation of the 2004 version of the Declaration.[55] It is therefore likely that the code of deontology refers to this latest version. Yet, a recent and very informative paper by Christoph Richter and Roswitha Bussar-Maatz, concerning the implementation of the Declaration of Helsinki in Germany, shows that there are serious differences in the way this document is referred to in the seventeen Federal States Medical Associations.[56] In Bayern, Berlin, Brandenburg, Mecklenburg-Vorpommern, Nordrhein-Westfalen and Rheinland-Pfalz, codes of deontology refer to the 1996 version, while in Baden-Württemberg and Bremen the reference is made without mentioning a specific version. In the nine other Länder, there is no reference to the Declaration in the codes of deontology. The author of the paper, Elmar Doppelfeld, chairman of the Working Group on Medical Ethics Committees in the Federal Republic of Germany (*Arbeitskreis Medizinischer Ethik-Kommissionen in der Bundesrepublik Deutschland*),[57] considers the reference to the Declaration in the present German Medical Association code of deontology unclear, and therefore void. The diverging opinion in the German medical profession is even more striking if one looks at the practice of the Research Ethics Committees (REGs). In the same paper, Richter and Bussar-Maatz provide the results of a questionnaire which they sent to fifty-six RECs in Germany. Of the forty-seven answers which they received, twenty-seven (57 per cent) mentioned that they refer to the 1996 version, and fifteen (31 per cent) that they follow the 2000 version. One REC worked with both version, and two refer to the 2000 version including the 2002 note of clarification. Two answers were unclear and one REC also mentioned that it is considering going back to the 1996 version. Not surprisingly, the authors called for a harmonisation of the RECs' practice as well as the Federal States Medical Associations code of deontology. This seems even more important as there is a discrepancy between the requirement of the drug regulation to adhere to the 1996 version of the Declaration of Helsinki and the fact that the majority of the RECs claim they follow the 2000 or other versions. The problem is more delicate than in Switzerland, as the Federal States Medical Associations' code of deontology has some legally binding force. In Germany, it may prove difficult to define which law should have the priority in the evaluation of a given project. In

---

54 "Ärztinnen und Ärzte beachten bei der Forschung am Menschen die in der Deklaration von Helsinki des Weltärztebundes niedergelegten ethischen Grundsätze für die medizinische Forschung am Menschen."

55 www.bundesaerztekammer.de/30/Auslandsdienst/99Handbuch2004.pdf.

56 Richter/Bussar-Maatz (2005), p. A-730 / B-616 / C-574.

57 www.ak-med-ethik-komm.de.

any case, the German example is certainly the most explicit regarding the problems raised by the numerous versions of the Declaration of Helsinki.

III.4.   France

France, being a member of the European Union, is also bound to implement directives 2001/20 and 2005/28. Indeed, in August 2004, the legislature amended the Law concerning the protection of persons involved in biomedical research of 20 December 1988.[58] In particular, article L. 1121-3 of the Public Health Code was modified as follows:

> "Biomedical researches on medicines are conducted in respect with the rules of good clinical practice as fixed by decree of the minister in charge of public health under proposition of the Health Products Safety Agency. For other types of research, recommendations of good practice are fixed by decree of the minister in charge of public health, under proposition of the Health Products Safety Agency for the products mentioned at article L. 5311-1".[59] (translated by the authors)

References to the Declaration of Helsinki could be made indirectly in those rules and recommendations. Yet, we found only one explicit reference to the Declaration in the French drug regulation. This relates to the implementation of the Commission Directive 2003/63/EC of 25 June 2003, amending Directive 2001/83/EC of the European Parliament and of the Council on the Community code relating to medicinal products for human use[60] that we analysed in Section III.1.1. By decree of the Ministry of Health and Social Protection, Annex 1 of that directive has been published in the French Official Journal.[61] As mentioned, this annex makes reference to the Declaration of Helsinki in relation to research conducted outside the European Union (see Section III.1.1).

According to the article L 4121-1 of the Public Health Code, the National Order of Physicians brings together in a binding way all doctors that are entitled to practice. Article L 4127-1 recognises the authority of the national council of the Order to adopt a code of medical deontology. This authority is strictly super-

---

58   Loi n. 2004-806 du 9 août 2004 relative à la politique de santé publique (J.O n. 185 du 11 août 2004, p. 1427).
59   "Les recherches biomédicales portant sur des médicaments sont réalisées dans le respect des règles de bonnes pratiques cliniques fixées par arrêté du ministre chargé de la santé sur proposition de l'Agence française de sécurité sanitaire des produits de santé. Pour les autres recherches, des recommandations de bonnes pratiques sont fixées par arrêté du ministre chargé de la santé, sur proposition de l'Agence française de sécurité sanitaire des produits de santé pour les produits mentionnés à l'article L. 5311-1. "
60   O.J. L. 159, 27.06.2003, p. 46.
61   Arrêté du 23 avril 2004 fixant les normes et protocoles applicables aux essais analytiques, toxicologiques et pharmacologiques ainsi qu'à la documentation clinique auxquels sont soumis les médicaments ou produits mentionnés à l'article L. 5121-8 du code de la santé publique, J.O n. 117 du 20 mai 2004, page 8960, texte n. 49.

vised.[62] After being adopted by the Order, the code is examined by the State Council and then signed by the Prime Minister.[63] The code of medical deontology has the value of a State council decree and is published in the regulatory part of the Public Health Code (articles R.4127-1 to 4127-112).

Article 15 of the code of medical deontology (or article R.4127-15 of the Public Health Code) deals with biomedical research. Although it does not explicitly refer to the Declaration of Helsinki, its "official" commentary, available on the website of the National Order of Physicians[64], states that:

> "The consent is an essential principle, a pillar both legal and deontological to the conduct of biomedical research involving human beings. This moral and legal requirement is expressed in several texts of which the oldest one is the Nuremberg Code (1947) followed by the declarations adopted by the World Medical Association in Helsinki and Tokyo".[65]

It is interesting to note that the commentary of article 15 of the code of medical deontology refers to the 1964 and 1975 versions of the Declaration, considering that this commentary was written in the late 1990s and is regularly revised. As in the Swiss and German cases, it shows a certain restraint of the medical profession when referring to the Declaration of Helsinki.

III.5.   United Kingdom

As Germany and France, the United Kingdom is a member of the European Union. It must also implement Directives 2001/20 and 2005/28 and it has done so by adopting the new Medicines for Human Use (Clinical Trials) Regulations 2004,[66] the annex of which refers to the 1996 version of the Declaration of Helsinki. We found another reference to the same version of the Declaration in the Medical Research Council (MRC) 1998 "guidelines for Good clinical practice in clinical trials".

The courts may use guidelines in resolution of civil disputes alleging medical negligence.[67] According to the Bolam case,[68] "a doctor is not guilty of negligence if he has acted in accordance with a practice accepted as proper by a responsible body of men skilled in that particular art". In another case,[69] the judge stated that

---

62   Terrier,(2003), p. 181.
63   Didier Frochot, Hiérarchie des normes dans le système juridique français, janvier 2002, in: www.defidoc.com.
64   www.conseil-national.medecin.fr/?url=deonto/article.php&offset=13.
65   Le consentement est en effet un principe essentiel, un pilier à la fois juridique et déontologique de la pratique de la recherche biomédicale sur l'homme. Cette exigence morale et juridique s'exprime à travers de nombreux textes dont le plus ancien est le Code de Nuremberg (1947) suivi des déclarations adoptées par l'Association Médicale Mondiale à Helsinki et à Tokyo.
66   Statutory Instrument 2004 no. 1031, in: www.opsi.gov.uk/si/si2004/20041031.html.
67   Hurwitz (1998), p. 27.
68   Bolam v. Friern Hospital Management Committee (1957 2 All ER 118-28).
69   Airedale NHS Trust v. Bland (Guardian ad litem) (1993 1 All ER 821-96).

"[...] if a doctor treating a PVS [Persistent Vegetative State] patient acts in accordance with the medical practice now being evolved by the Medical Ethics Committee of the BMA [British Medical Association], he will be acting with the benefit of guidance from a responsible and competent body of professional opinion, as required by the Bolam test".

However, a guideline itself may not be the subject of widespread consensus, and doctors should take reasonable steps to ascertain whether the guidance they are following is still current within the profession.[70] The consequences for deviating from such guidelines were discussed in a key judgement, Hunter v. Hanley[71], which mentioned that: "[...] such a deviation is not necessarily evidence of negligence". Three facts must be proven to establish medical negligence:

"First of all it must be proved that there is a normal practice; secondly it must be proved that the defendant has not adopted that practice; and thirdly (and this is of crucial importance) it must be established that the course the doctor has adopted is one which no professional man of ordinary skill would have taken if he had been acting with ordinary care".

The mere fact that the Declaration of Helsinki is mentioned in the MRC 1998 guidelines gives the Helsinki Declaration limited value in that it appears only as an indication of the professional standards that should be followed in biomedical research.

Professional committees seem sometimes to refer to Helsinki in their determination of what constitutes standard practice. In 2005 alone we found two cases considered by a Fitness to Practise Panel applying the General Medical Council's Preliminary Proceedings Committee and Professional Conduct Committee (Procedure) Rules 1988 that referred to the Declaration of Helsinki.[72] Both cases concerned physicians who conducted clinical trials for the pharmaceutical industry and, in doing so, failed to obtain the free and informed consent of the research subjects. The two decisions mention the physicians' obligation to act in accordance with the principles of the Declaration of Helsinki as part of the agreement they signed with the pharmaceutical company. Thus, the binding nature of the Declaration appears in those cases more as a matter of contractual obligation than of a professional duty. It would be interesting to see if there are other cases where the research protocol and the agreement with the sponsor made no reference to the Declaration and what conclusion the authorities reach in those cases. However, this is not an issue of legislative reference to the Declaration of Helsinki, but one of case-law which is not the focus of this chapter.

---

70 Document of the British Medical Association, Confidentiality and disclosure of health information, 14 October 1999, in: www.bma.org.uk/ap.nsf/Content/Confidentialitydisclosure ~other.
71 Hunter v. Hanley (1955 Session Cases 200-8).
72 Case Wilson, 21 October 2005, in: www.gmc-uk.org/concerns/decisions/search_database/ ftp_panel_wilson_20051021.asp; also Case Adams, 11 February 2005, in: www.gmc-uk.org/ concerns/decisions/search_database/ftp_panel_adams_20050211.asp.

III.6.   Canada

Canada does not have a uniform and comprehensive legislative or regulatory framework pertaining to research involving human subjects. The complexity of the constitutional division of powers in relation to health matters and the existing tension around potential encroachment of the federal parliament on provincial terrain is likely the reason why, despite frequent calls for coherent federal legislation, the federal government has never enacted a comprehensive statute focusing on research involving human subjects.[73] The federal government has jurisdiction over the regulation of drugs and medical devices, but provinces have general jurisdiction over health care and over the regulation of health care professionals. As in the United States, two different sets of documents are the main sources that govern research involving human subjects in Canada. One covers clinical trials that aim at testing new drugs or medical devices for approval in Canada. The other applies only in the context of federally funded research. To start with the latter: in 1996, the three major federal funding agencies enacted a new *Tri-Council Policy Statement: Ethical Conduct for Research Involving Humans* (TCPS).[74] The TCPS applies to all research funded by the funding agencies, but its ambit has also been expanded by the use of "memoranda of understanding". These memoranda of understanding are contractual agreements between the funding agencies and federally-funded academic institutions, in which these institutions agree to abide by the TCPS for all research that is being undertaken in the institution. Through the use of these contractual provisions, all research that is undertaken in federally funded institutions, including research sponsored by the industry, must respect the TCPS. Federal funding agencies could therefore request that research funds be reimbursed on the basis of breach of contract, if federally funded institutions do not respect the TCPS. Although this sanction has so far never been imposed, questions have been raised about the level of TCPS compliance by several federally funded institutions.[75]

The TCPS contains only two references to the Declaration of Helsinki. Art. 1.14 states that: "Rules pertaining to research abroad should be created and interpreted in the spirit of the Helsinki Accords [sic] and subsequent documents that encourage the free movement of researchers across national boundaries". In its discussion of the requirement of clinical equipoise, the TCPS also refers in a footnote to the Declaration of Helsinki's recognition of the "requirement that the health care of subjects should not be disadvantaged by research participation".[76]

---

73 See Lemmens (2005), pp. 39-50. Note, however, that the *Assisted Human Reproduction Act* (S.C. 2004, c. 2) introduces specific rules and a specific governance structure for research in the context of assisted human reproduction, including stem cell research.

74 Medical Research Council of Canada, Natural Sciences and Engineering Research Council of Canada & Social Sciences and Humanities Research Council of Canada (1998).

75 See Downie/McDonald (2004), pp. 159-181; Wilson (2005), pp. 9-11; Lemmens (2005).

76 See TCPS, supra note 74 at p. 7.1, footnote 2, which refers to Helsinki 1964, "as revised 1996, para. II.3."

With respect to clinical drug trials, Health Canada, the federal agency mandated to enforce the federal food and drug act, explicitly stipulates in its 2001 Clinical Trials Regulations that sponsors who want to test a new drug in a clinical trial must obtain an authorisation from Health Canada. This authorisation must include the name and contact information of the Research Ethics Board (REB) that approved the study (art. C.05.005 (c)(x)), as well as the name and contact information of any REB that previously rejected the protocol, with the reasons for this rejection (art. C.05.005 (d)).[77] The regulations further impose a general duty to "ensure that a clinical trial is conducted in accordance with good clinical practices" (C.05.010). The regulations themselves, however, do not contain any more details with respect to research ethics standards. Health Canada has introduced the full text of the ICH-GCP Guideline into its regulatory regime as a Guidance Document. However, this Guidance Document does not have the status of strict regulation. As Health Canada states: "Guidance documents are administrative instruments not having force of law and, as such, allow for flexibility in approach. Alternate approaches to the principles and practices described in this document may be acceptable, provided they are supported by adequate scientific justification".[78]

Although the ICH-GCP does not have the status of formal regulation, the Health Products and Food Branch of Health Canada sees it, nevertheless, as a fundamental part of the regulatory structure. The reference to good clinical practice standards in the Regulations is interpreted as providing the basis for potential regulatory sanctions against sponsors, researchers, or REBs that violate the ICH-GCP.[79] The regulatory authorities have started evaluating whether REBs are compliant with the ICH-GCP on the basis of this interpretation.

Interestingly, in the introduction to the Guidance Document, Health Canada states that "[c]ompliance with this standard provides public assurance that the rights, safety and well-being of trial subjects are protected, consistent with the principles that have their origin in the Declaration of Helsinki, and that the clinical trial data are credible".[80] As pointed out earlier, specific provisions of the ICH-GCP itself also refer to the Declaration of Helsinki. The Declaration of Helsinki is, in other words, only indirectly present in the Canadian regulatory practice, through a cross-reference in the ICH-GCP, which itself does not have the status of a directly enforceable regulation.

It seems unclear what legal sanctions would follow from violating provisions of the Declaration of Helsinki under Canada's drug regulatory regime. The Food

---

77 S.O.R./2001-203 [Clinical Trial Regulations].
78 Guidance for Industry, Good Clinical Practice: Consolidated Guideline ICH Topic E6, online: www.hc-sc.gc.ca/hpfb-dgpsa/tpd-dpt/e6_e.html.
79 Personal Communication with Jean Saint Pierre, coordinator, Good Clinical Practices Compliance Unit, Compliance and Enforcement Coordination Division, Health Products and Food Branch, Health Canada.
80 Guidance for Industry, Good Clinical Practice: Consolidated Guideline ICH Topic E6, online: www.hc-sc.gc.ca/hpfb-dgpsa/tpd-dpt/e6_e.html.

and Drug Regulations are accompanied by explicit and stringent regulatory sanctions. But any regulatory sanction based on a violation of a principle of the Declaration of Helsinki would likely be challenged on the basis that these principles are too remote and that the references are too vague to justify regulatory sanctions. Sanctions would be based on a general reference to good clinical practice in the clinical trials regulations, which would then point to the Guidance Document containing the ICH-GCP, which itself has a vague reference to "the principles of Helsinki".

Other more specific Guidance documents issued by Health Canada refer to Helsinki, highlighting how the Declaration is indeed seen as an expression of the core values of research involving human subjects. But the references are again too vague to have clear legal validity.[81]

While the direct enforceability of these documents and certainly of the Declaration of Helsinki is questionable, they can play a role in litigation, particularly in the absence of clear statutory and legal provisions. As in other common law jurisdictions such as the United Kingdom, when faced with a claim of negligence associated with an alleged violation of research ethics standards, the courts will have to determine whether there is indeed a violation of a standard of care. A court can use national, but also international research ethics codes and guidance documents as sources of information to determine such standard of care.[82]

The TCPS and the ICH-GCP are more widely used within Canada and are therefore more likely be seen as reflecting Canadian professional research standards than the Declaration of Helsinki or other international documents. That does not mean, however, that the Declaration of Helsinki will simply be discounted. As discussed earlier, the TCPS and the ICH-GCP documents refer vaguely to the Declaration and even point out that they originate in its principles. Moreover, as was mentioned in the context of the United Kingdom, contractual provisions in Canada often refer to the Declaration of Helsinki. This means that, as in the United Kingdom, the Declaration could be enforced as a contractual provision in Canada. In addition, since a multitude of contracts refer to the Declaration, it could be used to argue in court that the Declaration of Helsinki reflects the standard of care.

---

81 See e.g. Guidance to Establish Equivalence or Relative Potency of Safety and Efficacy of a Second Entry Short-Acting Beta$_2$-Agonist Metered Dose Inhaler (MDI) (February 1999), available online at www.hc-sc.gc.ca/dhp-mps/prodpharma/applic-demande/guide-ld/inhal-aerosol/mdi_bad_e.html. This guidance document obviously applies to only a very specific area of research. Moreover, the guidance, which was drafted back in 1992, still refers to the research ethics guidelines of the Medical Research Council, which no longer exists in Canada. This simply confirms the fact that this type of guidance document cannot be interpreted to have any significant legal value.

82 See Jutras (1993), p. 905; Campbell/Glass (2001), pp. 482-489; and Sossin/Smith (2003), pp. 867ff, in particular at p. 886, where they discuss why "[t]he legal status of ethical guidelines is ... murky".

Interestingly enough, in one of the rare Canadian cases involving medical research, a Quebec Superior Court referred in 1989 precisely to the Declaration of Helsinki, in its discussion of the meaning of the provisions of the Quebec Civil Code and the deontological code for physicians.[83] The court used the Declaration to determine the appropriate standard of disclosure of risk for physicians, without even mentioning the existence of national research ethics guidelines. At that time, the 1987 Guidelines on Research Involving Human Subjects of the Medical Research Council of Canada[84] applied to medical research funded by this federal funding agency and other research ethics guidelines did exist in Canada.[85]

IV.   Conclusion

The Declaration of Helsinki is undoubtedly an essential document in modern medical research ethics. We have seen the way in which this text has been gradually introduced, to various extents, into national and international legislation. This analysis certainly needs to be completed, not only to include a broader scope of national laws, but also to study each legal system in greater detail, especially in light of the principle of the rule of law. However, some general conclusions can still be drawn from these initial findings.

First, a so-called "direct dynamic reference" to the Declaration of Helsinki is most unlikely, since it would contradict the principle of legality or legal certainty. In fact, we have seen that such reference rarely occurs in the medical codes of deontology that we analysed. Even within the medical profession, there are serious controversies concerning the various versions of the Declaration. It is certainly important for the WMA to acknowledge this fact before considering any further revisions.

This leads us to a second remark. The most recent reference made to the Declaration of Helsinki in the laws is to the 1996 version. As we have seen, this can partly be explained by adherence to the ICH-GCP in the drug regulation, at least in Europe, Japan and the USA. Thus, the investigators are bound to follow that version in spite of more recent amendments. Some laws propose a solution to solve this potential conflict of norms: the investigator should respect in priority the provisions granting the greatest protection to the human subjects. This rule does not necessarily mean that the most recent version of the Declaration would

---

83   Weiss v. Solomon, (1989) R.J.Q. 731, 48 C.C.L.T. 280 (Sup. Ct.).
84   Medical Research Council of Canada (1987).
85   See, for example, Social Sciences and Humanities Research Council of Canada (1977). Whether a court would nowadays as easily ignore the existing national research ethics guidelines is doubtful. The TCPS and the ICH-GCP are much more established and widely used within the research community. Courts might still look at the Declaration of Helsinki, though, for example to spot inconsistencies with existing guidelines, or when the Declaration is explicitly mentioned in a research contract with the sponsor.

be applied. It imposes a case-by-case evaluation that is most likely going to take place *a posteriori*.

The solution of this conflict of norms will not only depend on the versions of the Declaration but also on what is understood by the "greatest protection of the human subjects". As noted by the Declaration of Helsinki paragraph 5: "In medical research on human subjects, considerations related to the well-being of the human subject should take precedence over the interests of science and society". This principle of the primacy of the individual is explicitly mentioned in other important documents at the international level. Article 2 of the 1997 Convention on Human Rights and Biomedicine[86], for example, states that: "The interests and welfare of the human being shall prevail over the sole interest of society or science". It is important to keep this principle in mind in view of the recent attempts to liberalise the rule on placebo-controlled clinical trials or when we think about the challenges created by the growing industrialisation and internationalisation of biomedical research.[87]

This then leads us to our third and final remark. More important than the reference to the Declaration of Helsinki itself is the fact that the regulations which we have analysed all refer to the fundamental and universal principles laid down in the Declaration. Whether someone refers to the first, 1964 version of the Declaration or to the latest one, the underlying principles have not changed. Although the WMA is often put under pressure by certain interest groups within or outside the medical profession, it has been able to maintain the integrity of the Declaration of Helsinki. This is an achievement of considerable importance, given that a weakening of the founding principles of the Declaration would automatically lead to a loss of legitimacy. The strength of the Declaration lies in its roots. Jay Katz showed great perceptiveness in 1969, when he questioned the so-called "improvement" of existing codes of professional ethics. It may be time to listen to him more carefully and redefine the priorities in research ethics, adapting the rules not to suit the needs of researchers or physicians, but to better protect human subjects and society. This will not necessarily require new rules, but more training of those who are involved in biomedical research. We wish to conclude with another premonitory statement by Jay Katz:

> "Education is a cornerstone for any meaningful attempt to construct a system of control of medical practice and experimentation. Once its importance is recognised, it has the virtue that something can be done about it. [...] The task of medical faculty is not limited to educating students, but extends to re-examining the entire structure of medical decision-making. New rules and procedures are especially needed, but can only be promulgated after their purposes

---

86 Convention for the Protection of Human Rights and Dignity of the Human Beings with Regards to the Application of Biology and Medicine: Convention on Human Rights and Biomedicine, Oviedo, 4 April 1997. conventions.coe.int/Treaty/en/Treaties/Html/164.htm; see Zilgalvis (2004), pp. 166ff; see also Roscam Abbing (1998), pp. 377-387.

87 On the placebo rule see Lemmens et al. (2004), pp. 153-74. On the industrialisation and internationalisation of research see Sprumont/Gytis (2005), pp. 245-267.

are clearly articulated. Here lessons from the past and present may serve as a guide to the future".[88]

Almost forty years later, one can only regret that too little progress has been achieved in that direction. Indeed, how many training programs for medical researchers today contain a solid mandatory component on research ethics that amounts to more than a token administrative requirement?

88   Katz (1970), p. 307.

References

Arnull, A. (1999): The European Union and its Court of Justice. New York: Oxford University Press.

Bachmann, K.-D./Heerklotz, B. (1994): Der Wissenschaftliche Beirat der Bundes-ärztekammer. Deutsches Ärzteblatt (1994), 10, p. A587.

Beschluss des Bundesverfassungsgerichts vom 9. Mai 1972, Neue Juristische Wochenschrift (1972), p. 1506.

Campbell, A./Glass, K.C. (2001): The Legal Status of Clinical and Ethics Policies, Codes, and Guidelines in Medical Practice and Research, McGill Law Journal 46 (2001), pp. 482-489.

Council of Europe (ed.) (2004): Biomedical Research. Strasbourg: Council of Europe Publishing.

Downie, J./McDonald, F. (2004): Revisioning the Oversight of Research Involving Humans in Canada, Health Law Journal 12 (2004), pp. 159-181.

Freund, P. E. (ed.) (1970): Experimentation with Human Subjects. New York: G. Braziller.

Gérard, M. (1992): Droit médical et déontologie: suggestions prudentes en faveur d'un rapprochement, in: Etudes offertes à Jean-Marie Auby. Paris: Dalloz.

Herranz, G. (1998): The Inclusion of the Ten Principles of Nuremberg in Professional Codes of Ethics: An International Comparison, in: Tröhler/Reiter-Theil (1998), pp. 127-139.

Hamann, P. A./Fenger, H. (2004): Allgemeinmedizin und Recht. Springer: Berlin.

Human, D./Fluss, S.S. (2001): The World Medical Associations's Declaration of Helsinki: Historical and Contemporary Perspectives. Unpublished manuscript.

Hurwitz, B. (1998): Clinical Guidelines and the Law, Negligence, Discretion and Judgment. Abingdon, Oxon: Radcliffe Medical Press.

Jutras, D. (1993): Clinical Practice Guidelines as Legal Norms, Canadian Medical Association Journal (1993), p. 905.

Katz, J. (1970): The Education of the Physician-Investigator, in: Freund (1970), p. 295ff.

Knoppers, B./Sprumont, D. (2000): Human Subjects Research, Ethics, and International Codes on Genetic Research, in: Murray/Mehlman (2000), pp. 566-576.

Laufs, A./Uhlenbruck, W. (1999): Handbuch des Arztrechts, 2nd ed. Munich: Beck.

Lemmens, T. et al. (2004): CIOMS' Placebo Rule and the Promotion of Negligent Medical Practice, European Journal of Health Law 11 (2004), pp. 153-174.

Lemmens, T. (2005): Federal Regulation of REB Review of Clinical Trials: A Modest but Easy Step Towards an Accountable REB Review Structure in Canada, Health Law Review 13 (2005), 2-3, pp. 39-50.

Louis, C. (1989): Communautés européennes. Paris: Dalloz.

Medical Research Council of Canada (1987): Guidelines on Research Involving Human Subjects. Ottawa: Medical Research Council of Canada.

Medical Research Council of Canada, Natural Sciences and Engineering Research Council of Canada & Social Sciences and Humanities Research Council of Canada (1998): Tri-Council Policy Statement: Ethical Conduct for Research Involving Humans. Ottawa: Public Works and Government Services Canada.

Murray, T. H./Mehlman, M. J. (eds.) (2000): Encyclopedia of Ethical, Legal, and Policy issues in Biotechnology. New York, Chichester: John Wiley & Sons.

Papadopoulou, R.-E. (1996): Principes généraux du droit et droit communautaire, origines et concrétisation. Athènes, Bruxelles: Sakkoulas & Bruylant.

Rawls, J. (1971): A Theory of Justice. Cambridge: The Belknap Press of Harvard University Press.

Richter, C./Bussar-Maatz, R. (2005): Deklaration von Helsinki: Standard ärztlicher Ethik, Deutsches Ärzteblatt 102 (2005), 11, pp. A-730, B-616, C-574.

Roscam Abbing, H. D. C. (1998): The Convention on Human Rights and Biomedicine. An Appraisal of the Council of Europe, European Journal of Health Law 5 (1998), pp. 377-387.

Social Sciences and Humanities Research Council of Canada (1977): Ethics Guidelines for Research with Human Subjects. Ottawa: Social Sciences and Humanities Research Council of Canada.

Sossin, L./Smith, C. W. (2003): Hard Choices and Soft Law: Ethical Codes, Policy Guidelines and the Role of the Courts in Regulating Government, Alberta Law Review 40 (2003), pp. 867ff.

Sprumont, D. (1999): Legal Protection of Human Research Subjects in Europe, European Journal of Health Law 6 (1999), pp. 25-43.

Sprumont, D./Gytis, A. (2005): The Importance of the National Laws in the Implementation of the European Legislation, European Journal of Health Law 11 (2005), pp. 245-267.

Terrier, E. (2003), Déontologie médicale et droit, thèse, Les Etudes hospitalières, Bordeaux.

Takis, T. (1999): The General Principles of EC Law. Oxford: Oxford University Press.

Tröhler, U./Reiter-Theil, S (eds.) (1998): Ethics Codes in Medicine: Foundations and Achievements of Codification since 1947, Aldershot (UK), Brookfield (USA), Singapore, Syndney (AUS): Ashgate.

Vesting, J.-W. (1998): Die Verbindlichkeit von Richtlinien und Empfehlungen der Ärztekammern nach der Musterberufsordnung 1997, Medizinrecht (1998), p. 169.

Wilson, M. (2005): Vulnerable Subjects and Canadian Research Governance, IRB: Ethics and Human Research (2005), pp. 9-11.

Zilgalvis, P. (2004): European Law and biomedical research, in: Council of Europe (2004), pp. 166ff.

Acknowledgements: The authors wish to thank Vincent Corpataux (scientific collaborator at the Institute of Health Law of the University of Neuchâtel, Switzerland) for research support and Linda Hutjens for careful editing. Dominique Sprumont took the overall lead, developing the conceptual framework and drafting various sections. Sara Girardin (European, French and German law) and Trudo Lemmens (Canadian Law) wrote the first drafts of specific sections and suggested changes to other sections. All authors signed off on the final version.

III.
History and Ethics of Research:
International Perspectives

Andreas Frewer

History of Medicine and Ethics in Conflict
Research on National Socialism as a Moral Problem

> "I solemnly pledge to consecrate my
> life to the service of humanity. [...]
> I make these promises solemnly,
> freely and upon my honour."[1]

I. Introduction

In September 1948, the second General Assembly of the World Medical Association (WMA) adopted the so-called "Declaration of Geneva", which was most
recently confirmed in May 2006 at a meeting in France.[2] The document, which
plays an important role in the history of medicine and medical ethics, was
formulated as a "new version" of the Hippocratic Oath.[3] It not only formulates a
number of central ethical principles but has to be understood as a direct response
to the experience of the Third Reich. Sentence number eight, for example, stated:
"I will not permit considerations of age, disease or disability, creed, ethnic origin,
gender, nationality, political affiliation, race, sexual orientation, social standing or
any other factor to intervene between my duty and my patient". During the Third
Reich and the Second World War in Germany, issues of "disability", "nationality", "political affiliation" and "race" posed fundamental problems for medicine
and society and led to some of the worst medical atrocities in modern history.
Other parts of the Geneva Declaration also reflected this historical context.[4]
    Although the Nuremberg Code is probably more widely known in the field of
research ethics, because of the informed consent principle, the Declaration of
Geneva is nonetheless of considerable importance. Since 1949, the Declaration is
quoted by the WMA in the "International Code of Medical Ethics". In Germany,
the relevance of the Geneva principles is underlined in a particular way. After the
war, the declaration was adopted as a preamble in the German professional code
of practice (*Musterberufsordnung*) as the *conditio sine qua non* for the reintegra-

---

1   First and last sentence of the Declaration of Geneva.
2   Geneva, Switzerland (September 1948), amended by the 22nd World Medical Assembly,
    Sydney, Australia, August 1968 and the 35th World Medical Assembly, Venice, Italy,
    October 1983 and the 46th WMA General Assembly, Stockholm, Sweden, September 1994
    and editorially revised at the 170th Council Session, Divonne-les-Bains, France, May 2005,
    the 173rd Council Session, Divonne-les-Bains, France, May 2006.
3   In the French Original: "Serment Hippocrate, formule du Genève".
4   See also Leven (1998).

tion of the German Working Committee of West German Medical Federations (*Arbeitsgemeinschaft Westdeutscher Ärztekammern*) into the international medical community. The declaration is part of the obligatory document for the licensing process as a German physician. Still, only few physicians know the historical context of the text.

This chapter intends to illustrate some of the historical problems and links between medical ethics and medical history in the 20th century. The focus is on the historiography of Nazi medicine and the extent to which research on this subject poses a moral problem with direct and indirect implications for the medical profession.

II.   History of Medicine and Medical Ethics

Issues of medical ethics were probably never as important as they have been throughout the 20th century. It is equally true that no other period in medical history has had such a profound impact on medical ethics than the period of National Socialism. This has to be understood *ex negativo*, given that medical abuses reached new levels in the Third Reich and during World War II. Key medical ethics codes of the 20th century were formulated in response to the crimes committed in that period. The Nuremberg Code, in particular, resulted from the revelations during the Doctors' Trial about criminal medical experiments and the 'euthanasia' programme. The ten principles of the Code were designed to serve as a landmark for research on human subjects in the future.[5] Those writing medical ethics codes after the war wanted to ensure that the tension between the rights of individuals and patients, on the one hand, and the interests of science, on the other, would never again result in "medicine without humanity" (*Medizin ohne Menschlichkeit*). The Declaration of Geneva as new *Serment Hippocrate, formule du Geneve* stood in relation to the best traditions in medicine since antiquity.

During the founding period of the WMA as the official representative of the international medical community, a number of problems occurred in relation to the role of medicine in the Third Reich. The continuity of personnel at the leading levels of the Federal Medical Board (*Bundesärztekammer*) repeatedly led to international irritations and concerns. At the end of the 1940s, members of the WMA discussed the readmission of a German delegation to the WMA which would have symbolised a rehabilitation of the German medical profession more generally. At first, feelers were put out to German officials through a number of informal talks. In October 1949, for example, WMA officials arranged a private meeting with representatives of the German medical profession. A couple of months later, in January 1950, a Swedish and a Swiss physician met with two representatives of the "Working Committee of West German Medical Federa-

---

5   See the contribution by Ulf Schmidt in this volume; also Frewer/Schmidt (2007). For the
     historical develpoment and the Journal "Ethics" (1922-1938) see Frewer (2000) and HAL.

tions".[6] The four doctors agreed to keep the content of the meeting confidential and not to release the results to the medical press.[7] The aim of the informal meeting was to forge closer relations between the German medical profession and the WMA, and to discuss the potential readmission of German membership into the WMA. Apart from the issue of reintegrating the German medical profession with the international medical community, one of the officials of the German "Working Committee", Dr Karl Haedenkamp, posed a significant problem for the readmission of German doctors to the WMA.

III. The Karl Haedenkamp Case

The WMA officials were concerned about the close relationship between Haedenkamp as a representative of the German medical profession and the Nazi state, and demanded a new beginning:

> "The employment of Dr. Haedenkamp has been deemed irreconcilable with the principles and views, expressed in the said declaration, which categorically disclaims all connections with Nazi ideology and condemns those members of the German medical profession, who took part in or tolerated acts against the noble tradition of medical men."[8]

The German doctors argued, on the other hand, that Haedenkamp's work was indispensable for the German medical profession; they justified his conduct in Nazi Germany by repeatedly pointing out that even leading Nazis had apparently no knowledge of the nature and extent of the crimes which had been committed by the regime during the war. Haedenkamp's leading role in the aryanisation of the German medical profession and in the dismissal of Jewish colleagues has in the meantime been well documented.[9] At the time, the two representatives of the German medical profession alleged that the Nazi leadership had acted alone and that leading physicians such as Haedenkamp had no insight knowledge into the crimes. The desire to rehabilitate the German medical profession through the readmission into the WMA was obviously very strong.[10] In Haedenkamp's case the existing facts spoke for themselves: Haedenkamp (1889–1955) became the leading representative of the German medical profession after the take-over of power by the Nazis in 1933. As the editor of the *Deutsches Ärzteblatt*, he wrote:

---

6   Dr Dag Knutson (Swedish physician) and Otto Leuch (Swiss physician) as well as Ernst Neuffer and Theodor Dobler as German representatives.
7   Interestingly, internal memoranda about this sensitive conference have survived in the Swiss archive of the WMA. See Report about the Conference in Stuttgart (1950), Lederer (2004) and the article by Susan Lederer in Frewer/Schmidt (2007).
8   Ibid.
9   See especially Schwoch (2001).
10   See Lederer (2004).

"The diverse changes in the admission process serve to cleanse, in the first place, through the elimination of those doctors whose continuing work in the public welfare sector are incompatible with the basic principles of today's policies of the medical profession."[11]

More than 5,000 doctors lost their jobs as a result of the wide-ranging "cleansing" process against Jews and political opponents. Many of them emigrated; others stayed, and were imprisoned, deported or killed as a result. Haedenkamp, on the other hand, advanced as the executive manager (*Hauptgeschäftsführer*) of the Federal Medical Board (*Bundesärztekammer*) after the war. His role throughout the Third Reich was either ignored or kept quite. Later, he was even awarded the Federal Service Cross (*Bundesverdienstkreuz*). After his death in 1955, the city of Cologne named the street in which the Federal Medical Board was located into "Haedenkampstraße" in his honour. Twenty years ago, and against the opposition of the Federal Medical Board, the street was renamed into "Herbert-Lewin-Straße" in recognition of one of the victims of the Nazi dictatorship.[12] The support for Haedenkamp was a particularly long and difficult case in the history of medicine in post-war Germany; it documents not only the problem of continuities in personnel but the inability for a fresh start by the medical profession. The Haedenkamp case was in many ways a "false start" for post-war German medicine.[13]

IV. History Reflected: The "Compulsory Oath"

At the beginning of the 1950s, the international community and representatives of the WMA demanded the recognition of German medical war crimes as a precondition for the readmission into the WMA. Following on from an intensive debate, the West German medical associations prepared a relevant statement in which the crimes during the Third Reich were admitted. The associations promised to do everything in their power to prevent any future transgression of the German medical profession.[14] The German Working Committee of West German Medical Federations specifically remarked that since 1947 all German doctors were obliged to swear the Hippocratic Oath through the Declaration of Geneva which had been formulated by the WMA.[15]

11 See Wert (1989), p. 94.
12 Herbert Lewin (1899-1982) worked in the Jewish Poly-Clinic in Berlin and, in 1937, became Head Physician at the *Israelitisches Krankenhaus* in Cologne. After being deported in 1941 – a policy which had been supported by some of the "coordinated" (*gleichgeschaltet*) representatives of the German medical profession like Haedenkamp – he worked as a physician in the ghetto of Lodz and in Auschwitz. Lewin survived and became the chairmen of the community of synagogues in Cologne in 1946. In 1949 – despite existing opposition and former Nazi sympathisers – he became the head of the gynaecological clinic in Offenbach. In 1952, Herbert Lewin was appointed to Professor and in 1955 he became the president of the regional association of Jewish communities in Hesse; see Wert (1989), p. 8, as well as Schwoch (2001) about Haedenkamp more generally. See also AHU (Berlin).
13 See Jütte (1997).
14 For the statement of Otto Leuch (1949) see also the contribution by Lederer in this volume.
15 The precise date is mentioned as 14 June 1947.

Despite these pledges, the German medical profession was determined to ignore, in some cases suppress, the content of the reports by the Nuremberg trial observers, especially the book "Science without Humanity" (*Wissenschaft ohne Menschlichkeit*)[16] as the new version of *Das Diktat der Menschenverachtung*[17] by Alexander Mitscherlich and Fred Mielke as well as the book "The Killing of the Mentally Ill" (*Die Tötung der Geisteskranken*)[18] by Alice Platen-Hallermund. Rather than using these reports about the development and extent of human experiments and the 'euthanasia' programme as a basis for an open and honest debate, some German physicians accused the authors of disloyalty (*Nestbeschmutzer*) and even threatened legal action.[19]

The silent introduction of the Declaration of Geneva was significantly easier. German officials used the text as the preamble for the professional code of practice (*Musterberufsordnung*) of the German medical profession. Not many people know, however, that the Declaration of Geneva was altered in an important way in the German version. The last sentence of the new oath was – contrary to other countries – slightly altered so as to change the meaning in not an insignificant manner. After recounting the new medical ethics cannon, doctors generally had to make the following declaration: "I make these promises solemnly, freely and upon my honour" (*"Je fais ces promesses solennellement, librement et sur l'honneur"*).[20]

However, in the German version of the Oath the word "freely" was deleted without a replacement. To compensate for the Nazi past, German doctors were faced with a paradox: A Code, a new Hippocratic Oath in the form of the Declaration of Geneva, was not given freely, but had been made compulsory for the German medical profession as a whole. The German version of the Oath turned into a contradiction in terms, given that an oath, which is not given freely, looses its credibility as measure for responsible action and limits its moral force in binding the doctor to the profession. It is paradoxical to force someone to take an oath; a true oath should only be taken after careful reflection and without any form of interference.

In 1951 – six years after the end of the Second World War and four years after the judgment in the Nuremberg Doctors' Trial – the General Secretary of the WMA finally discussed the readmission of the German and the Japanese medical profession with the various national medical associations. Significantly, twenty-

---

16   Mitscherlich/Mielke (1949). The later edition was called *Medizin ohne Menschlichkeit*; see also Mitscherlich/Mielke (1960).

17   See Mitscherlich/Mielke (1947).

18   Platen-Hallermund (1993).

19   For the row about documents at Göttingen (*Göttinger Dokumentenstreit*) and the attempts by Professor Sauerbruch, Professor Rein and Professor Heubner to white-wash their roles in the Nazi health system see especially Peter (1994) and Peter (2001).

20   See also the text which says: "I make these promises solemnly, freely and upon my honour". In the French version the section reads: "Je fais ces promesses solennellement, librement et sur l'honneur". In the German version: "Dies alles verspreche ich feierlich [und frei] auf meine Ehre".

eight out of thirty-one medical associations voted in favour to admit Germany into
the WMA, whereas thirty out of thirty-one associations voted in favour to readmit
Japan.[21] In this way, the West German medical profession was yet again integrated into the world community of doctors.[22]

The historical context of the Cold War may also have contributed to the
willingness to readmit Germany into the WMA, given that the Western states
needed the greatest possible unity to confront the growing tensions with the
Eastern block. This was already visible during the Doctors' Trial as the first of
twelve subsequent Nuremberg war crimes trials. In the West-German zones of
occupation the Allies increasingly tried to prevent any further destabilisation of
German society in post-war trials, or indirectly strengthen the Eastern block
through verdicts which could be seen as "victor's justice".

Although individual representatives of the German medical profession are
likely to have hoped for a genuine new beginning, historical research has shown
that there were significant continuities after the end of the Third Reich with regard
to personnel and political ideology.[23] The role and responsibility of professional
representatives such as Haedenkamp also became subsequently known. This did
not prevent the Federal Medical Board, as the representative organisation of West
German doctors, to honour and support Haedenkamp for a long time after the war.
The "case" did not only continue for a long time but it was agonisingly slow. The
naming of a street in honour of Haedenkamp lasted for total of thirty years, an
entire generation. This was one of many examples for the "inability to mourn", as
Alexander and Margaret Mitscherlich called it in their succinct socio-psychologi-
cal study by the same title. It soon became clear that the representatives of the
German medical profession had only paid lip-services in acknowledging the
crimes committed by German doctors, mainly to be readmitted to the WMA. The
way in which the profession dealt with the Nazi past revealed the extent to which
German doctors wanted to ignore their own share of responsibility and guilt.
When the role of Haedenkamp in the Third Reich could no longer be ignored, the
West German medical profession decided to rename the street, also as a symbol to
distance itself from this part of its professional history. The renaming of the
official address of the Federal Medical Board from "Haedenkamp Street" into
"Herbert-Lewin-Street" in the end took longer than expected, and the street kept
its name for some time on letter headings even after the city of Cologne had
officially renamed the address.[24]

21   See also the contribution by Susan Lederer in this volume.
22   Memorandum (1951), ibid.
23   See especially Godau-Schüttke (1998) for the Heyde-Sawade-Affair.
24   Wert (1989).

V. Moral Task: Documenting Medical Crimes for Compensation Purposes

The history of the Third Reich and the crimes against humanity which had been committed with the participation and leadership of doctors and scientists also influenced the early post-war period in another way: the Doctors' Trial, in particular, revealed the extent to which German medicine had been used for criminal means – witness reports, photographs and film clippings about medical crimes committed in concentration camps were published around the world. The international declarations, including the Nuremberg Code and the Declaration of Geneva, were meant to serve as a protection against barbarism and crimes in medical science. Apart from inculcating higher ideals within the medical profession, the doctors of the world were encouraged to tackle a range of pressing problems in the post-war world. In many places there was a need to care for the victims of the German dictatorship; refugees and other "displaced persons" had to receive medical attention and be integrated into society.

At the beginning of the 1950s, the World Health Organisation (WHO) approached the WMA in identifying and documenting the "number, location and condition of the survivors of concentration camps, who, under the Nazi regime, were victims of so-called scientific experiments".[25] The WMA tried to document the suffering of those concerned through international initiatives because the surviving victims had sought refuge in various countries of the world. One of the aims was to establish the basis for an appropriate compensation scheme. The plan was to collect all data about Nazi medical experiments and document them through the WHO.[26]

In Germany the process of coming to terms with the Nazi past was particularly difficult. Whereas former Nazi officials knew how to secure their former positions and pensions through the so-called *Persilscheine* (White-Wash-Certificates), there was a lack of political support to establish a coordinated programme to compensate the victims of the regime. In the papers of the psychiatrist and medical historian Werner Leibbrand, who worked in Erlangen and Munich, and who testified as the only German expert in the Nuremberg Doctors' Trial, an interesting contemporary document has survived which well illustrates the atmosphere of the time. In November 1947, the lawyer Borgmann sent Leibbrand some of his own personal reflections on the subject, entitled "Spotlight from the Lower Rhine" (*Streiflicht vom Niederrhein*), in which the atmosphere after the period of the Third Reich was described not only in the cities around Cologne:

> "Who today talks about the increasing numbers of victims of these monsters[?] And who at all risks to point out the true reasons for our misery? That is true in Bavaria with the natural brutality of that land, but has more recently also become a reality in these areas. *Pars pro toto*. A lawyer from Duisburg who in the spring of 1933 chased lots of judges and prosecutors and lawyers into the Nazi Party (harmless victims of his brutality are still today

---

25   Victims (1951), pp. 241-242; see the contribution by Lederer in this volume, too.
26   Annual Report by the WMA for the year 1952, ibid.

without position and income), has just received his political assessment elsewhere: Group 5".[27]

The critical comments of the lawyer about the difficulties in coming to terms with the past culminated in the sweeping conclusion to the medical historian:

> "Herr Professor Leibbrand: The injustice has increased to such an extent that it has to come out one day. The approximately 20,000,000 victims of the Hitler regime (Frankfurter Hefte, p. 1005, calculate an even greater number) will one day present their bill to the beati possidentes and the neo-fascists."[28]

At an international level the support for the compensation of the victims of Nazi medicine and the documentation of medical crimes in the name of a science without humanity was seen as a central task in the first phase of the establishment of the WMA. In Germany, the process of coming to terms with the past was fraught with particular problems.

VI. Nazi History as a Political Problem: Research and Opposition

Turning a blind eye to the crimes of the Nazi regime had different consequences for post-war German society; only since the 1960s a critical debate about the generation of Nazi perpetrators became possible. Various public controversies, including the famous "historians dispute" (*Historikerstreit*), had to be fought out in the Federal Republic in order to locate the Nazi period in its moral and political context of the 20th century. The issue of National Socialism continues to raise new problems of perspective and memoralisation.[29] Those interested in looking at the role of medicine in the Third Reich had to wait even longer, up until the early 1980s when the Berlin conference on health (*Berliner Gesundheitstag*) firmly placed the issue on the public agenda.[30] Although a number of critical studies on Nazi medicine existed at the time,[31] the subject itself has only been researched for about a quarter-of-a-century.[32] The people exposing the darker sides of Nazi medicine ranged from historians and experts in medical history, to doctors and health care personnel, to interested and engaged citizens. More and more publica-

---

27 Friedrich-Alexander-University Erlangen-Nürnberg (FAU), Institute for the History and Ethics in Medicine, Leibbrand papers (no page numbers), Borgmann to Leibbrand, 11 November 1947. "Group 5" means *without political guilt*.
28 Ibid.
29 For the literature on the culture of memorialisation see, for example, the studies by Jarausch/Sabrow (2002), Erler (2003), Eschebach (2005) and Gassert/Steinweis (2006).
30 See Baader/Schultz (1980).
31 See Dörner (1967), Hafner/Winau (1974).
32 As far as expert publications are concerned see the bibliographies by Beck (1995) and Ruck (1995). For the role of the subject of medical history see, for example, Meinel/Voswinckel (1994) and Kümmel (2001); on the subject of forced labour and medicine see Frewer/Siedbürger (2004) and Siedbürger/Frewer (2006).

tions, dissertations and edited volumes were published as a result of expert symposia and conferences.[33]

In 1983, a group of researchers also founded the 'Working Group to Research the History of "Euthanasia" and Compulsory Sterilisation' (*Arbeitskreis zur Erforschung der Geschichte der "Euthanasie" und der Zwangssterilisation*).[34] The focus of this group was the Nazi sterilisation programme in the context of eugenics and racial hygiene as well as the murder of patients under National Socialism. Whereas historical research on Nazi medical crimes became ever more broad, others continued to resist on a number of levels. Only a few examples can be mentioned here. By emphasising particularly difficult cases it is not the intention to create the impression that the research since the 1980s has not made substantial progress in a great variety of areas and in great depth.

In 1986, the paediatrician Hartmut Hanauske-Abel published – with reference to the Mitscherlich diagnosis – an article about the role of Nazi doctors in the British medical journal *The Lancet* under the title: "The Inability to Mourn: Educational Aims for Young German Doctors". Hanauske-Abel's critical publication resulted in the withdrawal of his licence to work as a doctor for the *Kassenärztliche Vereinigung* in accident and emergency cases. The then president of the Federal Medical Board, Karsten Vilmar,[35] even publicly accused the young physician and member of the organisation "International Physicians for the Prevention of Nuclear War" (IPPNW), who had been temporarily working as a paediatrician and Associate Professor in the United States,[36] that he was defaming German doctors collectively. The only person, however, who was dishonouring his profession with a mixture of ignorance and an attempt to play down Nazi medical atrocities was the representative of the medical profession himself. At he end of the 1980s – by the time Nazi medicine had already been researched for a decade – the highest ranking representative of the German medical profession still alleged that it had only been a minority of doctors who had participated in the injustices of the Nazi regime. Although national and international research had documented and exposed the role of doctors in the Third Reich, official representatives continued to gloss over and ignore the wide-spread support of doctors for the regime or the extent of their membership in the Nazi Party, SA, SS and the National Socialist Doctors' Association (*Nationalsozialistischer Deutscher Ärztebund*, NSDÄB).[37] A broad action programme by medical historians[38] had to show

33 The memorial sites in the former concentration camps, for example in Sachsenhasuen and Buchenwald, and in the former death camps in Hadamar, Pirna/Sonnenstein and Bernburg, also play an important role.

34 Wunder (2000), p. 251.

35 Professor Karsten Vilmar, born 24 April 1930 in Bremen, Surgeon. From 1978 to 1999, he was President of the Federal Medical Board (*Bundesärztekammer*) and the Annual German Medical Conference (*Deutscher Ärztetag*). Since 1992, he was the treasurer of the WMA.

36 Medical College, New York Hospital.

37 See, for example, Bareuther et al. (1998) and Kater (2000).

38 See also the article by Toellner (1998). Since the end of the 1980s, a number of newspapers and journals, for example the *Süddeutsche Zeitung* and *Deutsches Ärzteblatt*, published relevant articles and raised public awareness.

the participation and leadership of German doctors in policy measures which ranged from aryanisation and sterilisation to criminal human experiments and the Nazi 'euthanasia' programme.[39] Although the German Federal Court eventually declared the withdrawal of Hanauske-Abel's licence as invalid, it needed international protests and the continued public debate among the medical profession to force the German medical establishment to acknowledge that it had made a mistake, seven years after the beginning of the controversy and the campaign against the historically sensitive and critical physician.[40] Following the scandal surrounding the president of the Federal Medical Board, Vilmar, representatives of the German medical profession made genuine attempts to examine the history of the profession in the Third Reich in an adequate and transparent fashion; as a result, a number of articles and medical history books were published.[41]

Parallel to the debate about the Nazi past, the German medical profession became engulfed in yet another domestic and international scandal about one of its representatives, which is discussed below.

VII. The Sewering Scandal and the Nazi Past

The debate about the Nazi Past escalated into an international controversy in the case of Hans Joachim Sewering.[42] Born in 1916, Sewering, who worked as an internal practitioner in Dachau, near Munich, was one the most important representatives of the German medical profession and for a long time president of the Federal Medical Board. Since the establishment of the permanent committee of doctors of the European Community in 1959, Sewering had been a member of the German delegation and became the German representative for the General Council of the WMA in the same year. In 1966 he advanced to become a member of the board of the WMA and, in 1971, was appointed the treasurer of the WMA.

However, Sewering's nomination in 1993 to become the president of WMA sparked international protests, for of his role in the Nazi regime and because of allegations that he had played a part in the Nazi 'euthanasia' programme. On 26 October 1943, Sewering had apparently signed a "medical certificate" in the asylum of Schönbrunn, near Dachau, which authorised the transfer of the fourteen-year-old Babette F. to the Cure and Nursing Home Eglfing-Haar. Documents showed that the child was admitted on 1 November, and that it died in the institution shortly afterwards, on 16 November 1943. For the Eglfing-Haar's "Special Children's Ward" (*Kinderfachabteilung*) – the euphemistic cover for the killing centres for children – the case was just one of many.[43]

39   Schmuhl (1992), Frewer/Eickhoff (2000), Kater (2000).
40   See also Hanauske-Abel (1998).
41   See Bleker/Jachertz (1993) or Jütte (1997).
42   Professor Hans Joachim Sewering, born 30 January 1916. For recent historical work on the involvement of Sewering in the Nazi 'euthanasia' programme see Krischer (2006).
43   Apart from Babette F., about 1,500 children and young adults died from unnatural causes. Usually the children were given an overdose of the sedative luminal (Phenobarbitone) and

After 1945, the former SS member and pulmonary expert Sewering made a career in the professional organisations of German doctors as well as in a German conservative party (*Christlich Soziale Union*, CSU). Between 1955 and 1991 he was president of the Medical Board in the state of Bavaria and a member of the Board of the Federal Medical Board. From 1959 to 1973, Sewering represented the West German medical profession as the vice-president of the Federal Medical Board and the Annual German Medical Conference (*Deutscher Ärztetag*), and from 1973 to 1978 as the president. In 1991, two years prior to his application for the presidency of the WMA, the seventy-five-year-old became an honorary member of the Federal Medical Board.[44] Almost no-one had shown interest in his Nazi past and the list of his honorary positions became longer as time went by.[45] He was even able to receive important academic honours without problems. In 1968, he was given an honorary professorship in social medicine as well as for medical law and occupation, and, in 1985, an honorary doctorate from the Technical University of Munich. Revelations in the 1970s about financial irregularities in Sewering's Dachau practice let to a loss of trust in the medical profession for the president of the Federal Medical Board. When he eventually resigned in 1978 during the 81st German Medical Conference in Mannheim, the above-mentioned Karsten Vilmar became his successor. As a former member of the Nazi Party and the SS, Sewering was determined to be promoted to an international post: after years of active membership, he wanted to become the president of the World Medical Association (WMA).[46]

Individual doctors and institutions, especially the Jewish World Congress, eventually prevented the election of the former SS-doctor to the presidency of the WMA. Despite the protests from actively engaged and critical German doctors and medical organisations in the United States, Canada and Israel, a number of functionaries of the WMA, which to some extent relied on the financial resources from the German Medical Associations, defended Sewering as their candidate of choice for some time.[47] In 1993, Sewering finally resigned as the candidate who had been nominated by the Federal Medical Board's nominee to become the next president of the WMA.

Michael J. Franzblau, professor of dermatology at the University of San Francisco, who had lost more than twenty members of his family during the Third

veronal (sleeping tablets). As a result, they generally contracted pneumonia, bronchitis or other breathing deficiencies which eventually resulted in death. The second choice was morphium-scopolamine, the third death by starvation. The children did not die of poisoning, but from the medical complications caused by the overdose of a common medicine; see also Burleigh (1995), p. 103; Friedlander (1995), pp. 54-55.

44   Until today, Sewering is listed as an honorary member with a photograph but – compared to others – without his curriculum vitae on the official website of the Federal Medical Board; see www.bundesaerztekammer.de/25/40Fotos/10Vorstand/.

45   Sewering's decorations included the *Bayerischer Verdienstorden* (1962), the *Bundesverdienstkreuz Erster Klasse* (1969) and the *Großes Bundesverdienstkreuz* (1975).

46   See also Kater (1997).

47   Seidelman (1996), White (1996).

Reich, was particularly influential in bringing the scandal to the attention of the international public through large-scale notices in the American press, for example in the *New York Times*.[48] Sewering, on the other hand, denied any role in the 'euthanasia' killings. The German medical establishment continued – and in some cases continue – to support him, despite the occasional letter to the editors or critical commentary in the *Deutsches Ärzteblatt*. On his eightieth birthday in 1996, for example, it was reported in the column entitled "persons"[49] that Sewering had done a "great service" for the "formation of medical education" in Germany or that he had been actively engaged in the "preservation of ethics standards in medical practice through the creation of professional medical law". The historical or moral problems of the Nazi period and his role in the Third Reich was ignored, however. This not only led to a critical response from authors who demanded that the incomplete description of Sewering's career had to be "amended",[50] but also to rather naïve remarks that one should not prevent the "rehabilitation" of senior medical functionaries.[51] On an international level, the attempts to turn a blind eye to the Nazi past did not go unnoticed. In a letter to the editors, the Canadian medical historian William Seidelman remarked:

> "I am writing in response to the article [...] commemorating the 80th birthday of Professor Dr. Hans Joachim Sewering of Dachau. As a medical journal the Ärzteblatt is required to ensure that all important available information is included in an article pertaining to a particular subject. Unfortunately, the article documenting Professor Sewering's career omitted a number of important facts specifically."[52]

Seidelman once again listed the most important facts about Sewering's career:

> "In 1933, Prof. Sewering joined the SS: Membership 143 000. In 1934, Prof. Sewering joined the N-S Party: Membership 1 858 805. In 1943, Prof. Sewering worked as a physician at the Schönbrunn institution for the disabled where, on October 26 of that year, he signed an order transferring 14 year old Babette F[...] to the 'euthanasia' centre at Eglfing-Haar [...]."[53]

Seidelman also addressed the moral problems in dealing with the history of the medical profession in Germany:

> "Prof. Sewering maliciously blamed an international Jewish organization as the reason for his resignation. Prof. Sewering has yet to acknowledge the impact of his own past behaviour for his problem. The Ärzteblatt's omission of such critical information is equivalent to a radiologist neglecting to report the presence of suspicious radio-opacities on an X-ray or a pathologist failing to report the presence of malignant cells in a biopsy."[54]

---

48 See also www.abc7news.com: Nazi Hunter Update, 11 July 2002. Even the Bavarian state government was accussed of supporting a murderer over several decades.
49 Deutsches Ärzteblatt 93 (1996), 4 , pp. A-205 / B-177 / C-165.
50 Wandt (1996).
51 Deutsches Ärzteblatt 93 (1996), 17, pp. A-1082/B-902/C-844. Spektrum: Leserbriefe. There is also an "addition" to one of the letters to the editor by Dr H. Wandt in no. 10 (1996).
52 Seidelman (1996).
53 Ibid.
54 Ibid.

Since 1994, Sewering was prohibited from entering the United States because of his Nazi past, but, supported by influential circles in Germany, lives today – now in his nineties – in Dachau near Munich. Until recently, the Bavarian legal authorities saw no grounds to open investigative proceedings against the representative of the German medical profession.[55] Finally, the state prosecution announced that there were "no further grounds for an investigation" but that one would "continue to follow-up leads which can be taken serious".[56] For Sewering's ninetieth birthday, there was once again another article in the *Deutsches Ärzteblatt*, this time at least the critical aspects of his *curriculum vitae* were not omitted.[57] How does the medical profession deal with the German past as an integral part of its legacy? In what way is the subject of medicine under National Socialism being discussed today and communicated to future doctors?

VIII. The Culture of Memory and Education: Nazi Medicine in Medical Studies

Conducting a Survey with Medical Students on National Socialism[58] – this was the goal of a group of doctors and medical historians from Berlin. In a survey of 332 medical students from Berlin, the group wanted to examine the extent of their historical knowledge as well as their motivation and attitude to the Third Reich more generally.[59] The findings showed that in certain areas students have a lack of knowledge and education on the subject. The range of answers to questions such as "Who are Mitscherlich and Mielke?"[60] demonstrated, for example, significant deficits among the student generation. Only eight out of 332 students (2,4 %) knew that the psychoanalyst Alexander Mitscherlich and the medical student Fred Mielke had been observers at the Nuremberg Doctors' Trial and were the authors of the documentation "Medicine without Humanity".[61] Whereas the issue of National Socialism is generally been discussed in schools, it appears that the

---

55 The journal *Der Spiegel* commented: "Sewering: A clean slate. In time for the medical conference in Mannheim, the Deutches Ärzteblatt described once again the professional career of the controversial President of the Federal Medical Board Sewering – but their description was incomplete". See *Der Spiegel* (1978), 21 [The Doctors' Leader Sewering and the 'euthanasia' programme].

56 Stiller (2002), p. 51.

57 See Hibbeler (2006). Sewering's role is even mentioned in the American literature; see the book by Lilly Brett (1998).

58 The original title of the project was "Asking Medical Students about National Socialism".

59 The questionaire consisted of a total of 35 questions: 12 questions were there to test knowledge and 23 questions to assess attitudes. The aim was to assess the basic knowledge in the following subjects: general knowledge on National Socialism, the role of medicine during the Nazi period, motivation and critical understanding in the field of Nazi medicine as well as attitudes to current and controversial topics.

60 See Langkafel et al. (2002).

61 Almost three-quarter of the students did not know either of the names (73 per cent). 13 per cent of those questioned were of the opinion that the two men had been doctors in the concentration camp of Buchenwald. See Langkafel et al. (2002).

knowledge of medical students on this subjects is sometimes rather limited.[62] Paradoxically, in some cases, they do not show much interest in debating this subject in any great depth.

In a study entitled "The Horror Wears Off" (*Der Schrecken nutzt sich ab*), the theologian Markus Zimmermann-Acklin showed in detail the range of cultural problems which exist in Germany in relation to remembering the crimes of the regime and, especially, the Nazi 'euthanasia' programme.[63] The dimensions of the Third Reich's policy of annihilation fades further into the background in the memory of the people. Yet not only the knowledge that Nazi crimes pose a specific moral challenge fades into the background, but there is evidence which suggests that the transfer of general historical knowledge about the Nazi period becomes increasingly more difficult. To gain a general understanding about specific subjects of Nazi history is likewise difficult to obtain.

A similar pictures emerges at the top of the educational hierarchy. How do the highest representatives of the medical profession or even medical experts respond to sensitive questions that relate to medical history and medical ethics under National Socialism? The above mentioned Vilmar is a case in point, to say the least: if even a president of the Federal Medical Board continues to argue by the late 1980s that the Nazi medical profession had been ignorant and innocent then that says it all. There are certainly a range of very good projects and activities which are supported by the representatives of the medical profession and carried out;[64] but even among experts, who, one would assume, should be well informed as part of their professional perspective about the history and ethics under National Socialism, one can obviously find, in certain cases, a substantial lack of general knowledge and a limited understanding of the reception and core content of Nazi medical history.[65] On the whole, one can increasingly find the attitude that – in a metaphorical sense – "the cover of the history books about the Nazi period should finally be closed". This is not only counter-productive but also not appropriate from a scientific perspective, given that there are still major studies which

---

62   In my own seminars and lectures about the history of the 'euthanasia' programme, which I have delivered over the last ten years, I have noted that the knowledge of students about the number of victims is often rather limited. In general, the students' estimate is far too low ("10,000") but there have also been instances where students have given an estimate of "60 million".

63   Cf. Zimmermann-Acklin (2000), title, see also Kaiser et al. (1992).

64   See also the long-term engagement by the Berlin Medical Board for this subject (*Berliner Ärztekammer*) or, more recently, the new project organised by the Federal Association of Medical Insurers (*Kassenärztlichen Bundesvereinigung*) in Berlin.

65   Prof. C. Wiesemann, President of the Academy for Ethics in Medicine, and the official representative of the subject medical history at the University of Göttingen, refered for instance repeatedly to "Julius Moser" [sic] in a paper at the expert symposium in Tübingen in 1998, and was seemingly surprised when members of the audience corrected her. Some of the attending medical historians were quite taken aback by this and other mistakes of her. To germanise the name of the most important social democratic health politician during the Weimar Republic, Julius Moses, who as a Jewish member of parliament lived through the horrors of the Nazi period and who died in 1942 in the concentration camp of Theresienstadt, is symptomatic of the lack of knowledge among certain "experts".

were only recently produced or important research work which has not yet been completed.[66] On a national as well as local level and for individual towns and faculties there is still a significant amount of work to do if we want to understand the history of Nazi Germany better.[67] Of course, sophisticated knowledge about the various historical dimensions on Nazi Germany does exist, on an national and international level, and diverse research work has been carried out[68] and relevant exhibitions have been organised.[69]

On the whole, the history of medicine under National Socialism is extraordinarily multifaceted, and there is probably no other subject and period which has been researched in such a comprehensive fashion, and which continues to be researched in Germany. The emphasis on certain difficult cases should not hide the fact that every year numerous medico-historical dissertations on all aspects of the history of medicine in the Third Reich are being produced; here institutes for medical history have an important role to play in relation to research, education and knowledge transfer. In some places there are significant discrepancies between the theory and practice of historical study. To illustrate this point, I would like to return to the above-mentioned example to work towards a just "compensation" of the victims of National Socialism which is actually internationally supported, and which originally had been one of the primary objectives of the international medical community and subject of research and documentation.

IX. The Politics of Coming to Terms with the Past: 'Pure Science' in the Göttingen Research Scandal

One of the most heated debates in Germany and in the wider world on the history of the Third Reich relates to the problem of the injuries and "compensation" of forced and slave labourers during the Second World War.[70] As part of the public discourse about this aspects of Nazi history, the federal authorities established the

---

66 See, for example, Voswinckel (2002) and the excellent project to update the "Encyclopedia of Doctors" (*Ärztelexikon*) by Isidor Fischer with information about those Jewish colleagues, who had to emigrate or were deported, as well as with those colleagues from the whole of Europe, who had been forgotten as a result of the Nazi period.

67 In some places the history of the faculties has been well researched. Some universities, however, still need to conduct research about the withdrawal and disallowing of doctorates, the employment of forced and slave labourers, the continuity of personnel and the lack of denazification.

68 In the case of Julius Moses even through dissertations; see, most recently, for example Reuland (2004); see also Nadav (1985).

69 See, for example, the travelling exhibition "without conscience – conscientious" (*gewissenlos gewissenhaft*); see Ley/Ruisinger (2001) or the American exhibition "Deadly Medicine" which is currently shown in Dresden. There was also an exhibition project about Julius Moses by the Friedrich-Ebert-Stiftung, see Schneider (2006).

70 See especially Herbert (1999) and Spoerer (2001). To discuss the general aspects of the history of forced and slave labourers would go beyond the purview of this article; with regard to the role of medicine, see Frewer/Siedbürger (2004) and Siedbürger/Frewer (2006).

Trust "Memory, Responsibility, Future" which was meant to contribute to the
financial support of the survivors. The Trust was the result of an initiative between the German government and industry to come to terms with particular
aspects of German history.[71] Historical research was subsequently advanced by
hundreds of experts and specially appointed historians in various regional projects
and through the work of active citizens. On a special mailing list called "NS-
Zwangsarbeit" (Nazi Forced and Slave Labour)[72] questions, reports and expert
information are posted on a daily basis in order to support historical research and
the documentation of those affected. Despite the lack of sources and long delays,
there will soon be few subjects on Nazi history which have been so well documented in such a detailed fashion through the range of reports and publications.
German historians and historically interested citizens have actively promoted a
transparent way of coming to terms with their own past in a broad spectrum
ranging from experts, institutions and companies to workshops and even schools.
Often survivors were invited in order to bring to life this part of German history,
especially for the younger generation of Germans. However, in some places, there
is also a certain degree of opposition: not all companies and not all public institutions had the same interest in coming to terms with their past. Time and time
again there are reports where research projects have been hampered. It seems
questionable, to say the least, if interested pupils, together with their teacher, have
to enforce the release of files and access to archival material from the mayor of a
south-German town through a court injunction.[73] There have also been problems
in the medical field and the town of Göttingen even had to face up to a scandal of
international proportions.

Since 2000, a group of researchers and students from the Göttingen University
Clinics wanted to examine the extent to which forced and slave labourers were
employed and exploited in their successor institution.[74] Historians subsequently
identified more than 120 persons in the "personnel files" who were directly
employed in the university clinics of Göttingen: their employment ranged from
laboratory assistants and carers, to boilermen, gardeners and messengers but also
as "Resident Pregnant Women" (*Hausschwangere*) for examinations in the gynaecological clinic.[75] Moreover, it was possible to identify the personal information
of hundreds of forced and slave labourers – which are important supporting
documents for their employment records and compensations claims – and document the entire system of medical politics (*Behandlungspolitik*) at the clinics.[76]
The facts are neither particularly surprising nor particularly dramatic in compari-

---

71 See, for example, the webpage www.stiftungsinitiative.de.
72 See www.zwangsarbeit-forschung.de (the mailing list is being administered by Dr B. Brem-
    berger from Berlin).
73 These were very engaged pupils from the Paul-Klee-School in Gersthofen; for further back-
    ground material, see also http://www.zwangsarbeit-gersthofen.de.
74 See, for example, Wormer (2002) and Abbott (2003).
75 See Frewer et al. (2004).
76 See Frewer et al. (2006) and the contributions in Bruns et al. (2007)..

son to other hospitals in Germany.[77] What made the research in Göttingen so difficult was the general attitude of the leading personalities of the medical institution:
it took more than one-and-a-half years alone until a research project was
supported with personnel and resources, and the more the working group uncovered the more obstructive the official position became. Access to an archive containing the papers from the department of neurology and psychiatry was denied
without reasonable grounds. It took another one-and-a-half years to determine
whether the historical work would violate issues of "medical confidentiality",
despite the fact that expert reports from historians, the data protection officer and
the head of the city archive existed[78] and parallel work on a number of patient
files was being conducted. A particular problem arose with regard to publications
which had to be signed off and agreed internally as well as the issue of whether
the clinic should contribute to the above-mentioned Trust initiative which is based
on voluntary contributions and not linked to any legal claims of those affected.
Although the leading personalities of the institution had specifically been invited,
they repeatedly did not attend the seminars which had been organised by experts
and students of the faculty in 2001 and 2002. Researchers at the Göttingen Institute for Ethics and History of Medicine were told over many years that the leadership of the clinic was in talks with the Ministry of Science of Lower Saxony.
Later the press office of the clinic reported that the information had been incor-
rect.[79] What was more depressing was the fact that an initial initiative to collect
donations was nipped in the bud on the grounds that there was no hard evidence
whether the institution had employed forced and slave labourers in the Third
Reich, although detailed reports existed to this effect already. Only when students
from the Göttingen faculty handed the relevant minister for science a leaflet
during the festivities of the 25th anniversary of the new clinic,[80] and after the national and international press had drawn the attention of the public to this matter,
it was possible that the project was extended and the files finally were released.

Leaving aside all the difficulties in coming to terms with the past, the suppres-
sion of files and the attempted cover-up at the level of the leadership of the
institution, one of the most problematic aspects remained the behaviour of, and
argumentation by specific individuals. One the one hand, the embattled dean of
the faculty, Professor Manfred Droese, a former pathologist, advised students in a
letter that they should not discuss too hastily this subject in public[81] or proposed
during a meeting of the faculty that actively engaged students might want to post
themselves by the roadside to collect donations. On the other hand, the deputy
dean, Professor Claudia Wiesemann, remarked repeatedly that one should concentrate on "pure research" and not spend time with uncovering documentation which

77   See Gottschalk et al. (2003), Frewer/Siedbürger (2004) and Frewer et al. (2001).
78   Letter by the Director of the City Archive Göttingen, Dr E. Boehme, 25 November 2002.
79   Oral and written statement from members of the press office of the Göttingen clinic.
80   On 29 November 2002.
81   The subject had by then been brought to the attention of the public through the publication of
     a number of articles on a regional and national level; M. Droese to B. Lache (representative
     of medical students), 10 December 2001.

would help survivors for their compensation claims: *Scientific research is more important for those affected than the 500 Euro compensation* [sic].[82] This was a depressing state of affairs in the history of medicine under National Socialism, because Wiesemann and others yet again used the argument of "pure science" which apparently had precedence over the justified claims of those who had been affected by the Nazi regime.[83] Moreover, Wiesemann managed that the Institutional Review Board (*Ethikkommission*) of the faculty did not discuss a written request on research ethics on this subject.[84]

On a more positive side, the students from the University of Göttingen should be named who voluntarily researched and debated this part of their institution's history in seminars and special lectures and showed engagement and courage at the level of the board of faculty.[85] Of concern, however, is the way in which the institution conducts its politics of memory. On the one hand, medical students have to swear an oath on the Declaration of Geneva for the last two years, but, on the other, students receive manuscripts in the seminars of the local Institute for Ethics and History of Medicine which not only violate existing copyrights[86] but which also specifically ignore the more problematic aspects of the institutions' history and how it is dealing with the past.[87]

In the meantime, extensive research work was conducted in the town and county of Göttingen[88] and efforts were made to commemorate the suffering of forced and slave labourers. In May 2003, a memorial stone was officially unveiled in the presence of some of Göttingen's former forced and slave labourers from the Ukraine.[89] Since 2000, various initiatives have repeatedly proposed the unveiling

82 Minutes of the Board of Faculty (16 December 2002) as well as statement by several of those who attended the meeting This statement was repeated several times with degrees of variation to those historians working on this topic and in different contexts; see Bruns et al. (2007).

83 This was especially shameful, because Wiesemann, as a professor of medical history, should have had a more historically and ethically differentiated view on the subject, but had apparently been entagled in her obedience for authority and a conflict of interest with regard to her own career. It was not surprising, however, that it was someone like Wiesemann who had referred to "Moser"; see footnote 65.

84 See, for example, letter by C. Wiesemann to R. Rüther (Head of IRB) and the members of the Institutional Review Board, 21 February 2003. See Bruns et al. (2007).

85 See Flugblatt "NS-Zwangsarbeit am Klinikum Göttingen – Endlich das Schweigen brechen [NS-Forced Labour at the University Hospital Göttingen – Finally break the silence] (29 November 2002), see Bruns et al. (2007), Frewer et al. (2004) and Gottschalk et al. (2002).

86 See also the written report by the experts on copyright which concluded that the head of the department for Ethics and History in Medicine had intentionally carried this out or had at least acted in grave negligence. See Bruns et al. (2007).

87 In a 60-page manuscript, which was designed as teaching material for an official seminar on the subject of "History, Theory, Ethics in Medicine" at the faculty of Göttingen, certain chapters were used without permission from the book *Medizin und Zwangsarbeit im Nationalsozialismus*, see Frewer/Siedbürger (2004), but the chapter dealing with the clinic in Göttingen was omitted and not given to the students of Göttingen.

88 See especially the work by Tollmien (2000), Schörle (2000), Siedbürger (2004) and others.

89 The text of on the memorial stone is as follows: "To commemorate the people in the whole of Europe who were abducted by the Nazis from their home and who had to work as forced and

of a plaque by the university clinics of Göttingen but until today this has not been carried out. Although having been planned for a long time, and repeatedly proposed as a form of reconciliation, the survivors have not yet been invited by the clinics to come to Göttingen.[90]

X. History and Ethics: Concluding Remarks

The representative body of the medical profession has learned important lessons from its past and has in the meantime supported a whole range of historical projects and publications or, like in the case of forces and slave labourers, has publicly made a call for donations.[91] On the whole, the constant reminder of historical memory and moral responsibility remains a sensitive field which demands persistent activity, especially when central medical qualities are thereby put into practice and people not only pay lip service to declarations and medical ethics standards.

In the Sewering-controversy, the Canadian doctors and the medical historian Seidelman raised sensitive issues with regard to German history:

> "By omitting critical details of Sewering's personal and professional history the Ärzteblatt and the Bundesärztekammer cause serious damage to the reputation of the German medical profession. One might explain the omission of these facts on the basis that they would be inappropriate in an article celebrating a person's 80th birthday. But one cannot ignore either the fact that Babette F[...] will never celebrate an 80th birthday or the reasons why."[92]

In the same way this applies to the attitude of certain medical faculties to the Nazi period or to the above-mentioned politics of memory on the subject of forced and slave labourers. Medicine, contemporary history and ethics have significant effects on each other. The understanding of "pure research" and the belief that "scientific research" would be much more useful than the personal compensation of the victims is not only a cynical but a fatal error. Two generations after the end of the Second World War, this approach does not help those victims, who have in the meantime died or who have not been compensated. It only shows how

---

slave labourers in Göttingen in the period between 1939 to 1945. The City of Göttingen" ("*Zum Gedenken an die von den Nationalsozialisten aus ihrer Heimat verschleppten Menschen aus ganz Europa, die von 1939-1945 in Göttingen Zwangsarbeit leisten mussten. Stadt Göttingen*").

90 Although the case of Göttingen may seem extraordinary, given its extent, there were also problems in other places with regard to research and the politics of memory. See, for example, the information about the clinic in Tübingen: http://www.medizin.uni-tuebingen.de/persrat/infos/infozeitung/04_00/zwangsarbeit.html.

91 The current president as well as the general secretary and other members of the Federal Medical Board are all engaged in the same way and have shown considerable historical as well as ethical expert knowledge about the subject. There is also substantial expertise about the role of medicine under National Socialism in the editorial board of the *Deutsches Ärzteblatt*.

92 Seidelman (1996).

important the various activities by medical historians and active citizens are,[93] and how relevant conferences such as the one on "Medicine and Conscience" (*Medizin und Gewissen*) – which is the third of its kind[94] – or the current American exhibition in Dresden on "Deadly Medicine" can be for the culture of memory about the role of medicine under National Socialism.[95]

93 The ongoing educational work on the memorial sites should be especially highlighted at this point.
94 For the conferences "Medizin und Gewissen" see Kolb et al. (1998). See also Ley/Ruisinger (2001) for the German exhibition "gewissenlos gewissenhaft" on Nazi Medicine.
95 See the exhibition which has been borrowed from the US-Holocaust Museum in 2006.

References

Abbott, A. (2003): University Faces Up to Wartime use of Slaves, Nature 422 (2003), p. 792.

Abderhalden, E. (1939): Rasse und Vererbung vom Standpunkt der Feinstruktur von blut- und zelleigenen Eiweißstoffen aus betrachtet, Halle (Saale): Deutsche Akademie der Naturforscher Leopoldina.

Abderhalden, E. (1947): Gedanken eines Biologen zur Schaffung einer Völkergemeinschaft und eines dauerhaften Friedens. Zürich: Rascher.

Aly, G. (ed.) (1987): Die „Aktion T4". Die „Euthanasie"-Zentrale in der Tiergartenstraße 4. Berlin: Edition Hentrich.

Annas, G. J./Grodin, M. A. (eds.) (1992): The Nazi Doctors and the Nuremberg Code. Human rights in human experimentation. Oxford: Oxford University Press.

Ärztekammer Berlin (ed.) (1989): Der Wert des Menschen. Medizin in Deutschland 1918-1945. Berlin: Edition Hentrich.

Ärzte warnen vor dem Atomkrieg/IPPNW (ed..) (1987): Medizin unter dem Nationalsozialismus. Rundbrief herausgegeben von Ärzte-Initiativen und Kollegen. Sondernummer. November 1987.

Baader, G./Schultz, U. (eds.) (1980): Medizin im Nationalsozialismus. Tabuisierte Vergangenheit – Ungebrochene Tradition? Berlin-West: Verlagsgesellschaft Gesundheit.

Bareuther, H./Brede, K./Ebert-Saleh, M./Gründberg, K./Hau, S. (eds.) (1998): Medizin und Antisemitismus. Historische Aspekte des Antisemitismus in der Ärzteschaft. Münster: Literatur-Verlag.

Baur, E./Fischer, E./Lenz, F. (1921): Grundriß der menschlichen Erblehre und Rassenhygiene. München: Lehmanns.

Beauchamp, T. L./Childress, J. F. (2001): Principles of Biomedical Ethics. New York, Oxford: Oxford University Press.

Beck, C. (1995): Sozialdarwinismus, Rassenhygiene und Vernichtung „lebensunwerten" Lebens. Eine Bibliographie zum Umgang mit behinderten Menschen im "Dritten Reich" - und heute. Bonn: Psychiatrie Verlag.

Becker, H./Dahms, H.-J./Wegeler, C. (eds.) (1998): Die Universität Göttingen unter dem Nationalsozialismus. München: Saur.

Becker, P. E. (1988): Zur Geschichte der Rassenhygiene. Wege ins Dritte Reich, Teil I und II. Stuttgart: Thieme.

Beushausen, U./Dahms, H. U./Koch, T./Massing, A./Obermann, K. (1998): Die Medizinische Fakultät im Dritten Reich, in: Becker et al. (1998), pp. 183-286.

Binding, K./Hoche, A. (1920): Die Freigabe der Vernichtung lebensunwerten Lebens, ihr Maß und ihre Form. Leipzig: Meiner.

Bleker, J./Jachertz, N. (eds.) (1993): Medizin im „Dritten Reich" (2., erweiterte Auflage). Köln: Deutscher Ärzteverlag.

Burleigh, M. (1995): Death and Deliverance, 'Euthanasia' in Germany, 1900-1945. Cambridge, New York: Cambridge University Press.

Brett, L. (1998): Einfach so. [Just like that]. Aus dem Engl. von Anne Lösch. Vienna, Munich: Deuticke.

Bruns, F./Frewer, A./Siedbürger, G. (eds.) (2007): Zwangsarbeit, Medizin und Geschichte. Erlangen, Jena: Palm & Enke (in press).

Bromberger, B./Mausbach, H./Thomann, K.-D. (1985): Medizin, Faschismus und Widerstand. Frankfurt am Main: Mabuse-Verlag.

Cahill, L. S. (1994): Lessons We Have Learned?, in: Michalczyk (1994), pp. 213-216.

Caplan, A. (1992): The Doctors' Trial and Analogies to the Holocaust in Contemporary Bioethical Debates, in: Annas/Grodin (1992), pp. 258-275.

Caplan, A. (1992): The Relevance of the Holocaust to Bioethics Today, in: Michalczyk (1994), pp. 3-12.

Catel, W. (1962): Grenzsituationen des Lebens. Beitrag zum Problem der begrenzten Euthanasie, Schriften aus dem Kreis der Besinnung. Nürnberg: Glock und Lutz.

Deichgräber, K. (1955): Der hippokratische Eid. Stuttgart : Hippokrates-Verlag.

Diepgen, P. (1938): Die Heilkunde und der ärztliche Beruf. Eine Einführung. München, Berlin: Lehmann.

Dörner, K. (1967): Nationalsozialismus und Lebensvernichtung. Nach dem Krieg gegen die psychisch Kranken, Vierteljahreshefte für Zeitgeschichte 15 (1967), pp. 121-152.

Dörner, K. (1988): Tödliches Mitleid: zur Frage der Unerträglichkeit des Lebens oder: die Soziale Frage: Entstehung, Medizinisierung, NS-Endlösung, heute, morgen. Gütersloh: Jakob van Hoddis.

Dörner, K./Ebbinghaus, A./Linne, K. (eds.) (1999): Der Nürnberger Ärzteprozeß 1946/47. Wortprotokolle, Anklage- und Verteidigungsmaterial, Quellen zum Umfeld, Deutsche Ausgabe. München: Saur.

Dörner, K./Haerlin, C./Rau, V./Schernus, R./Schwendy, A. (eds.) (1980): Der Krieg gegen die psychisch Kranken. Nach „Holocaust": Erkennen – Trauern – Begegnen. Gewidmet den im „Dritten Reich" getöteten psychisch, geistig und körperlich behinderten Bürgern und ihren Familien. Rehburg-Loccum: Psychiatrie-Verlag.

Ebbinghaus, A./Dörner, K. (eds.) (2001): Vernichten und Heilen. Der Nürnberger Ärzteprozeß und seine Folgen. Berlin: Aufbau.

Edelstein, L. (1969): Der hippokratische Eid. Zürich, Stuttgart : Artemis-Verlag.

Elkeles, B. (1996): Der moralische Diskurs über das medizinische Menschenexperiment im 19. Jahrhundert, Medizinethik, Band 7. Stuttgart: Gustav Fischer.

Erler, H. (ed.) (2003): Erinnern und Verstehen. Der Völkermord an den Juden im politischen Gedächtnis der Deutschen. Frankfurt am Main, New York: Campus.

Eschebach, I. (2005): Öffentliches Gedenken. Deutsche Erinnerungskulturen seit der Weimarer Republik. Frankfurt am Main, New York: Campus.

Ethik. Sexual- und Gesellschafts-Ethik (1926-1938): Edited by Geheimrat Prof. Dr. E. Abderhalden, Halle a. d. Saale [successor of: „Ethik, Pädagogik und Hygiene des Geschlechtslebens" (1922) and „Sexualethik" (1925)].

Faulstich, H. (1998): Hungersterben in der Psychiatrie 1914–1949. Mit einer Topographie der NS-Psychiatrie. Freiburg im Breisgau: Lambertus.

Feral, T./Brunswic, H./Henry, A. (eds.) (1998): Médecine et nazisme. Considérations actuelles. Paris, Montréal (Qc): Harmattan

Fischer, I. (ed.) (1932): Biographisches Lexikon der hervorragenden Ärzte der letzten 50 Jahre. Berlin, Wien: Urban & Schwarzenberg.

Frewer, A. et al. (eds.) (1999): Medizinverbrechen vor Gericht. Das Urteil im Nürnberger Ärzteprozeß gegen Karl Brandt und andere sowie aus dem Prozeß gegen Generalfeldmarschall Erhard Milch. Bearbeitet und kommen-tiert von U.-D. Oppitz. Mit einem Beitrag von Thure von Uexküll, Erlanger Studien zur Ethik in der Medizin, Band 7. Erlangen, Jena: Palm & Enke.

Frewer, A. (2000): Medizin und Moral in Weimarer Republik und National-sozialismus. die Zeitschrift „Ethik" unter Emil Abderhalden, Frankfurt am Main, New York: Campus.

Frewer, A./Bruns, F. (2003): „Ewiges Arzttum" oder „neue Medizinethik" 1939-1945? Hippokrates und Historiker im Dienst des Krieges, Medizinhistorisches Journal 3/4 (2003), pp. 313-336.

Frewer, A./Eickhoff, C. (eds.) (2000): „Euthanasie" und die aktuelle Sterbehilfe-Debatte. Die historischen Hintergründe medizinischer Ethik, Frankfurt am Main, New York: Campus.

Frewer, A./Gottschalk, K./Mälzig, U. et al. (2001): Zwangsarbeit und Medizin im „Dritten Reich", Deutsches Ärzteblatt 98 (2001), 44, pp. A 2866-2868.

Frewer, A./Neumann, J. N. (eds.) (2001): Medizingeschichte und Medizinethik. Kontroversen und Begründungsansätze 1900-1950. Frankfurt am Main, New York: Campus.

Frewer, A./Schmidt, U. (eds.) (2007): Standards der Forschung. Historische und ethische Probleme klinischer Studien. Frankfurt am Main: Lang.

Frewer, A./Schmidt, U./Wolters, C. (2004): Hilfskräfte, Hausschwangere, Unter-suchungsobjekte. Der Umgang mit Zwangsarbeitenden in der Universitäts-frauenklinik Göttingen, in: Frewer/Siedbürger (2004), pp. 341-362.

Frewer, A./Siedbürger, G. (eds.) (2004): Medizin und Zwangsarbeit im National-sozialismus. Einsatz und Behandlung von „Ausländern" im Gesundheits-wesen. Frankfurt am Main, New York: Campus.

Frewer, A./Siedbürger, G./Bremberger, B. (eds.) (2007): Der „Ausländereinsatz" und das Gesundheitswesen. Stuttgart: Steiner (in press.).

Friedlander, H. (1995): The Origins of Nazi Genocide: From Euthanasia to the Final Solution. Chapel Hill, London: The University of North Carolina Press.

Friedlander, H. (1997): Der Weg zum NS-Genozid. Von der Euthanasie zur Endlösung. Berlin: Berlin-Verlag.

Friedrich, H./Matzow, W. (eds.) (1992): Dienstbare Medizin. Ärzte betrachten ihr Fach im Nationalsozialismus. Göttingen: Vandenhoeck & Ruprecht.

Galinski, D./Glinsmann I. (1989): Das Geheimnis der Versöhnung heißt Erinnerung, Ausstellungskatalog. Hamburg: Körber-Stiftung.

Gassert, P./Steinweis, A. E. (eds.) (2006): Coping with the Nazi Past. West German Debates on Nazism and Generational Conflict, 1955-1975. New York, Oxford: Berghahn Books.

Gerst, T. (1994): Der Auftrag der Ärztekammern an Alexander Mitscherlich zur Beobachtung und Dokumentation des Prozeßverlaufs, Deutsches Ärzteblatt 91 (1994), pp. 1037-1046.

Godau-Schüttke, K.-D. (1998): Die Heyde-Sawade-Affäre. Wie Juristen und Mediziner den NS-Euthanasieprofesor Heyde nach 1945 deckten und straflos blieben. Baden-Baden: Nomos-Verlagsgesellschaft.

Gottschalk, K./Frewer, A./Zimmermann, V. (2002): Zwangsarbeit und Gesundheitswesen im Nationalsozialismus. Fachliteratur und Forschungsperspektiven, Deutsche Medizinische Wochenschrift 127 (2002), 11, pp. 573-575.

Gruber, G. B. (1948): Arzt und Ethik. Berlin: de Gruyter.

Gruber, G. B. (1953): Über asklepische Pflichten, Niedersächsisches Ärzteblatt 7 (1953), pp. 67-70, and pp. 111-116.

Guckes, B. (1997): Das Argument der schiefen Ebene: Schwangerschaftsabbruch, die Tötung Neugeborener und Sterbehilfe in der medizinethischen Diskussion. Stuttgart: Gustav Fischer.

Grün, B./Hofer, H.-G./Leven, K.-H. (eds.) (2002): Medizin und Nationalsozialismus. Die Freiburger Medizinische Fakultät und das Klinikum in der Weimarer Republik und im „Dritten Reich". Frankfurt am Main: Lang.

Habermas, J. (1987): Vom öffentlichen Gebrauch der Historie. Das offizielle Selbstverständnis der Bundesrepublik bricht auf, Historikerstreit (1987), pp. 243-255.

Hafner, K.-H./Winau, R. (1974): Die Freigabe der Vernichtung lebensunwerten Lebens, Medizinhistorisches Journal 9 (1974), pp. 227-254.

Hanauske-Abel, H. (1998): Von Anbeginn eine tiefe Beziehung: Nationalsozialismus und Ärzteschaft im Jahre 1933, in: Kolb et al. (1998), pp. 52-67.

Hanauske-Abel, H. M. (1986): From Nazi holocaust to Nuclear Holocaust: A Lesson to Learn?, Lancet 2 (1986), 8501, pp. 271-273.

Hanauske-Abel, H. M. (1996): Not a Slippery Slope or Sudden Subversion: German Medicine and National Socialism in 1933, British Medical Journal 313 (1996), 7070, pp. 1453-1463.

Hastings Center (ed.) (1976): Biomedical Ethics and the Shadow of Nazism. A Conference on the Proper Use of the Nazi Analogy in Ethical Debate, Hastings Center Report, Special Supplement (August 1976). New York.

Hegselmann, R./Merkel, R. (eds.) (1992): Zur Debatte über Euthanasie. Beiträge und Stellungnahmen. Frankfurt am Main: Suhrkamp.

Helmchen, H./Winau, R. (eds.) (1986): Versuche mit Menschen, Berlin: de Gruyter.

Herbert, U. (1999): Fremdarbeiter. Politik und Praxis des "Ausländer-Einsatzes" in der Kriegswirtschaft des Dritten Reiches. Bonn: Dietz.

Heß, M. (2000): Zur Geschichte der Entschädigung von "Euthanasie"-Opfern: Gedenken und Handeln: in: Frewer/Eickhoff (2000), pp. 370-382.

Hibbeler, B (2006): Sewering wird 90 Jahre: Verdient, aber umstritten, Deutsches Ärzteblatt 103 (2006), pp. A-209, B-181, C-177.

Historikerstreit (1987): Die Dokumentation der Kontroverse um die Einzigartigkeit der nationalsozialistischen Judenvernichtung. München, Zürich: Piper.

Jachertz, N. (ed.) (1997): Gestalten statt verwalten – Aufgaben und Selbstverständnis der Bundesärztekammer 1947-1997. Köln: Deutscher Ärzteverlag.

Jarausch, K./Sabrow, M. (eds.) (2002): Verletztes Gedächtnis. Erinnerungskultur und Zeitgeschichte im Konflikt. Frankfurt am Main, New York, Campus.

Jütte, R. (ed.) (1997): Geschichte der deutschen Ärzteschaft. Organisierte Berufs- und Gesundheitspolitik im 19. und 20. Jahrhundert. Köln: Deutscher Ärzteverlag.

Kaiser, J. C./Nowak, K./Schwartz, M. (1992): Eugenik. Sterilisation. „Euthanasie". Politische Biologie in Deutschland 1895-1945. Eine Dokumentation. Berlin: Buchverlag Union

Kater, M. H. (1987): The Burden of the Past. Problems of a Modern Historiography of Physicians and Medicine in Nazi Germany, German Studies Review 10 (1987), pp. 31-56

Kater, M. H. (1989): Doctors under Hitler. Chapel Hill, London: The University of North Carolina Press.

Kater, M. H. (1997): The Sewering Scandal of 1993 and the German Medical Establishment, in: Junker (1997), pp. 213-234.

Kater, M. H. (2000): Ärzte als Hitlers Helfer. Hamburg: Europa-Verlag.

Katz, J. (1994): The Concentration Camp Experiments: Their Relevance for Contemporary Research with Human Beings, in: Michalczyk (1994), pp. 73-86.

Katz, J. (1998): Menschenopfer und Menschenversuche. Nachdenken in Nürnberg, in: Kolb et al. (1998), pp. 225-243.

Klee, E. (1986): Was sie taten – Was sie wurden. Ärzte, Juristen und andere Beteiligte am Kranken- oder Judenmord. Frankfurt am Main: Fischer.

Klee, E. (1997): Auschwitz, die NS-Medizin und ihre Opfer. Frankfurt am Main: Fischer.

Klee, E. (2001): Deutsche Medizin im Dritten Reich. Karrieren vor und nach 1945. Frankfurt am Main: Fischer.

Koch, G. (1984): Euthanasie, Sterbehilfe. Eine dokumentierte Bibliographie, Bibliographica genetica-medica. Erlangen, Jena.

Kolb, S./Seithe, H./IPPNW (eds.) (1998): Medizin und Gewissen. 50 Jahre nach dem Nürnberger Ärzteprozeß, Kongressdokumentation. Frankfurt am Main: Mabuse-Verlag.

Krischer, M. (2006): Kinderhaus. Leben und Ermordung des Mädchens Edith Hecht. München. Deutsche Verlagsanstalt.

Kümmel, W. F. (2001): Geschichte, Staat und Ethik: Deutsche Medizinhistoriker 1933-1945 im Dienste "nationalsozialistischer Erziehung", in: Frewer/Neumann (2001), pp. 167-203.

Langkafel, P./Drewes, T./Müller, S. (2002): Medizinstudium: Mitscherlich und Mielke – wer sind die?, Deutsches Ärzteblatt 99 (2002), 13 pp. A-834, B-693, C-647.

Lederer, S. E. (2004): Research without Border: The Origins of the Declaration of Helsinki, in: Roelcke/Maio (2004), pp. 199-217.

Leven, K.-H. (1997): Der Hippokratische Eid im 20. Jahrhundert, in: Toellner/ Wiesing (1997), pp. 111-129.

Leven, K.-H. (1998): Der historische Ort des Genfer Gelöbnisses, Ärzteblatt Baden Württemberg 53 (1998), Beilage Ethik in der Medizin 63 [also in: Wiesing, U. (ed.) (2003): Diesseits von Hippokrates. 20 Jahre Beiträge zur Ethik in der Medizin. Stuttgart: Gentner, pp. 253-257].

Leven, K.-H. (2002): „Diese gelassene Verleugnung von Schuld" – die Medizin und ihre nationalsozialistische Vergangenheit, in: Grün et al. (2002), pp. 15-33.

Ley, A./Ruisinger, M. M. (eds.) (2001): Gewissenlos – Gewissenhaft. Menschenversuche im Konzentrationslager. Erlangen: Specht.

Lifton, R. J. (1989): Ärzte im Dritten Reich. Frankfurt am Main: Sigmund-Freud-Institut.

Meinel, C./Voswinckel, P. (eds.) (1994): Medizin, Naturwissenschaft, Technik und Nationalsozialismus. Kontinuitäten und Diskontinuitäten. Stuttgart: Verlag für Geschichte der Naturwissenschaft und Technik.

Michalczyk, J. J. (ed.) (1994): Medicine, Ethics and the Third Reich. Historical and Contemporary Issues. Kansas: Sheed & Ward.

Mitscherlich, A./Mielke, F. (1947): Das Diktat der Menschenverachtung. Eine Dokumentation. Heidelberg: Schneider.

Mitscherlich, A./Mielke, F. (1949): Wissenschaft ohne Menschlichkeit. Medizinische und eugenische Irrwege unter Diktatur, Bürokratie und Krieg. Heidelberg: Schneider.

Mitscherlich, A./Mielke, F. (1960): Medizin ohne Menschlichkeit. Dokumente des Nürnberger Ärzteprozesses. Frankfurt am Main, Hamburg: Fischer-Bücherei.

Nadav, D. S. (1985): Julius Moses (1868-1942) und die Politik der Sozialhygiene in Deutschland. Gerlingen: Bleicher.

Peter, J. (1994): Der Nürnberger Ärzteprozeß im Spiegel seiner Aufarbeitung anhand der drei Dokumentensammlungen von A. Mitscherlich und F. Mielke. Münster: Literatur-Verlag.

Peter, J. (2001): Unmittelbare Reaktionen auf den Prozeß. Die Kontroverse in der „Göttinger Universitätszeitung", in: Ebbinghaus/Dörner (2001), pp. 473-475.

Platen-Hallermund, A. v. (1993): Die Tötung Geisteskranker in Deutschland, [Reprint], Mit einem Vorwort der Autorin und einem Geleitwort von Klaus Dörner. Bonn: Psychiatrie Verlag.

Ramm, R. (1943): Ärztliche Rechts- und Standeskunde. Der Arzt als Gesundheitserzieher. Berlin: de Gruyter.

Reich, W. T. (ed.) (1978): Encyclopedia of Bioethics (4 vols.). New York London: Free Press.

Reich, W. T. (ed.) (1995): Encyclopedia of Bioethics (5 vols.), New York London: Macmillan.

Reuland, A. J. (2004): Menschenversuche in der Weimarer Republik. Norderstedt: Book on Demand GmbH.

Roelcke, V./Maio G. (eds.) (2004): Twentieth Century Ethics of Human Subject Research. Historical Perspectives on Values, Practices, and Regulations. Stuttgart: Steiner.

Ruck, M. (ed.) (1995): Bibliographie zum Nationalsozialismus, Köln: Bund-Verlag.

Sass, H.-M. (1983): Reichsrundschreiben 1931: Pre-Nuremberg German Regulations Concerning New Therapy and Human Experimentation, Journal of Medicine and Philosophy 8 (1983), pp. 99-111.

Schlaudraff, U. (1990): Ethik im Schatten des Holocaust, Ethik in der Medizin 2 (1990), pp. 47-48.

Schmierer, K. (1996): Medizingeschichte und Politik: Die Karrieren des Fritz Lejeune (1892-1966), Diss. med., Berlin.

Schmuhl, H.-W. (1992): Rassenhygiene, Nationalsozialismus, Euthanasie. Von der Verhütung zur Vernichtung „lebensunwerten Lebens" 1890-1945. Göttingen: Vandenhoeck und Ruprecht.

Schneider, M. (ed.) (2006): Julius Moses. Schrittmacher der sozialdemokratischen Gesundheitspolitik in der Weimarer Republik. Vorträge anläßlich der Ausstellungseröffnung am 15. Dezember 2005 in der Friedrich-Ebert-Stiftung, Berlin. Historisches Forschungszentrum. Bonn: Friedrich-Ebert-Stiftung.

Schörle, E. (2000): Gutachten zur Situation von Zwangsarbeitern bei der Firma Schneeweiß in Göttingen während der Zeit des Nationalsozialismus, Göttingen, [unpublished].

Schulze-Lenzen, M. (2000): Versuche mit Kindern. Abgründig: Emil Abderhalden und die Zeitschrift „Ethik", Frankfurter Allgemeine Zeitung (2000), p. N 6.

Schwoch, R. (2001): Ärztliche Standespolitik im Nationalsozialismus. Julius Hadrich und Karl Haedenkamp als Beispiele. Abhandlungen zur Geschichte der Medizin und der Naturwissenschaften. Husum: Matthiesen Verlag.

Seidelman, W. E. (1996): Vergangenheit: One Cannot Ignore […]. Leserbrief, Deutsches Ärzteblatt 93 (1996), 17, pp. A-1082, B-902, C-844.

Siefert, H. (1973): Der hippokratische Eid und wir? Plädoyer für eine zeitgemäße ärztliche Ethik: Ein Auftrag an den Medizinhistoriker. Frankfurt am Main: Feuchtwangen.

Siedbürger, G. (ed.) (2004): Chiampo, Giuseppe: Überleben mit Stift und Papier. Aus dem Tagebuch eines Italienischen Militärinternierten im Zweiten Weltkrieg in Hilkerode/Eichsfeld. Göttingen: Schmerse.

Siedbürger, G./Frewer, A. (eds.) (2006): Zwangsarbeit und Gesundheitswesen im Zweiten Weltkrieg. Einsatz und Versorgung in Norddeutschland. Hildesheim, Zürich, New York: Olms.

Spoerer, M. (2001): Zwangsarbeit unter dem Hakenkreuz. Ausländische Zivil-
arbeiter, Kriegsgefangene und Häftlinge im Deutschen Reich und im
besetzten Europa 1939-1945. Stuttgart, München: Deutsche Verlags-Anstalt.

Stiller, M. (2002): Süddeutsche Zeitung (2002), p. 51.

Süß, W. (2003) Der "Volkskörper" im Krieg: Gesundheitspolitik, Gesundheitsver-
hältnisse und Krankenmord im nationalsozialistischen Deutschland 1939-1945,
München: Oldenbourg.

Toellner, R. (1998): Der blinde Spiegel. Über das Verhältnis der deutschen Ärzteschaft zum Nürnberger Ärzteprozeß in seiner epochalen Bedeutung, in: Kolb
et al. (1998), pp. 288-303.

Toellner, R./Wiesing, U. (eds.) (1997): Geschichte und Ethik in der Medizin. Von
den Schwierigkeiten einer Kooperation, Jahrbuch Medizin-Ethik, Band 10,
Stuttgart, Jena: Fischer.

Tollmien, C. (1999): Nationalsozialismus in Göttingen (1933-1945). Univ. Diss.,
Göttingen.

Tröhler, U./Reiter-Theil, S. (1997): Ethik und Medizin 1947-1997. Was leistet die
Kodifizierung von Ethik?. Göttingen: Wallstein Verlag.

Victims of So-Called Experimentation Under Nazi Regime (1951), WMA
Bulletin 3 (1951), pp. 241-242.

Voswinckel, P. (ed.) (2002): Biographisches Lexikon der hervorragenden Ärzte
der letzten fünfzig Jahre, hrsg. und bearb. von Isidor Fischer. Teil: 3. Nach-
träge und Ergänzungen: Aba – Kom. Bearbeitet und herausgegeben von Peter
Voswinckel. Hildesheim, Zürich, New York: Olms.

Wandt, H. (1996): Vergangenheit: Ergänzung, Deutsches Ärzteblatt 93 (1996),
pp. A-573, B-481, C-457.

White, L. W. (1996): The Nazi doctors and the medical community, honor or
censure? The case of Hans Sewering, Journal of Medical Humanities 17, 2
(1996), pp.119-35.

Wormer, H. (2002): Akten unter Verschluss. Ärztekammerpräsident Jörg-Dietrich
Hoppe fordert zu Spenden auf – doch gelegentlich werden die Nachfor-
schungen erschwert, Süddeutsche Zeitung 297 (2002), p. 9.

Wunder, M. (2000): Medizin und Gewissen: Die neue Euthanasie-Debatte in
Deutschland vor dem historischen und internationalen Hintergrund, in:
Frewer/Eickhoff (2000), pp. 250-275.

Zimmermann-Acklin, M. (2000): "Der Schrecken nutzt sich ab". Zur Wechselwir-
kung von Geschichte und Ethik in der gegenwärtigen Euthanasiediskussion,
in: Frewer/Eickhoff (2000), pp. 448-470.

Archives

AHU: Archives of the Humboldt University of Berlin, Berlin.

FAU: Institute for the History of Medicine and Medical Ethics, Friedrich-
Alexander University Erlangen-Nuremberg, Leibbrand papers, Erlangen.

HAL: Hallisches Archiv der Leopoldina, Abderhalden papers, Halle (Saale).

WMA: World Medical Association, Archives, Geneva, Switzerland.

Ulf Schmidt

Medical Ethics and Human Experiments at Porton Down: Informed Consent in Britain's Biological and Chemical Warfare Experiments[1]

I.   Introduction

By the end of the Second World War the advancing allied forces discovered a new nerve gas in Germany. It was called Tabun. Codenamed GA, it was found to be extremely toxic. British experts were immediately dispatched to examine the agent. On arrival, they discovered that German scientists had also developed even more toxic nerve agents, including Sarin, known as GB.[2] The first organised testing of Sarin on humans began in October 1951 at Porton Down in Wiltshire, Britain's biochemical warfare establishment since the First World War. In February 1953, volunteer number 562 experienced the first recorded serious adverse reaction. Testing continued. Two months later, on 27 April, six subjects were given 300 milligrams of Sarin. One of the volunteers, a man named Kelly, suffered serious ill effects, fell into a coma, but then recovered. Although asked by their superiors to reduce the amount tested to the "lowest range of dosage" – which would have been somewhere in the region of 10-15 milligrams – Porton's scientists continued their tests with a "lower" dosage, reducing it from 300 to 200 milligrams.[3]

On 6 May 1953, tests were carried out on a further six subjects. Number 745 was Leading Aircraftsman Ronald Maddison. All six men went into the chamber at around 10 a.m. All were wearing respirators. Each had two pieces of uniform, serge and flannel tied loosely over the forearm. 200 milligrams of pure Sarin was applied onto the layers of cloth, on the inside of the left forearm. Maddison was

<hr/>

1   In 2004, the author was appointed historical expert to Her Majesty's Coroner for Wiltshire and Swindon in the Inquest looking into the death of Ronald George Maddison. Unless stated otherwise, the material presented derives from the "Exhibits" that were supplied to the interested parties and from the Inquest "Transcript". The following abbreviations apply: Maddison-Inquest-Exhibit = "Exhibit", and Maddison-Inquest-Transcript = "Transcript". The author also used the following report: Exhibit, MNJ/20/1, vol. 2A, pp. 84-142, Report of a Court of Inquiry. Reference AY. 1030. Chemical Defence Experimental Establishment, Porton, Wilts., May 1953 (in the following referred to as: Report of a Court of Inquiry 1953); for the discovery of German nerve agents see Exhibit, MNJ/20/3, X1501, G. Brunskill, Attachment 10, Physiological Observers for Porton, 28 May 1945, p. 149; see also Schmidt (2006).

2   Exhibit, MNJ/20/3, X1501, G. Brunskill, Attachment 10, Physiological Observers for Porton, 28 May 1945, p. 149.

3   Transcript, Day 1.

the fourth of the six to be contaminated at 10.17 a.m. Each was to remain in place for thirty minutes from the time of contamination. But at 10.40 a.m. he said he felt "pretty queer". Maddison was sweating and sent from the chamber. His respirator and the contaminated cloth were removed and he walked to a bench about 30 yards away, still sweating. After two minutes an ambulance was called, a minute later Maddison said he could not hear. He was given an injection of Atropine Sulphate intravenously, and then a further injection, intramuscularly. Maddison became unconscious shortly after he said he could not hear. At 10.47 a.m. he arrived at the Porton medical centre. He was put to bed and given oxygen. But shortly afterwards his respiration became irregular. He was gasping. Resuscitation attempts immediately began. At 11 a.m. his colour had become ashen grey and no pulse could be found. Anacardone was injected and further dosages of Atropine. As a last resort, he was given adrenaline, injected directly into his heart. At 1.30 p.m. Maddison was pronounced dead.[4] Days later, the Coroner received a telephone call from the Home Office: "Home Secretary says essential inquest should be held in-camera on grounds of national security. Must not be published".[5] And the Secretary of the Coroner's Society told the Coroner: "At the present moment, the motto seems to be least said, soonest mended".[6] Now, fifty-three years later, records have been made publicly available that can clarify what really happened at Porton Down.

My aim is to provide a historical analysis of the ethical, political and legal dimensions of Britain's biochemical warfare programme in the early stages of the Cold War. So far the debate on non-therapeutic human experiments carried out at Porton in the 1950s and 1960s has been characterised by a lack of historical focus and a medical ethics context. A number of basic questions are central to understanding the events: Did the subjects give voluntary consent? How was consent obtained? Were the risks explained to the subjects? What safeguards were taken? The chapter examines the nature of Britain's Cold War research on humans at Porton in order to come to a better understanding about the extent to which medical ethics standards, including the Nuremberg Code, formulated in 1947 in response to Nazi medical atrocities, were communicated and introduced, as well as ignored, by the British authorities and the research community. I argue that Maddison's case study, and other human experiments at Porton from that period, can highlight some of the central dilemmas of human experimentation, especially regarding the issue of informed consent. I will address the tension that existed during the Cold War, and indeed thereafter, between the use of warfare agents as part of national defence policies, on the one hand, and the principles of human research ethics, on the other. I will first examine how the concept of informed consent developed and was understood in the UK before and after the promulgation of the Nuremberg Code. What, for example, was the level of consent that was generally required in experimental research, and within the

4   Transcript, Day 1.
5   Ibid.
6   Ibid.

specific and secretive military milieu at Porton? Secondly, I will look at the role that consent played in the experimental programme at Porton Down. (A full analysis of the discrepancy between the expectation of informed consent as it was understood in principle, and research practice in the UK, lies outside the purview of this chapter.) Finally, I will look at Maddison's legacy, and assess the extent to which the history of Porton may influence the way in which Britain is beginning to face up to her Cold War past.

Porton's biochemical warfare programme, in which Maddison died, can only be understood in the context of the Cold War. Recently declassified material seems to suggest that in some cases Britain's national security interests overrode individual human rights and accepted standards of research ethics. Over the last decade, a similar picture has emerged for the US' human radiation experiments.[7] The Cold War was, above all, a period of substantial rearmament, arms development, and weapons testing. As the world began to learn the destructive potential of nuclear weapon systems, chemical warfare agents were seen as "outmoded" and generally ineffective for military use. However, given the experience of the Second World War, the British authorities were acutely aware that chemical weapons could cause substantial damage and panic among the population. Britain's threat of retaliation may have prevented Nazi Germany from using chemical weapons. Yet, the scale of the German chemical warfare programme only became apparent after German scientists had been interrogated and chemical weapon arsenals were discovered. Germany produced 12,000 tons of the nerve agent Tabun during the war. The advantage of the "G" agents (Tabun [GA], Sarin [GB], Soman [GD], Ethyl Sarin [GE] and Cyclo Sarin [GF]) lay in the fact that they were significantly more toxic than earlier chemical agents, could cause death quickly, and could be disseminated more easily. Research to explore the full potentialities of the agents in the 1950s and 1960s was not only influenced by the perceived threat that the Soviet Union might use these weapons, but also by the experience of the Second World War. The war had changed the degree of risk scientists were willing to take when conducting experiments on humans. The Cold War and its perceived urgency provided Porton and other Allied research establishments with the strategic and moral justification for the testing of radiological, chemical and biological substances on man.[8]

Porton's nerve agent experiments were unique in several respects. They were by far one of the largest nerve agent trials ever performed, involving more than 1,500 subjects.[9] The specific group that was exposed to Sarin, and to which

7   United States Advisory Committee on Human Radiation Experiments (1996); Moreno (1999).

8   For the United States see United States Advisory Committee on Human Radiation Experiments (1996), also Pechura/Rall (1993), Lederer (1995), Vilensky (2005). For the United Kingdom see Harris/Paxman (1982, reprint 2002), Carter (1992), Goodwin (1998), Bud/Gummett (1999), Carter (2000), Care (2000a), Care (2000b), Evans (2000), Balmer (2001), Hammond/Carter (2002).

9   H. Cullumbine, Head of the Physiology Section at Porton, stated in May 1953 that "in all, some 1,726 subjects have been tested" with nerve gases (see Report of a Court of Inquiry

Maddison belonged, included almost 400 subjects.[10] The Porton experiments were also unusual in the magnitude of the risks. An increasing number of subjects were exposed to an increasingly high dosage of the nerve agent Sarin,[11] which was known by the principal investigators to be highly toxic and potentially lethal in minute concentrations.[12] Porton's investigators knew the great risks involved in the exposure of human subjects to nerve agents.[13] They were also reminded of this fact by the adverse reactions some of the servicemen had to Sarin exposure.[14] Porton's scientists appear to have carried out a series of dangerous experiments on Maddison and other subjects, which demanded, given the nature of the experiments, that the highest degree of safety and the most rigorous standards of research ethics known at the time should have applied. In summary, Maddison's death was an accident waiting to happen which resulted from an inadequate level of disclosure and an understatement of risks, despite the fact that there was widespread consensus in the UK that the principles of the Nuremberg Code should govern these types of experiments. The material presented also shows that the principle of informed consent was in place in UK legal doctrine and medical practice from at least 1933 onwards, long before the promulgation of the Nuremberg Code.

II.   Informed Consent in the United Kingdom

Consent and discussions about the issue of consent in experimental, non-therapeutic research played a considerable role in the UK and abroad throughout the 19th and the first half of the 20th century.[15] Not all experiments on humans, whether therapeutic or non-therapeutic, required the informed consent of the subject. But most scientists accepted the need for volunteers (and their informed consent), particularly when there was a possibility of harm. Since 1830 English law was understood to require that a physician had to obtain the informed consent of the research subject, even if the experiment was for therapeutic purposes. Doctors failing to do so risked litigation.[16] Earlier, in 1767, an English court had decided in *Slater v. Baker and Stapleton* that the defendants would be held liable because they had operated on the patient "without consent" and without telling the

---

1953, p. 50). An internal Porton statistic, Note no. 119, on the "History of the Service Volunteer Observer Scheme at C.D.E.E." gives the following figures: 34 (1945/46); 242 (1948/49); 159 (1949/50); 234 (1950/51); 384 (1951/52); 531 (1952/53). This makes a total of 1,584 subjects who were exposed to nerve gas.

10   A total of 396 men were contaminated with varying doses of liquid GB. Exhibit, MNJ/17, Porton Technical Paper 373; Exhibit, MNJ/30, Porton Technical Paper 399.

11   See Report of a Court of Inquiry 1953, p. 74.

12   Ibid., p. 73.

13   Ministry of Supply (1952a); Ministry of Supply (1952b).

14   Exhibit, MNJ/17, Porton Technical Paper 373, p. 70.

15   Sass (1983); Grodin (1992); Vollmann/Winau (1996); Hazelgrove (2002); Hazelgrove (2004).

16   Willcock (1830), pp. 109-110.

patient "what is about to be done to him".[17] "From 1767, therefore", as Ian Kennedy has pointed out, "it has been clear ... that the general principles of our judicial negligence-based regulatory system will apply to the medical malpractice claim".[18]

One of the oldest medical ethics codes, formulated by William Beaumont in 1833, already contained many of the principles – although most of them by implication – which would later inform the Nuremberg Code in 1947. According to Beaumont, researchers should conduct experimental work only if the information could not be obtained by other means, for example through animal experimentation, and if the investigators were conscientious and responsible in their work. They had to abstain from random trials, obtain the voluntary consent from the subject and had to be prepared to discontinue the experiment if it caused distress to the subject.[19]

Claude Bernard's medical ethics code from 1865 is another case in point in that the Hippocratic principle of *primum non nocere* (first of all, to do no harm) mattered when it came to non-therapeutic research on humans. In his famous text, *An Introduction to the Study of Experimental Medicine*, Bernard claimed that human experiments "that can only do harm are forbidden, those that are harmless are permissible, and those that may do good are obligatory".[20] He also stated that

"The principle of medical and surgical morality was never to perform on a human subject an experiment whose outcome could only be harmful in some degree, even though the results might be highly advantageous to science, i.e. to the health of others".[21]

Yet the language in which most medical ethics codes were written, especially those within the Anglo-Saxon tradition, was often vague and subject to general interpretation in order to leave investigators with the freedom of discretion, for example the Code of Ethics of the American Medical Association which was adopted in 1847.[22]

Ironically, the country that began to develop the most stringent and clearly defined medical ethics regulations at the end of the 19th century was Germany. As early as 1891 the Prussian Ministry of the Interior issued a regulation that ensured that tuberculin would "in no case be used against the patients' will" for the treatment of tuberculosis. Three years later, in 1894, the German Supreme Court stressed that surgical and other potentially life-threatening treatments needed the consent of the patient. In 1900, the Prussian Ministry of Religious, Educational and Medical Affairs issued a legal directive that non-therapeutic interventions on humans were "absolutely prohibited" if the subject "has not declared unequivocally that he consents to the intervention" and if "the declaration has not been made

---

17 Faden/Beauchamp (1986), p. 115; see also Katz (1972), p. 526; Kennedy/Grubb (1994), p. 526; Berg et al. (2001), pp. 42f.
18 Kennedy/Grubb (1994), p. 527.
19 Beecher (1970), Appendix A, p. 219.
20 Ibid., p. 234.
21 Quoted from Katz (1992), p. 229.
22 Grodin (1992), pp. 124f; see also Katz (1984), Appendix A, pp. 230-236.

on the basis of a proper explanation of the adverse consequences that may result from the intervention".[23] The requirement for voluntary informed consent was officially recognised as "fundamental to ethically sound experimentation".[24]

Similar views were advanced in the American and British context since the beginning of the 20th century. The famous clinician William Osler, who later taught as a Regius Professor at Oxford, did not prohibit non-therapeutic experiments *per se*, like Bernard had done, but demanded that investigators should obtain the informed consent from the subject. In 1907 Osler stated that "for the human being absolute security and full consent are the conditions which make such test [non-therapeutic research] permissible".[25] In 1916 the *Journal of the American Medical Association* warned doctors that the potential knowledge gained from experiments did not justify even harmless interventions without consent. The *Journal* (probably the editors) stated that it was "a generally recognised" ethical standard of the medical profession that subjects should have a right to control "the uses to which his own body is put". Operations "for the satisfaction of the operator" or the "immediate benefit of others" were not permissible, unless "the consent of the person on whom the operation is to be performed has previously been obtained".[26]

At the end of the 1920s a series of unethical and in some cases fatal experiments on children in the north-German city of Lübeck prompted further public debate about medical ethics standards.[27] In February 1931, the Reich Ministry of the Interior issued the "Regulations Concerning New Therapy and Human Experimentation".[28] The directives were among the most comprehensive research rules by any standard at the time and some elements were even more elaborate than the principles of the Nuremberg Code. Contentious issues, such as individual autonomy, beneficence, informed voluntary consent or therapeutic and non-therapeutic research, were formulated to protect the rights and dignity of patients. In § 12, which is concerned with non-therapeutic research, the 1931 Reich Regulations stated that "experimentation shall be prohibited in all cases where consent has not been given".[29]

In the UK, discussions on the ethics of human experimentation in the 1930s led to the formulation of a legal position by the Treasury Solicitor. Indeed, the position of the current UK government is largely based on the advice given at the time. In June 1933, the British Medical Research Council (MRC) asked the Treasury Solicitor for advice on experimental research into the causation of influenza. On 21 June 1933, the Treasury Solicitor, after consulting the Director of Public Prosecution, advised the MRC on the subject:

---

23   Grodin (1992), p. 127; also Vollman/Winau (1996), p. 1446.
24   Grodin (1992), p. 128.
25   Rothman (1997), p. 79.
26   Anonymous (1916), pp. 1372-1373.
27   Frewer (2000), pp. 139-145; also Maio (2002); Winau (1996), pp. 25f.
28   Sass (1983); Grodin (1992); Katz (1997), p. 410.
29   Grodin (1992), p. 131.

"As regards civil liability I am of opinion that the consent of the person on whom the experiment is made would afford a complete answer to any claim for damages either by himself or by his dependents. I assume, of course, that the nature of the risk which the person in question was being invited to incur would be explained to him, and that the experiment itself would be conducted with all due care and that all precautions suggested by medical science would be taken.

As regards criminal responsibility the position is, from a theoretical point of view, more difficult to define in precise language. Although consent is a complete answer to a civil claim for damages it is not necessarily so in the case of criminal proceedings. If therefore the death of a patient should unfortunately occur, the fact that it was the result of some act to the performance of which he gave his consent would not of itself be a complete defence in the event of proceedings of a criminal nature being instituted against the person performing the act in question".[30]

The Treasury Solicitor also told the MRC that the risk of a criminal charge against the MRC was so remote as to be negligible if the patient had given his full consent and if all the risks of the experiment had been explained.[31] The Treasury Solicitor assumed, of course,

"that the person responsible for performing the experiment would be able to show that it had been conducted with the full consent of the patient, given after proper appreciation of the risks involved, and that it had been performed with all due care and skill. Evidence to this effect would exclude any issue of criminal negligence".[32]

Although few documented cases involve informed consent, contemporary judicial practice in the UK reaffirms the position of the Treasury Solicitor.[33] Other contemporary documents show that the MRC took the Treasury Solicitor's position on board and advised researchers accordingly.[34] Whilst accepting that research subjects could be exposed to some risk for the benefit of society, the MRC advised scientists to produce evidence that would show that the experiment had been conducted with the "full consent of the patient, given after proper appreciation of the risks involved, and that it had been performed with all due care and skill".[35]

More generally, scientists accepted that research on humans had to be ethical in order to be permissible long before the Nuremberg Code. This is not surprising, given that one of the universal principles of medical ethics demands that a physician-scientist should not do harm, either to a patient or to a research subject. Those investigators who wanted to search for new knowledge, which would not necessarily benefit the patient-subject, were required to inform the subject about the risks involved and obtain the subject's consent. Indeed, the advice of the MRC

---

30   The National Archives, London (TNA), TS27/398, Gwyer (Treasury Solicitor) to MRC, 21 June 1933.

31   TNA, TS27/398, Gwyer (Treasury Solicitor) to MRC, 21 June 1933.

32   Ibid.

33   Kennedy/Grubb (1994), pp. 90f.

34   TNA, FD1/428. MRC to Krebs, 29 August 1945. MRC to Eiringer, 8 December 1947. MRC to Davidson, 14 December 1951. MRC to Spiers, 26 May 1952

35   TNA, FD1/428, MRC to Erich Eiringer, 8 December 1947.

was to obtain confirmation of this in specific cases by using a written consent form as early as 1945.[36]

Following the Second World War, the Allies decided to prosecute a number of doctors who were involved in Nazi medical atrocities. As part of the judgement in the Nuremberg Doctors' Trial, the judges issued a ten-point medical ethics code, which laid down the human rights of patient-subjects and the duties of physician-researchers for experiments on humans.[37] The aim of the Code was to find a solution to resolve one of the most fundamental conflicts in human experimentation: to balance the need for the advancement of medical science for the benefit of human society with the right of the individual to personal inviolability, autonomy and self-determination. The decision to include the Code into the judgement meant that, for the first time, written guidelines for permissible research on humans were incorporated into the canon of international law. The Code established fundamental human rights in medicine, and placed the welfare of the patients in the foreground of medical practice. In the Nuremberg Code neither medicine, nor science, nor society, nor any kind of collective or utilitarian ethics has priority over the protection of the individual to remain physically and psychologically unharmed. A person's right to self-determination and inviolability cannot be calculated against the need for medical progress, or any other claim that society and science may or may not have to trump individual rights of its citizens.

Principle one of the Code has been of importance for the history of medical ethics which reaches far beyond Nuremberg. The principle links the experiment to the voluntary consent of the experimental subject. That means that the experiment can only be carried out after the "voluntary, personal consent" has been obtained, and only after the subject has been clearly informed about the risk involved in the best possible manner. The Code makes it categorically clear that the person involved in the experiment has to have the legal capacity to give a voluntary consent. Moreover, prior to obtaining consent, the exact nature, duration and objective of the experiment, the applied methods and means as well as all potential implications of the experiment for the health of the person have to be made clear. The experimental subject has to have sufficient knowledge of, and capacity to comprehend, the subject matter in order to make an enlightened and informed decision. This was meant to protect unconscious and mentally handicapped persons or humans who, because of their specific illness, may be unable to give voluntary consent.

Whatever the immediate effects of the Code, which for the first decade was mostly seen as "a good code for barbarians but an unnecessary code for ordinary physician-scientists", it had significant implications for contemporary medical

---

36   TNA, FD1/428. MRC to Krebs, 29 August 1945. Issue of provision of consent by volunteers in human experiments. Appended draft of consent form; TNA, TS27/398. MRC to Prendergast, 29 August 1945; Prendergast to MRC, 30 August 1945; Prendergast to MRC, 5 September 1945; draft of consent form, 7 September 1945.

37   For a discussion about the history and legacy of the Nuremberg Code, see Schmidt (2004); see also the article by Ulf Schmidt in this volume.

ethics and ethics regulations.[38] The principles laid down in the Code were embodied, in one form or another, in various national and international conventions regulating the use of human subjects in biomedical research, for example in Article 7 of the International Covenant on Civil and Political Rights, which states that "no one shall be subjected without his free consent to medical or scientific experimentation".[39] Moreover, the Code helped to shape the four Geneva Conventions of 1949, providing basic protection against criminal human experiments in times of war. In 1953, the US military confirmed the legal validity of the Nuremberg Code in a "top secret" memorandum about the "Use of Human Volunteers in Experimental Research".[40] Since then the Code has served many times as a point of reference in civilian tort actions involving non-therapeutic experiments.[41] The Code also became a model for subsequent international agreements which placed human rights at the centre of human experimentation.[42] Even though researchers ignored, and in some cases violated, the principles of the Code throughout the 1950s and 1960s, research institutions and medical scientists seem to have been aware of its legal and ethical implications.[43] Indeed, there is fresh evidence that British scientists and the MRC accepted the Code as the guiding principle in non-therapeutic research at the time.[44]

Even before the Nuremberg Code was promulgated, British physicians conducted a debate about the ethics and quality of the German experiments which had been carried out on non-volunteers. The debate was triggered in November 1946 in the British journal, *The Lancet*, and followed up by the *British Medical Journal*.[45] In January 1947, the Secretary of the British Medical Sciences Committee stated that he considered investigators who "performed harmful experiments on human beings without their consent" to be "guilty of a crime", independent of their national or cultural context:

> "The actions performed are admittedly criminal in any system of national and international law, and scientists are as subject to the law as other persons; they can claim no personal immunity on the grounds that their crimes are committed for disinterested motives".[46]

Similarly, in 1948, one year after the promulgation of the Nuremberg Code, L. J. Witts commented about Nazi medical experiments in the *British Medical Journal* (BMJ):

---

38   Katz (1996), pp. 1662-1666.
39   Perley et al. (1992), pp. 149-173, at p. 153.
40   Annas/Grodin (1992), pp. 343-345.
41   Proctor (2000), pp. 15-16.
42   Arnold/Sprumont (1998), pp. 84-96.
43   Schmidt (2004), pp. 264-297.
44   TNA, FD9/855, Draft – Council memorandum "Experiments on Man: Conditions for Conduct", including statement on the "Condition on which experiments can be conducted on man", 2 January 1956.
45   Anonymous (1946); Mellanby (1946); Layton/Nelson-Jones (1946); Hilton (1947); Herbert (1947).
46   Herbert (1947), pp. 84-85.

"The plain fact is that few researchers would willingly inoculate themselves with jaundice, and it is an absolute rule of clinical research that one should never do to others what one would not do to oneself. Once break this rule and one is on the slippery slope that led so many Nazis to the abyss. Moreover, it is a moot point whether a healthy citizen is within his legal rights in volunteering for a dangerous experiment ... [which] are rarely wise in peace-time".[47]

The Nuremberg Code slowly but gradually raised a critical awareness of the international medical community and found entry into international codes of practice to which the United Kingdom had subscribed.[48] In 1946 the World Medical Association (WMA) was founded at the headquarters of the British Medical Association in Tavistock House, London. In its 1949 report on German Medical War Crimes the WMA published the Nuremberg Code in full, thereby making it available to all physicians and scientists of the world, including those of the British Medical Association.[49] In February 1952 the "1942 Club", a group of eminent UK medical scientists, held its thirteenth meeting at the Royal College of Surgeons to discuss "The Problem of Human Experiment".[50] In line with Hippocratic medical ethics, Professor Gardner, Regius Professor of Medicine at the University of Oxford, believed that the "moral issue" was evident: "the doctor must be sure that no harm is done to the individual".[51] Another scientist had considered the problem together with legal advisors. UK medical scientists were told that

"no civil action can follow an experimental observation if the consent of the patient has first been obtained, if the nature of the risk has been explained to the patient and all due care has been taken in the experiment. A satisfactory answer to these three questions would not necessarily prevent a criminal charge, but if the three could be answered adequately, it is thought that the risk of a conviction is negligible".[52]

In the mid-1950s, UK scientists and editors of medical journals increasingly expressed concern about the ethics of human experimentation.[53] British research-ers knew that the greater the potential risks to subjects, the more comprehensive the necessary disclosure for valid informed consent had to be. A February 1955 editorial, "Experiments on Human Beings", in the *BMJ* discussed these issues.[54] The editor asked "What safeguards should the medical profession erect to protect the public and to preserve its traditional *mores*?". The journal then stated that "Mr. B. Shimkin considers that the clearest rules for guidance were those laid down at the Nuremberg trials".[55] Nine months later, in November 1955, the MRC came to

---

47 Quoted from Ministry of Defence (2006), pp. 383f; see also Witts (1948), p. 458.
48 See also Hazelgrove (2002), pp. 116ff.
49 United Nations War Crimes Commission (1949).
50 Exhibit, CCB/4; X2862, Minutes of the Thirtieth Meeting of the "1942 Club", 1 February 1952; see also Hazelgrove (2002), footnote 75.
51 Exhibit, CCB/4; X2862, Minutes of the Thirtieth Meeting of the "1942 Club", 1 February 1952.
52 Ibid.
53 Anonymous (1955), pp. 526-527.
54 Ibid., pp. 526-527.
55 Ibid., p. 527; see also Shimkin (1953), pp. 205-207.

the conclusion, after consulting key members of the British medical profession, that the Nuremberg Code should serve as the main point of reference in experimental research on humans in the UK.[56] The MRC had come to this conclusion after holding a conference in September 1955 to consider the "Conditions on which experiments can be conducted on man".[57] In the revised and agreed minutes of the meeting, the MRC and some of the leading representatives of the British medical community, stated:

> "It was axiomatic that full consent must always be obtained before an experiment was conducted on man, that the conditions drawn up by the Nuremberg Tribunal (copy attached) set out adequately the requirements which should be satisfied before the consent could be termed full and also the other conditions which should regulate the conduct of the experiment".[58]

The material shows that the British medical establishment recognised the principles of the Nuremberg Code prior to the formulation of the 1964 Declaration of Helsinki[59] by the WMA, or the 1967 ethics guidelines from the Royal College of Physicians. Sections of the medical community, however, resisted the introduction of the Code, and experiments continued to be conducted that were open to professional criticism by men such as Henry K. Beecher in the US or by Maurice H. Pappworth in the UK.[60]

---

56 TNA, FD9/855, MRC minutes of "Meeting on 27.9.55 to consider "Conditions on which experiments can be conducted on man", 18 November 1955.
57 Ibid.
58 TNA, FD9/855, Draft – Council memorandum "Experiments on Man: Conditions for Conduct", including statement on the "Condition on which experiments can be conducted on man", 2 January 1956.
59 See the article by Susan Lederer in this volume.
60 Schmidt (2004), pp. 284-287.

III.   Porton Down and Human Experimentation

The UK was clearly no moral and ethical "wasteland" and UK government
agencies were generally committed to uphold international standards of medical
morality and individual justice. UK medical scientists were also aware of and
committed to honouring the ethical principles of the Nuremberg Code at the time
of the Porton experiments. Experiments that involved a significant risk and were
non-therapeutic demanded the *highest* standards of research ethics, not the *lowest*
or those that were *generally* applied in UK medical practice and research. In 1925,
the War Office reassured the Commander-in-Chief, Southern Command,
Salisbury, about servicemen under his command who were given the opportunity
to volunteer for experiments involving the exposure to mustard gas at Porton, that
the risk involved in the tests was negligible.[61]

In November 1930 the War Office received a copy of the recently revised
"regulations in force at Porton for the protection of observers who are submitted to
gas test for experimental purposes". The War Office was told that

> "the most scrupulous care is taken to ensure that tests are so conducted that not only no injury
> is incurred, but that only the minimum of discomfort is caused. Nobody but volunteers are
> submitted to these tests …".[62]

One month later, in December 1930, the Secretary of State for War told Parliament that since January 1929 some 520 servicemen had taken part in experiments
with mustard gas, and that all relevant precautions had been taken to ensure that
the servicemen would not be harmed.[63] In January 1931, Colonel Look,
Commandant at the Experimental Station, Porton, told the War Office that "the
question of the experiments on volunteers from outside Units should now be
reopened". Look specifically addressed the issue of "information" that was
provided to the servicemen:

> "Great care is taken to ensure that observers from outside Units understand the object of each
> particular test, and it is considered that there is no risk of such observers getting a wrong
> impression as to the efficiency of their respirators or false ideas as to what is being done".[64]

Research that was considered harmful to the subjects was refused. In 1926, the
Chief Superintendent from the Chemical Defence Research Department at the
War Office declined to grant permission for breathing tests with toxic smoke at
Porton, believing that "the proposal might prove very far reaching in the long run
and possibly result in difficulties as regards injury to health…".[65] In 1932,
research at Porton was again proposed in which servicemen would breathe in a

---

61   TNA, WO286/11 (Police Ref. X61), H. J. Creedy (War Office) to the General Officer,
     Commanding-in-Chief, Southern Command, Salisbury, 30 July 1925.
62   Exhibit, MNJ/20/2, X1501, Expanded Statement (B), 19 November 1930, pp. 136-138.
63   TNA, WO286/11 (Police Ref. X61), Parliamentary Question no. 170, 18 December 1930.
64   Exhibit, MNJ/20/2, X1501, Colonel R.F. Look, Commandant, Experimental Station Porton,
     to the Chief Superintendent, Chemical Defence Research Department, War Office, 24
     January 1931, p. 142.
65   Ibid.

small amount of toxic smoke. The Army Council, however, refused permission for the tests. Given that the UK government was about to ratify the "Geneva Protocol for the Prohibition of the use in war of Asphyxiating, Poisonous or other Gases, and of Bacteriological Methods of Warfare", which had been drawn up by the League of Nations in 1925, officials were reluctant to permit chemical warfare experiments that involved any risk. One official noted: "I consider that nothing of this kind, involving some risk, however small, should be carried out while the conference is sitting at Geneva".[66]

The outbreak of war in 1939 may have altered the situation. With the country at war, government officials were more likely to take greater risks in understanding the efficiency of certain agents the enemy might employ. On 23 April 1940, the War Committee produced a memorandum which stated that Porton had again asked to expose human subjects to toxic smoke, and stressed the "difference between peace and war conditions and the increase in the importance of the experimental work being carried on sternutators".[67] One official noted:

> "I do not consider there is any objection on medical grounds to the application put forward. These tests would be carried out under expert supervision and with adequate precautions. I therefore support the application".[68]

In considering informed consent at Porton, we have to acknowledge that Britain's discovery of large stocks of nerve gas in Germany in 1945 substantially changed the nature of the experiments at Porton. The existence and testing of nerve gas introduced a new and unknown risk to those servicemen who participated in the research, yet Porton does not seem to have modified its experimental procedure accordingly. In May 1945, a British military official noted that "our investigation of German chemical warfare has revealed the existence of large stocks of a novel type of poison gas that they were intending to use from air and ground weapons".[69] The official felt that since the testing of the new substance

> "is simply an extension of the normal routine it should not involve any additional administrative problems ... Porton, of course, are responsible for seeing that the men are not exposed to any concentration of gas which would do them permanent harm".[70]

Some British scientists, however, began to feel uneasy about human experiments. In October 1952 R. J. V. Pulvertaft, Professor of Clinical Pathology at the University of London, drew attention to the fact that UK servicemen might easily be encouraged into participating in potentially hazardous experiments without knowing the full risks involved:

66   Exhibit, MNJ/20/2, X1501, Memorandum by the War Committee, "Employment Of Observers From The Services On Physiological Tests Involving Exposure To Sternutators", 23 April 1940, pp. 146-147.
67   Ibid.
68   Ibid.
69   Exhibit, MNJ/20/3, X1501, G. Brunskill, Attachment 10, Physiological Observers for Porton, 28 May 1945, p. 149.
70   Ibid.

"[...] Now that service is compulsory for all, they [the medical services of the Armed Forces] must be prepared to resist any tendency to find a useful reservoir of clinical experiments in this group of healthy young men – especially since, in a disciplined force, the 'volunteer' can easily be encouraged by sanctions or privileges".[71]

In January 1953, three-and-a-half months before Maddison's death, American officials, seeking to carry out similar experiments at Edgewood Arsenal, Maryland, inquired of their British counterparts: "What advance information as to the nature of the tests is given to the men in their units before they are asked to volunteer?"[72] On 11 February 1953, S. A. Mumford, Chief Superintendent at Porton, replied:

"No advance information as to the nature of the tests is given to the men in their Units before they are asked to volunteer beyond the attached Appendix A to W.O. memo 112/mix/580 AG1 (A) copy attached".[73]

The Americans chose to ignore this advice as they went on to insist that the consent of volunteers had to be obtained in writing and according to the Nuremberg Code. The evidence suggests that throughout the 1930s and 1940s it was considered important to explain to the subjects at Porton what was meant by gas, and inform the subjects of the nature of the tests. However, those responsible for the experiments in the early 1950s do not seem to have explained to volunteers the nature of the substances to which they would be exposed, or to have fully informed them about the risks. Some of Porton's subjects seem to have been exposed to escalating doses of toxic, even lethal, substances. The risks significantly increased with nerve-gas testing, but the level of consent which was obtained from the subjects, and the information that was provided to them, seem instead to have generally decreased in the climate of the Cold War, or at best remained the same.

Contemporary correspondence about informed consent at the time of Maddison's death includes witness statements for the Coroner's Inquest and the Court of Inquiry by the Ministry of Supply at the time. The Court of Inquiry wanted to know, for example, "what information" was provided to the subjects concerning the experiment. One witness stated that the subjects were "given a general idea" of the tests. They were told of "the possible effects" and that they could "withdraw" if they wanted to.[74] Asked by the Court whether the subjects were "given" any "written questions", another witness stated that the subjects

---

71   Pulvertaft (1952), pp. 839ff.
72   Exhibit, MNJ/20/3, X1502, D. C. Evans to S.A. Mumford, 23 January 1953, p. 300.
73   Exhibit, MNJ/20/3, X1502, S. A. Mumford to D.C. Evans, 11 February 1953, pp. 298-299. The Appendix "A" to War Office Memorandum 112/Misc/5860/AG1 (A) dated 6th November 1950 stated: "1) The physical discomfort resulting from tests is usually very slight. Tests are carefully planned to avoid the slightest chance of danger, and are under expert medical supervision. 2) During their stay at Porton, volunteers do not undertake any military duties or fatigues, and are free every evening. 3) Extra pay is given which normally brings each volunteer some ten to fifteen shillings a week".
74   See Report of a Court of Inquiry 1953, p. 53.

were "asked if they wanted to ask any questions".[75] The answer suggests that the scientists shifted the responsibility of obtaining information about the experiment to the research subjects themselves. The subjects were then "told briefly" what the test would be.[76]

The scientists appear to have misled the subjects by providing them with only a general idea about the experiments, and by understating the dangers involved. The witness Stanley Mumford stated that research subjects were "given a broad idea and they are told by the Medical Officer *that there is no risk* [emphasis added]".[77] Internally, however, after one of the men had fallen into a coma, Porton conceded that there were hazards involved in the tests.[78] Porton officials seem to have been concerned that if they were to supply the subjects with more detailed information, some, if not many, might refuse to participate in the experiments. As one Porton scientist stated: "If you advertised for people to suffer agony you would not get them".[79] Given the known health risks, the information provided was misleading. The Court of Inquiry acknowledged this: "to say there is not the slightest danger is a mis-statement as you are in fact dealing with a dangerous substance".[80] The Court also felt that the subjects "should be told quite clearly what risks they are going to take" before they undertook the journey from the parent units, something that had apparently not been done.[81]

In May 1953, H. Woodhouse, the Treasury Solicitor's representative, also came to the conclusion that the subjects had been misled at Porton, and that the government should accept responsibility for Maddison's death. Woodhouse realised that there was a significant discrepancy between the procedures which Porton was using in recruiting volunteers, including the information that was provided to them, and the level of actual risk to which the subjects were exposed:

> "[…] in dealing with a dangerous but largely unknown substance like G.B. [Sarin] it would be difficult to show that there had been no negligence (a very high degree of care being required in relation to dangerous substances), and partly because the terms of the information to be brought to the notice of personnel to encourage them to volunteer … terms indicating that there was not the slightest element of danger, have proved [to be] somewhat misleading".[82]
> (The author discovered this correspondence on 17 October 2003 in the headquarters of "Operation Antler" in Devizes, Wiltshire)

With regard to future experiments on humans, Woodhouse suggested that the Minister should pay appropriate compensation and should not seek to adopt a system of indemnities or "blood chits" which would place the responsibility upon the person volunteering for the experiments. Given that the servicemen had

---

75 See Report of a Court of Inquiry 1953, p. 65.
76 Ibid.
77 Ibid, p. 86 and p. 93.
78 Ibid, p. 84.
79 Ibid, p. 86.
80 Ibid, p. 87.
81 Ibid, p. 88.
82 TNA, WO286/11 (Police Ref. X61), H. Woodhouse (for the Treasury Solicitor), to Legal 1 (Mr. Griffith-Jones), Ministry of Supply, 15 May 1953.

received misleading information for experiments which included "a definite element of unknown danger", Woodhouse proposed to change the wording to recruit volunteers in the future:

> "I suggest that the wording of the information to be brought to the attention of personnel to encourage them to volunteer ought to be altered. The sentence: 'Tests are carefully planned to avoid the slightest chance of danger' has proved misleading. Indeed it is difficult to see how it was ever possible to say truthfully that tests with lethal gases did not contain 'the slightest chance of danger'. The true position, I take it, is that the tests are arranged so as to eliminate all foreseeable danger, but that as the tests are designed for the purpose of obtaining further information about substances the properties and performance of which are to some extent unknown, there is always some possibility (even it be exceedingly remote) of a danger being discovered".[83]

By July 1953, officials had followed the advice of the Treasury Solicitor. Instead of saying that "Tests are carefully planned to avoid the slightest chance of danger", the notice now read: "The physical discomfort resulting from tests is usually very slight. Tests are arranged so as to eliminate all foreseeable danger, and are under expert medical supervision".[84] The change of wording occurred as a direct result of Maddison's death. Instead of providing the subjects with more information about the risks involved, officials decided to phrase the invitation in such a way as to provide even less information. The new statement may not have been misleading, at least not to the same extent, but it does not appear to have been a fair representation of the nature, purpose and risk of experiments that were subsequently carried out on human volunteers at Porton.

On 13 July 1953, Woodhouse again took up the issue of human experiments at Porton. Maddison's death had clearly raised a number of important ethical and legal issues. He noted that the Service Departments of the British military had at the time given their permission for the recruitment of volunteers for the testing of mustard gas, but not for the significantly more dangerous nerve agents:

> "It seems [...] [t]hat the arrangement for service volunteers at Porton were originally made at a time when the experiments related principally if not entirely to mustard gas and that these arrangements have continued over the years without any clear acceptance by Service Department of the fact that the present experiments involve the use of substances which are more lethal and more uncertain in operation than mustard gas".[85] (This correspondence was discovered by the author on 17 October 2003 in the headquarters of "Operation Antler" in Devizes, Wiltshire)

Woodhouse identified the main shortcoming in Porton's experimental procedures. His comments show that the procedures for recruiting volunteers, and for providing them with information about the nature and risk of the experiments, and for obtaining their consent, effectively derived from a time when the Service

---

83 TNA, WO286/11 (Police Ref. X61), H. Woodhouse (for the Treasury Solicitor), to Legal 1 (Mr. Griffith-Jones), Ministry of Supply, 15 May 1953.

84 TNA, WO286/11 (Police Ref. X61), Appendix 'A' to 86/Chemical/899(SW1), dated 9th July, 1953.

85 TNA, WO286/11 (Police Ref. X61), H. Woodhouse (for the Treasury Solicitor), to Legal 1 (Mr. Griffith-Jones), Ministry of Supply, 13 July 1953.

Departments were concerned about the testing of mustard gas, that is from after the First World War. In short, the procedures for recruiting research subjects at Porton, and for obtaining their consent, appear not to have been updated in order to take account of the higher degree of risk to which the subjects were exposed in the early 1950s.[86] Given this state of affairs, the Treasury Solicitor advised the Minister of Supply on 1 August 1953 that the Crown or the Minister was, in all likelihood, liable for Maddison's death, and that Section 10 of the Crown Proceedings Act from 1947 had no application.[87]

Whereas civil servants and other officials acknowledged the legal and ethical problems which Maddison's death raised, politicians were given a somewhat different picture. On 7 May 1953, twenty-four hours after Maddison died, Duncan-Sandys, who was responsible for Porton Down as the Minister of Supply (1951-54), informed Prime Minister Churchill about the death of an RAF. [Royal Airforce] serviceman at Porton. Duncan-Sandys told Churchill that "these tests are of an exceedingly mild type and are conducted under strict medical supervision".[88] The same information was given to the Home Secretary, Sir David Maxwell-Fyfe, who had been the Deputy Chief Prosecutor in the Nuremberg Trials (1945-1946), to the Minister for Defence and the Secretary of State for Air. A draft statement about the "fatal accident" at Porton, prepared by the Ministry of Supply, noted: "In every case the nature of the test and the anticipated result was described to the volunteer prior to the test so that he could withdraw if he so wished".[89] It may well be, given what we know today, that Duncan-Sandys was rather economical with the truth on this occasion, something that was later reflected in the information provided to Parliament. In November 1953, the Parliamentary Secretary at the Ministry of Defence was asked whether he was satisfied that "when National Service men volunteer their offer of service should be accepted? Would he not agree that, since many of them are under age, their status is different from that of a man who is making the Services his career?" In his reply, the Parliamentary Secretary stated: "The men are volunteers and the nature of the experiment is clearly explained to them and they are then given a chance to withdraw. There has been only one fatal accident since 1922."[90] The official government position contrasted with the information that was given to the research subjects.[91]

86 See Report of a Court of Inquiry 1953, p. 54.
87 TNA, WO286/11 (Police Ref. X61), H. Woodhouse (for the Treasury Solicitor), to Legal 1 (Mr. Griffith-Jones), Ministry of Supply, 1 August 1953. The author discovered this correspondence on 17 October 2003 in the headquarters of "Operation Antler" in Devizes, Wiltshire. As a result, the UK Ministry of Defence (MoD) has decided not to rely on Section 10(2) of the Crown Proceedings Act 1947 as a defence in cases involving nerve agents.
88 Exhibit, MNJ/20/3, X1501, Duncan-Sandys to Churchill, 7 May 1953, pp. 226-227.
89 Exhibit, MNJ/20/3, X1501, Fatal Accident at the Chemical Defence Experimental Establishment, Porton, Near Salisbury, on 6th May, 1953, Statement by the Ministry of Supply, Fifth Draft, pp. 196-197.
90 TNA, WO286/11 (Police Ref. X61), House of Commons, Official Report 17th November, 1953, Cols. 1567/8, Experimental Work (Service Volunteers).
91 See Report of a Court of Inquiry 1953, p. 86, and p. 93.

IV.   The Testimony of Former Servicemen

The existing witness statements obtained by "Operation Antler"[92] of former servicemen who attended Porton Down in the early 1950s, together with oral history interviews conducted by the author, confirm that subjects were not properly informed about the experiments.[93] In evaluating the statements of former servicemen caution obviously needs to be exercised which the passage of time may have had on their personal recollections. Renver Charles Brant, who attended Porton as an Army participant at the end of April 1953, stated:

> "I had never heard of Porton Down and consequently I had no idea of what they did there … I did have knowledge of mustard gas and the dangers of inhaling it … I suppose the fact that you were there as a volunteer indicated that you consented to take part in the experiments … I had no knowledge of nerve agents at that time so I don't suppose it would have meant anything to me even if they had told me this at the time".[94]

Kenneth Earl attended Porton at the same time as Maddison and participated in the same kind of Sarin experiment as Maddison, but two days earlier, on 4 May 1953. Earl stated:

> "The main test and the one I remember more about was a test, which took place inside a heated chamber. I cannot remember being given any other information in relation to this test and in fact if I had been told (as I know now) what this test involved me coming into contact with, then I would have without doubt have said 'no' to the test".[95]

In another statement Earl stated: "I would reiterate that I had no idea that I was going to be testing nerve gas when I went to Porton Down".[96] Earl, like many of the Porton servicemen, does not recall having "any knowledge of nerve gas or their effects" before he went to Porton.[97]

James Patrick Kelly, who attended Porton in April 1953, also had no knowledge of nerve gas or nerve agents but knew of the effects of mustard gas.[98] He believed that he was participating in a "Gas Warfare Course" and that he would "receive tuition on the details of Gas Warfare". He recalled that he "expected to attend lectures, have demonstrations and be bombarded with information to learn … I had a real thirst for knowledge".[99] Instead, Kelly participated in a Sarin experiment and appears not to have been informed about it: "I had no idea at the

---

92   In July 1999, the Wiltshire Constabulary began to investigate allegations made by a former serviceman, who stated that during his National Service he took part in research into finding a cure for the Common Cold at Porton. As a result of this and other allegations the Force initiated a major enquiry, called "Operation Antler". The purpose of the investigation was to examine the role of the Service Volunteer Programme at Porton Down in relation to chemical and biological warfare experiments during the period 1939-1989.

93   See also Lee et al. (2004) p. 19.

94   Statement of Renver Charles Brant, 23 October 2002.

95   Statement of Kenneth Earl, 15 May 2000.

96   Statement of Kenneth Earl, 16 November 2000.

97   Ibid.

98   Statement of James Patrick Kelly, 2 May 2003.

99   Ibid.

time what the liquids were that I was testing. I certainly was not told what the liquids were, or that there would be any short or long term health risks".[100] He also stated that in one of the experiments a drop of clear liquid was placed onto the inside of his wrist, but "was not told what this droplet was".[101] In another experiment "the liquid was dispensed from a small eyedropper, and again I was not told what it was".[102] In another statement Kelly stated:

"No one explained the substances that they were using, or the purpose of the test. We received no formal briefing or explanation about Porton Down, or the work they were doing there. The tester never asked us if we were happy to take part. We were told to take part in certain test, we had no option to do one test or another".[103]

Kelly also recalls that he was "confused" by the experience because he could not understand how the experiments related to Gas Warfare Training, but felt that being a soldier he could not speak up.[104]

Frederick Henry John Moules attended Porton in March 1953. He knew that Porton was a "Chemical-testing place". He also believed that he received "a briefing that the test was with a nerve agent of some kind". Once the liquid was placed on his arm Moules "collapsed" and was taken to Porton's hospital where he was "drifting in and out of consciousness for about three days".[105] Moules statement seems to suggest that the information which he received, if he received it, must have been general and did not inform him about the potential effects of the experiments.[106]

John Leonard Newbury, who attended Porton between 27 April and 1 May 1953, stated that he had

"absolutely no idea what I was going to Porton Down for and Chemical/Biological warfare experiments never came into my mind. If I had any idea of what I was going to Porton Down for involved Chemical or Biological Warfare experiments I would not have volunteered to go".[107]

On arrival at Porton, however, Newbury appears to have been told that he would be experimented on with "nerve gas" and later was told that he would be exposed to "radioactive nerve gas".[108] This came as a "complete shock" to him and others. Although some of the men were concerned, they were told that the experiments posed no risk: "Many of our course expressed concerns and this man reassured us by saying dilute amounts would be used and it was totally safe".[109] Newbury also

100 Statement of James Patrick Kelly, 18 November 1999.
101 Ibid.
102 Ibid.
103 Statement of James Patrick Kelly, 2 May 2003.
104 Ibid.
105 Statement of Frederick Henry John Moules, 5 June 2000.
106 Ibid.
107 Statement of John Leonard Newbury, 29 April 2003.
108 Statement of John Leonard Newbury, 22 March 2000.
109 Ibid.

felt that his "mere presence there as a volunteer was construed as consent",[110] and that he was "definitely not given the option of pulling out of the experiment".[111]

Peter George de Carle Parker attended Porton at the same time as Maddison and participated in the same Sarin experiment as Maddison, but was not in the chamber with him on 6 May. He believed that Porton was "an experimental place for gases, but the teargas types nothing more than that".[112] Parker feels that he did not give consent at the time to be experimented on with nerve gas: "As far as consent was concerned, yes I consented to having tear gas, but not a nerve gas".[113] He recalls that "the whole process was very casual and we were reassured all the time and told there was nothing to worry about". On 4 May 1953 Parker also participated in the same kind of experiment as Maddison: "Again we were not told about exactly what was being applied on us".[114] Parker, like Kenneth Earl, stated that he would not have consented to the Porton experiment had he been informed that he would be exposed to nerve gas.[115]

Granville Popplewell, who attended Porton at the end of April 1953, recalls that the notices asking for volunteers had "no mention of nerve gases".[116] Popplewell believed that he had consented to the experiments "because the bottom line being I volunteered for the tests". In one set of experiments he was exposed to mustard gas and was told that he would be exposed to mustard gas. In another set of experiments he was given five drops of a liquid on the inside of both his lower arms, but was not told what it was, nor was he told what the possible effects of the substance could be: "I didn't know what the chemical was. I did, however, trust them".[117] His statement seems to suggest that the investigators were happy to reveal details about experiments with mustard gas, but held back information involving tests with nerve agents, perhaps for reasons of national security in the climate of the Cold War.

Peter John Sammons attended Porton in February 1953 as a Royal Navy participant. His knowledge of nerve agents was "very limited" and he

> "had never heard of Sarin or any other nerve agent. I thought that the gas that my father was exposed to during the First World War, was a nerve agent. I really had no idea. When I saw the notice asking for volunteers for Porton Down, the words 'nerve gas' didn't mean anything to me".[118]

Sammons recalls that he was not informed about the experiment or about the risks involved: "At no time did any of the scientists tell us what it was that they were going to test on us." As a result of one of the experiments Sammons collapsed and was hospitalised for several days. The experience left him so frightened that he

110 Statement of John Leonard Newbury, 22 March 2000.
111 Statement of John Leonard Newbury, 29 April 2003.
112 Statement of Peter George de Carle Parker, 7 June 2000.
113 Ibid.
114 Ibid.
115 Statement of Peter George de Carle Parker, 13 December 2001.
116 Statement of Granville Popplewell, 20 December 2000.
117 Ibid.
118 Statement of Peter John Sammons, 2 May 2003.

"informed the scientists that [he] was no longer willing to take part in any other experiments".[119] After leaving Porton, Sammons appears to have been "ordered" back to Porton several times. Each time he informed the investigators that he "didn't want to take part in any more tests".[120] In August 1953 Sammons was called back to Porton yet again. There a person, whom Sammons described in his statement as the "head-man",

"tried to persuade me to take part in more tests. He advised me of how I had let them down by not completing all of the experiments. I was generally made to feel that I had not done everything that was expected of me. I was also told by this 'head man' that I was not to discuss any of my visits to Porton with anyone".[121]

Although the existing witness statements seem to suggest that in general no duress was exercised by Porton's staff, Sammons statement raises the issue of coercion and undue persuasion. His statement is of concern and raises questions as to the existing ethical culture at Porton.

Alan John Bangay, who attended Porton at the same time as Maddison but did not participate in the same Sarin experiment as Maddison, had "never heard of nerve gas although [he] had heard of mustard gas". He remembers that the notices asking for research subjects were making "no references to either of these substances". Bangay recalls that he was not informed about the tests:

"We were given no information about the tests we were going to undergo and I do not recall anybody asking any questions. We were not given the option of withdrawing from any tests, although I do remember being told to ask questions if I didn't understand any instructions".[122]

Bangay's recollections seem to confirm that the scientists placed the responsibility for obtaining information about the experiments on the shoulders of the experimental subjects.

Douglas Michael Gray, who attended Porton twice as a Royal Navy participant in 1952 and in 1953, remembered that the investigators placed "some form of liquid" on his arm: "I was not told what this liquid was".[123] Gray recalled that "on leaving Porton I still had no idea what the liquid was that had been placed on my arm".[124] In January 1953, he returned to Porton to participate in yet another experiment: "Again on this occasion we were given virtually no information about the experiment or what substance it involved".[125] In 1996 he was informed that he had been exposed to the nerve agent Cyclo Sarin (GF) in 1952 and Sarin (GB) in 1953. "Had I been told this at the time and been aware of the dangers involved I

---

119 Statement of Peter John Sammons, 7 December 2000.
120 "Although I was recalled to Porton, I was determined not to take part in any further tests. My experiences had scared me to death. I was so frightened by it that I was able to refuse requests by senior officers who wanted me to take part in further tests. I would not ordinarily have refused a senior officer's requests", Statement of Peter John Sammons, 2 May 2003.
121 Statement of Peter John Sammons, 7 December 2000.
122 Statement of Alan Bangay, 4 May 2000.
123 Statement of Douglas Michael Gray, 17 February 2003.
124 Ibid.
125 Ibid.

do not believe I would have consented to taking part. Had I just been told it was a nerve agent but not warned of any dangers I may ".[126]

Derek Melbourne Johns, who attended Porton in April and May 1953, had "no idea whatsoever of what went on there".[127] Johns recalled that "none of our intake seemed to really know why we were there".[128] He also recalled that it is possible that the word "nerve gas" may have been mentioned in conjunction with the forthcoming experiments, but that it had no meaning because he did not know what nerve gas was and was not informed about the possible risks:

> "Although I have said that I think they may have said that a nerve gas would be in the chamber that didn't really mean a lot to me at that time. I didn't know much about nerve gases if anything".[129]

Derrick Henry Johnson attended Porton in 1953. He "didn't know where Porton Down was, in fact I had never heard of it and didn't know what they did there". Johnson recalled that in the notice asking for research subjects "there was a very long word[130] on it that I couldn't understand or pronounce. It meant nothing to me". Johnson recalls that he was told about some of the substances the investigators would be testing, but was not informed about their effects or potential risks to his health:

> "On the first day, they told us that we would be doing gas tests. I think they told me what sort of gas but it did not mean anything to me. Later on in the week, I think someone from the military told us the names of a couple of gases that we would be testing but I did not know anything about them. The only gas I had heard of was mustard gas".[131]

John Dudley Shepherd attended Porton at the same time as Maddison. He recalled "having an introduction talk, and being lined up and photographed naked".[132] Shephard said of himself: "I was (and still am) the type of person to question facts, and I was certainly not adverse to questioning authority".[133] His statement suggests that those subjects who wanted to know what was about to happen to them, could find out by asking the questions: "I was told that the scientists were in the late stage of investigating side effects of a very low dose of a nerve gas of some type by using radioactive tracer label".[134] Shephard was apparently not told what the substance was he would be exposed to: "To this day I do not know exactly what the substance given to me was, but I suspect it was a low level dose of radioactive nerve agent".[135]

Geoffrey Mervin Thorne, who attended Porton in 1953, recalled:

126 Statement of Douglas Michael Gray, 17 February 2003.
127 Statement of Derek Melbourne Johns, 21 January 2003.
128 Ibid.
129 Ibid.
130 Johnson might refer to the word "physiological" which appears to have been on the notices asking for research subjects.
131 Statement of Derrick Henry Johnson, 6 February 2003.
132 Statement of John Dudley Shepherd, 13 July 2000.
133 Ibid.
134 Ibid.
135 Ibid.

"We were told absolutely nothing. The only thing we were told was what was the actual task they wanted us to do. We were not told why we were doing it or what they were trying to ascertain".[136]

He also does not recall that they were "given any formal briefings by the staff as to why we were there or what we were doing. It really was a case of we just did what we were told to do".[137] Three years ago Thorne was informed that he had been exposed to the nerve agent Sarin. The information "came as a total shock" to him.[138] The above evidence is a sample of statements made by witnesses who attended Porton at around the time of Maddison's death. It supports the proposition that

1) many, if not most, of the servicemen were told that there was no risk in the experiments and that the tests were "totally safe".

2) many, if not most, of the servicemen had little or no knowledge of what nerve agents or nerve gases were.

3) many, if not most, had received little or no information of what would happen to them at Porton Down.

4) many, if not most, would probably have refused to participate in the experiments had they known that they would be exposed to nerve agents, had they been given information what nerve agents were and told of their potential hazards.

5) some of them were told at Porton that they would be exposed to nerve agents but were not given any detailed information about nerve agents or about the risks involved in the tests.

6) some of them were *not* told at Porton that they would be exposed to nerve agents and were not given any detailed information about nerve agents or about the risks involved in the tests.

7) many of them are likely to have associated or confused nerve agents and nerve gases with mustard gas which they knew from the Second World War or from the experiences of their relatives.

8) some of them felt that they were not given any options or any say in the experiments, for example to choose in which of the experiments they wanted to take part or to pull out of the experiment.

9) in at least one instance some form of coercion and undue persuasion appears to have been applied to an experimental subject.

Porton's scientists obtained consent only partially and in a generally "roundabout" way. Moreover, the information given to the subjects was inadequate to make an informed decision. The scientists knew that nerve gases were highly toxic in minute quantities, and that exposure entailed significant risk.[139] They were

---

136 Statement of Geoffrey Mervin Thorne, 13 January 2003.
137 Ibid.
138 Ibid.
139 See Exhibit, MNJ/39, Porton Memorandum no. 34 from 30 June 1949 and Exhibit, MNJ/19, Porton Memorandum no. 39 from 2 August 1950.

knowingly increasing exposure to levels that were dangerous to the subjects.[140] In 1952 and 1953, six experimental subjects were hospitalised as a result of exposure to nerve agents.[141] The Kelly incident in April 1953, in which one of the service-men fell into a coma, was the clearest indication that the experiments posed a significant risk. It was a clear warning that from that moment onwards the most rigorous safeguards and standards of medical ethics needed to be applied if the scientists decided to continue with the experiments. It was a warning to pursue the experiment, if at all, only under extreme caution. The record suggests that more rigorous safeguards were not introduced and that more rigorous ethical standards were not applied. The Kelly incident was a warning flag, and a chance to reassess the entire experimental programme. This, we know, was not done.

After Maddison died, procedures came under scrutiny. As the Treasury Solicitor pointed out: "Misleading statements in an invitation of this sort, even if made in complete innocence, are always apt to give rise to criticism when anything has gone wrong". [142] And something had gone wrong indeed. According to a hand-written document from 5 May 1953,[143] and a typed version from 8 May 1953,[144] the object of the experiments was to "discover the dosage of GB [Sarin], GD [Soman] and GF [Cyclo Sarin] which when applied to the clothed or bare skin of men would cause incapacitation or death". A report about the experiments from 1954 repeated this objective.[145] None of the evidence that I have seen indicates that any of the experimental subjects, including Maddison, was ever informed about the specific objective of the experiments, and I believe it to be rather unlikely that any man in his right mind would have volunteered for such an experiment.[146] The consent, which may have been obtained from Maddison, would not have qualified as having been "informed". His consent, if it were obtained, was therefore invalid.

V.   Maddison's Legacy

The Porton experiments were non-therapeutic, and therefore qualitatively different from medical treatment research. By definition, none of the Porton nerve agent experiments was conducted in order to benefit the subjects or carried out in their best interest. Since the experiments were not intended to benefit the subjects, the subjects possessed the fundamental right to decide whether or not they were prepared to participate in the experiment. That is why the issue of consent is of

140 See Report of a Court of Inquiry 1953, p. 74.
141 Exhibit, MNJ/17, Porton Technical Paper 373, p. 70.
142 TNA, WO286/11 (Police Ref. X61), H. Woodhouse (for the Treasury Solicitor), to Legal 1 (Mr. Griffith-Jones), Ministry of Supply, 13 July 1953.
143 Exhibit, CEB/16/2, 7 Page hand written document titles 'The Percutaneous Toxicity of the G Compounds', 5 May 1953.
144 Exhibit, JJH/187/5, The Percutaneous Toxicity of the G Compounds, 8 May 1953.
145 Exhibit, MNJ/30, Porton Technical Paper 399.
146 See also Witness Statement of FJ Verallo, 17 March 2000.

such importance. Already in 1946, General Telford Taylor, the chief prosecutor in the Doctors' Trial, had stated in his opening address:

> "Whatever book or treatise on medical ethics we may examine, and whatever expert on forensic medicine we may question, will say that it is a fundamental and inescapable obligation of every physician under any known system of law not to perform a dangerous experiment without the subject's consent".[147]

Research over the last decade, however, has shown that many Anglo-American medical scientists did not abide by the Nuremberg Code or its informed consent principle during the Cold War. This applied to therapeutic as well as to non-therapeutic experiments. According to Jay Katz, government officials and their advisers at best paid lip service to the principle of informed voluntary consent.[148] One former physician remarked that in the 1940s and 1950s "the doctor was king or queen. It never occurred to a doctor to ask for consent for anything".[149] Another doctor commented:

> "I am aware of no investigator (myself included) who was actively involved in research involving human subjects in the years before 1964 who recalls any attempts to secure 'voluntary' and informed consent according to Nuremberg's standards".[150]

In an environment dominated by a paternalistic doctor-patient relationship, it was often left to individual doctors to inform their patients about the nature and purpose of the experiment. Physicians, so it seems, were less concerned about the issue of informed consent in therapeutic research, both in the US and UK, except, perhaps, where there was a significant level of risk involved.

For non-therapeutic experiments that involved the possibility of harm, informed consent was an essential requirement long before the Porton experiments. The principle of informed consent was recognised before the 1960s and certainly before any kind of bioethics movement was on the horizon. For the UK, in particular, the principle of informed consent was recognised among the legal and medical establishment from at least 1933 onwards. The fact that scientists in the UK, and elsewhere, may have ignored this[151] – including in the Porton Down experiments – does not change the fact that it was widely considered wrong if scientists had not obtained fully informed consent in non-therapeutic research.

Maddison was a member of the Armed Forces and his death occurred at the hand of the state. In 2002, Judge Woolf, the High Court judge who quashed the original inquest, pointed out:

> "That death should occur in such a situation is a matter of real public concern. There can be no doubt in this case that the concerns which existed as to how Mr Maddison should have been put in a position where he was subject to an experiment which risked his life are still alive today and are still matters of public interest".[152]

---

147 Schmidt (2004), p. 175.
148 United States Advisory Committee on Human Radiation Experiments (1996), p. 544.
149 Katz (1996), p. 1665.
150 Ibid.
151 Schmidt (2004), pp. 264-297.
152 Transcript, Day 1.

In November 2004, after a sixty-four day trial, the Inquest jury ruled that Maddison was "unlawfully killed", and that the cause of death was a chemical warfare agent used in a non-therapeutic experiment. Many lawyers and experts see this not only as a significant moment in legal history but also one that may have profound and long-term implications on hundreds of servicemen who were exposed to chemical agents over the years (including the Gulf-War veterans). There have also been steps to call for a full public inquiry into the tests carried out at Porton Down.[153] No Coroner has ever been required to investigate a death that took place so long ago and the investigation has faced significant problems. The ethical, legal and indeed symbolic implications of the Inquest, however, are largely undisputed. Maddison's death and the legacy of the recent Inquest are likely to become part of a gradual process by which Britain is beginning to face up to her Cold War past.

---

153 Hansard (Westminster Hall), 22 February 2005, Column 32WH, Porton Down; see also Care (2005), p. 15.

References

Annas, G. J./Grodin, M. A. (eds.) (1992): The Nazi Doctors and the Nuremberg Code. Human Rights in Human Experimentation. New York, Oxford: Oxford University Press.

Annas, G. J./Grodin, M. A. (1999): Medical Ethics and Human Rights: Legacies of Nuremberg, Hofstra Law & Policy Symposium 3 (1999), pp. 111-123.

Anonymous (1916), "The Right and Wrong of Making Experiments on Human Beings", Journal of the American Medical Association 67 (1916), pp. 1372-1373.

Anonymous (1946): A Moral Problem, The Lancet, 30 November 1946.

Anonymous (1955): Experiments on Human Beings, British Medical Journal (1955), pp. 526-527.

Alexander, L. ([1947] 1976): Ethics of Human Experimentation, Psychiatric Journal of the University of Ottawa 1 ([1947] 1976), pp. 40-46. Reprint.

Arnold, P./Sprumont D. (1998): The "Nuremberg Code": Rules of Public International Law, in: Tröhler/Reiter-Theil (1998), pp. 84-96.

Balmer B. (2001): Britain and Biological Warfare: Expert Advice and Science Policy 1930-65. Basingstoke: Palgrave.

Beecher, H. K. (1966): Ethics in Clinical Research, New England Journal of Medicine 274 (1966), pp. 1354-1360.

Beecher, H. K. (1970): Research and the Individual. Human Studies. Boston: Little, Brown.

Berg, J. W./Appelbaum, P. S./Parker, L. S./Lidz, C. W. (2001): Informed Consent: Legal Theory and Clinical Practice. Oxford: Oxford University Press.

Bud, R./Gummett P. (1999): Cold War, Hot Science: Applied Research in Britain's Defence Laboratories, 1945-1990. Amsterdam: Harwood Academic Publishers.

Care, A. (2000a): Poisoned by their own People, The Independent, 3 October 2000.

Care A. (2000b): The Porton Down Human Guinea Pigs – Gassed without Consent, Association of Personal Injury Lawyers 12 (2000), 2.

Care, A. (2005): After the Inquest: Porton Down revisited, Association of Personal Injury Lawyers 15 (2005), 1, p. 15.

Carter G. B. (1992): Porton Down: 75 Years of Chemical and Biological Research. London: HMSO.

Carter G. B. (2000): Chemical and Biological Defence at Porton Down, 1916-2000. London: HMSO.

Davidson, M. (1957): Medical Ethics. A Guide to Students and Practioners. London: Lloyd-Luke.

Deutsch, E. (1997): Der Nürnberger Kodex. Das Strafverfahren gegen Mediziner, die zehn Prinzipien von Nürnberg und die bleibende Bedeutung des Nürnberger Kodex, in: Tröhler/Reiter-Theil (1997), pp. 103-114.

Drinan, R. F. (1992): The Nuremberg Principles in International Law, in: Annas/Grodin (1992), pp. 174-182.

Dörner, K./Ebbinghaus, A. (eds.) (1999): The Nuremberg Medical Trial 1946/47. Transcripts, Material of the Prosecution and Defense, Related Documents. Munich: Saur, Microfiche.

Elkeles, B. (1996): Der moralische Diskurs über das medizinische Menschenexperiment im 19. Jahrhundert. Stuttgart: Gustav Fischer.

Evans R. (2000): Gassed: British Chemical Warfare Experiments On Humans at Porton Down. Thirsk: House of Stratus.

Faden, R. R./Beauchamp, T. L. (eds.) (1986): History and Theory of Informed Consent. New York: Oxford University Press.

Frewer, A. (2000): Medizin und Moral in Weimarer Republik und Nationalsozialismus. Die Zeitschrift 'Ethik' unter Emil Abderhalden. Frankfurt am Main, New York: Campus.

Frewer, A./Neumann, J. N. (eds.) (2001): Medizingeschichte und Medizinethik. Kontroversen und Begründungsansätze 1900-1950. Frankfurt am Main, New York: Campus.

Goodwin B. (1998): Keen as Mustard: Britain's Horrific Chemical Warfare Experiments in Australia. St Lucia, Old., Australia: University of Queensland Press.

Grimley Evans, J./Beck, P. (2002): Informed Consent in Medical Research, Clinical Medicine 2 (2002), pp. 267-272.

Grodin M. (1992): Historical Origins of the Nuremberg Code, in: Annas/Grodin (1992), pp. 121-144.

Hammond P./Carter, G. B. (2002): From Biological Warfare to Healthcare. Porton Down 1940-2000. Basingstoke: Palgrave.

Harris R./Paxman, J. (1982, reprint 2002): A Higher Form of Killing. The Secret History of Gas and Germ Warfare. New York: Chatto & Windus.

Hazelgrove, J. (2002): The Old Faith and the New Science: The Nuremberg Code and Human Experimentation Ethics in Britain, 1946-73, Social History of Medicine 15 (2002), pp. 109-135.

Hazelgrove, J. (2004): British Research Ethics after the Second World War: The Controversy at the British Postgraduate Medical School, Hammersmith Hospital, in: Roelcke/Maio (2004), pp. 181-197.

Herbert, D. (1947): A Moral Problem, The Lancet (1947), pp. 84f.

Hilton, S. H. (1947): A Moral Problem, The Lancet (1947), p. 43.

Honigman, P. (1997): Zur Legitimität medizinischer Ethik-Kodizes aus britischer Sicht, in: Tröhler/Reiter-Theil (1997), pp. 249-256.

Ivy, A. C. (1947): Nazi War Crimes of a Medical Nature, Federation Bulletin 33 (1947), pp. 133-146.

Jones, J. J. (1981): Bad Blood, The Tuskegee Syphilis Experiments. London: Collier Macmillan Publishers.

Katz, J. (1972): Experimentation with Human Beings. The Authority of the Investigator, Subject, Profession, and State in the Human Experimentation Process. New York: Russell Sage Foundation.

Katz, J. (1984): The Silent World of Doctors and Patient. London: Collier Macmillan Publishers.

Katz, J. (1992): The Consent Principle of the Nuremberg Code: Its Significance Then and Now, in: Annas/Grodin (1992), pp. 227-239.

Katz, J. (1996): The Nuremberg Code and the Nuremberg Trial: A Reappraisal, Journal of the American Medical Association 276 (1996), 20, pp. 1662-1666.

Katz, J. (1997): Human Sacrifice and Human Experimentation: Reflections at Nuremberg, Yale Journal of International Law 22 (1997), pp. 401-418.

Kennedy, I./Grubb, A. (1994): Medical Law: Text with Materials. London: Butterworths.

Kidd, A. M. (1953): The Problem of Experimentation on Human Beings: III. Limits of the Right of a Person to Consent to Experimentation on Himself, Science 117 (1953), pp. 211-212.

Layton, T. B./Nelson-Jones, A. (1946): A Moral Problem, The Lancet (1946), p. 882.

Lederer, S. E. (1995): Subjected to Science. Human Experimentation before the Second World War. Baltimore: John Hopkins University Press.

Lederer, S. E. (2004): Research without Borders: The Origins of the Declaration of Helsinki, in: Roelcke/Maio, pp. 199-217.

Lee, H. A./Gabriel, R./Bale, A./Welch, D. (2004): Clinical findings in 111 ex-Porton Down volunteers, Journal of the Royal Army Medical Corps 150 (2004), pp. 14-19.

Macklin, R. (1992): Universality of the Nuremberg Code, in: Annas/Grodin (1992), pp. 240-257.

Maehle, A.-H. (1998): Werte und Normen: Ethik in der Medizingeschichte, in: Paul/Schlich (1998), pp. 335-354.

Maehle, A.-H. (1999): Professional Ethics and Discipline: The Prussian Medical Courts of Honour, 1899-1920, Medizinhistorisches Journal 34 (1999), pp. 309-338.

Maehle, A-H. (2000): Assault and Battery, or Legitimate Treatment?, Gesnerus 57 (2000), pp. 206-221.

Maio, G. (1996): Das Humanexperiment vor und nach Nürnberg, in: Wiesemann/Frewer (1996), pp. 45-78.

Maio, G. (2002): Ethik der Forschung am Menschen: Zur Begründung der Moral in ihrer historischen Bedingtheit. Stuttgart-Bad Cannstatt: Frommann-Holzboog.

McCance, R.A. (1957): The Practice of Experimental Medicine, in: Davidson (1957), pp. 140-150.

Medical Research Council (1957): MRC 53/649: Clinical Investigations, in: Davidson (1957), pp. 151-153.

Mellanby, K. (1946): A Moral Problem, The Lancet (1946), p. 850.

Ministry of Defence (2006): Historical Survey of the Porton Down Service Volunteer Programme 1939-1989. Unpublished manuscript.

Ministry of Supply (1952a): Chief Characteristics of Nerve Gas, Lancet (1952), 6728, pp. 286-287.

Ministry of Supply (1952b): Chief Characteristics of Nerve Gas, The British Medical Journal (1952), 4779, pp. 334-335.

Moll, A. (1902): Ärztliche Ethik. Die Pflichten des Arztes in allen Beziehungen seiner Thätigkeit. Stuttgart: Enke.

Moreno, J. D. (1996): The Only Feasible Means: The Pentagon's Ambivalent Relationship with the Nuremberg Code, Hastings Center Report 26 (1996), pp. 11-19.

Moreno, J. D. (1997): Reassessing the Influence of the Nuremberg Code on American Medical Ethics, Journal of Contemporary Health Law and Policy 13 (1997), pp. 347-360.

Moreno J. D. (1999): Undue Risk. Secret Experiments on Humans. New York: W. H. Freeman.

Pappworth, M. H. (1967): Human Guinea Pigs. Experimentation on Man. London: Routledge & K. Paul.

Paul, N./Schlich, T. (eds.) (1998): Medizingeschichte: Aufgaben, Probleme, Perspektiven. Frankfurt am Main, New York: Campus.

Pechura, C. M./Rall, D. P. (1993): Veterans at Risk: The Health Effects of Mustard Gas and Lewisite. Washington, D.C.: National Academy Press.

Perley, S./Fluss, S. S./Bankowski, Z./Simon, F. (1992): The Nuremberg Code: An International Overview, in: Annas/Grodin (1992), pp. 149-173.

Popper, S. E./McCloskey, K. (1995): Ethics in Human Experimentation: Historical Perspectives, Military Medicine 160 (1995), pp. 7-11.

Proctor, R. N. (2000): Expert Witnesses Take the Stand. Historians of Science can Play an Important Role in US Public Health Litigation, Nature 407 (2000), pp. 15-16.

Pulvertaft, R. J. V. (1952): The Individual and the Group in Modern Medicine, Lancet (1952), 6740, pp. 839-842.

Roelcke, V./Maio G. (eds.) (2004): Twentieth Century Ethics of Human Subject Research. Historical Perspectives on Values, Practices, and Regulations. Stuttgart: Steiner.

Rothman, D. J. (1997): Der Nürnberger Kodex im Licht früherer Prinzipien und Praktiken im Bereich der Humanexperimente, in: Tröhler/Reiter-Theil (1997), pp. 75-88.

Sass, H.-M. (1983): Reichsrundschreiben 1931: Pre-Nuremberg German Regulations Concerning New Therapy and Human Experimentation, The Journal of Medicine and Philosophy (1983), 8, pp. 99-111.

Schmidt, U. (2001): Der Ärzteprozeß als moralische Instanz? Der Nürnberger Kodex und das Problem "zeitloser Medizinethik", in: Frewer/Neumann (2001), pp. 334-373.

Schmidt, U. (2004): Justice at Nuremberg. Leo Alexander and the Nazi Doctors' Trial. Basingstoke, Macmillan/Palgrave.

Schmidt, U. (2006): Cold War at Porton Down: Informed Consent in Britain's Biological and Chemical Warfare Experiments during the Cold War, Cambridge Quarterly for Healthcare Ethics 15 (2006), 4, pp. 366-380.

Shevell, M. I. (1998): Neurology's Witness to history: Part II. Leo Alexander's Contribution to the Nuremberg Code (1946 to 1947), Neurology 50 (1998), pp. 274-278.

Shimkin, M. I. (1953): The Problem of Experimentation on Human Beings: I. The Research Worker's Point of View, Science 117 (1953), pp. 205-207.

Shuster, E. (1997): Fifty Years Later: The Significance of the Nuremberg Code, The New England Journal of Medicine 337 (1997), 20, pp. 1436-1440.

Shuster, E. (1998): The Nuremberg Code: Hippocratic Ethics and Human Rights, Lancet 351 (1998), pp. 974-977.

Smith, R. G. (1994): Medical Discipline: The Professional Conduct Jurisdiction of the General Medical Council, 1858-1990. Oxford: Clarendon Press.

Tröhler, U./Reiter-Theil S. (eds.) (1997): Ethik und Medizin: 1947-1997. Göttingen: Wallstein.

Tröhler U./Reiter-Theil S. (eds.) (1998): Ethics Codes in Medicine: Foundations and Achievements of Codification since 1947. Aldershot, Brookfield, Singapore, Sydney: Ashgate.

Tusa, T./Tusa, J. (1995): The Nuremberg Trial. London: BBC books.

United Nations War Crimes Commission (1949): German Medical War Crimes. A Summary of Information. London: HMSO.

United States Advisory Committee on Human Radiation Experiments (1996): Advisory Committee on Human Radiation Experiments Final Report. Washington, D.C: Supt. of Docs., U.S. GPO.

Vilensky, J. A. (2005): Dew of Death. The Story of Lewisite, America's World War I Weapon of Mass Destruction. Bloomington: Indiana University Press.

Vollmann, J./Winau, R. (1996): Informed Consent in Human Experimentation before the Nuremberg Code, British Medical Journal (1996), 313, pp. 1445-1447.

Winau, R. (1996): Medizin und Menschenversuch. Zur Geschichte des "informed consent", in: Wiesemann/Frewer (1996), pp. 13-29.

Wiesemann, C./Frewer, A. (eds.) (1996): Medizin und Ethik im Zeichen von Auschwitz. Erlangen, Jena: Palm & Enke.

Willcock J. W. (1830): The Laws Relating to the Medical Profession with an Account of the Rise and Progress of its Various Order. London: Clarke.

Witts, L. J. (1948): The Problems of Clinical Research, British Medical Journal (1948), 2, pp. 455-459.

Wood, J. R. (1950): Medical Problems in Chemical Warfare, Journal of the American Medical Association 144 (1950), 8, pp. 606-609.

World Medical Association (1970): Principles for Those in Research and Experimentation, in: Beecher (1970), p. 240.

Acknowledgements: The chapter was written as part of a Wellcome Trust-funded project on "Cold War at Porton Down: Medical Ethics and the Legal Dimension of Britain's Biological and Chemical Warfare Programme, 1945-1989". It is an extended version of the article on "Cold War at Porton Down: Informed Consent in Britain's Biological and Chemical Warfare Experiments during the Cold War" which I published in Cambridge Quarterly for Healthcare Ethics in 2006. I would like to thank the Wellcome Trust for its generous support.

John R. Williams

The Declaration of Helsinki
The Importance of Context[1]

I. Introduction

This chapter will focus on a feature of the Declaration of Helsinki (hereafter DoH) that is crucial for an understanding of this and related documents, namely, the context of research ethics and, more broadly, of medical research in general. Context as understood here includes many aspects: scientific, political, commercial, professional, socio-cultural and ethical. The other contributors to this volume deal with some of these topics but their insights can benefit from synthesis and elaboration. The thesis of this chapter is that the context of medical research has undergone significant change since the DoH was first developed and adopted and therefore research ethics has had to change as well. Whether this has involved a change in the principles of the DoH will be discussed below.

II. Science

As Ulrich Tröhler points out, medical research has a long, and somewhat chequered, history. At least since the 16th century in Europe, the medical community has always been on the lookout for better ways to treat or prevent diseases. The 20th century witnessed a great leap forward in systematic medical research, although it was misused terribly by physicians from many countries, most notably Germany and Japan, in the 1930s and 1940s.

By today's standards, medical research in the 1950s was still at a relatively primitive stage. However, it was developing rapidly, especially in the use of controlled clinical trials of new pharmaceutical products. Whereas new products had previously been tested mostly on those affected by the disease the product was intended to treat, in the hope that it could benefit the research subject (so-called "therapeutic research"), phase one trials now used healthy subjects ("volunteers") for testing the safety of new products. Once safety was demonstrated, there was a need to determine efficacy, and it was felt that the best way to do this was to test the product against a placebo, which required blinding both research subjects and the physician investigators. Of course this meant that those receiving the placebo

---

1   The views expressed in this chapter are those of the author and not necessarily those of the World Medical Association.

could not benefit from the research intervention. As with healthy volunteers, this methodology called into question the premise that the interests of the research subject should prevail over those of the researchers, science or the community at large.

As Susan Lederer points out, during the 1950s and 1960s clinical research was developing most rapidly in the U.S.A. There the need for healthy subjects for phase one studies was met primarily by prisoners and, for vaccines, by institutionalized children. Despite European objections to the use of such individuals, whose ability to provide freely informed consent was so obviously compromised, the American approach prevailed in the 1964 DoH.

Medical research continued its rapid development after 1964. Povl Riis notes that clinical trials became widely accepted in Europe in the late 1960s, resulting in a need to recruit large numbers of research subjects. Clinical trials have since spread across the globe. Moreover, other types of medical research besides drug and vaccine development – diagnostics, surgery, epidemiology, public health – have expanded and these too require research subjects. More recent research areas include genetics, informatics and nanotechnology. Other health professions besides medicine – nursing and dentistry, for example – have become involved in research involving human subjects. The ever-increasing amount of scientific knowledge, so readily available through the Internet, has resulted in the need for individual researchers to focus on highly specialized topics and, at the same time, to participate in teams and networks that coordinate and integrate their micro-studies.

To sum up, medical research has evolved significantly since the time of the first DoH. It is no wonder that research ethics has had to evolve as well, given this change of context. Whether this evolution has resulted in a change of principles or simply of the application of unchanging principles will be discussed below.

III. Politics

Whereas science is constantly evolving and expanding, politics is depressingly resistant to positive change. Nevertheless, changes do occur and some of these have significant influence on medical research and research ethics. Here we will consider the politics both of governments and of medical associations.

One constant factor in governmental politics during the past century, and indeed much farther back, has been the predominance assigned to national security, and especially the military, in medical research. Till Bärnighausen shows how this played out both in Japan from 1932 to 1945 and subsequently in the U.S.A. where political and military considerations coalesced in the decisions to cover up the war crimes of Japanese military researchers and to make use of their "tainted" data. Many other, similarly reprehensible, instances of military influence on medical research have been uncovered, and no doubt these are just the tip of the iceberg. Despite condemnation of physician involvement in biological and chemical weapons development by the World Medical Association and other professional bodies, many governments do not hesitate to skew their support of medical research in favour of potential military applications. When the end of the Cold War no longer justified such research priorities, it was soon replaced by the War on Terror.

One way in which the political context of medical research has changed since the 1960s is with regard to the regulation of research activities. The requirement of ethics committee approval of research involving human subjects that was introduced in the 1975 version of the DoH has been replicated in numerous governmental and intergovernmental documents, including the two that arguably have had the most influence on medical research practices globally – the International Conference on Harmonization (ICH) Good Clinical Practice Guidelines and the European Union Clinical Trials Directives. As Dominique Sprumont et al. point out, political authorities in many countries have adopted laws dealing with medical research that include requirements related to ethics. However, since politicians are subject to many and diverse influences, it is not surprising that these laws sometimes reflect the interests of certain powerful lobbying groups rather than the highest ethical standards.

Susan Lederer shows that medical associations are by no means immune from political pressures even when dealing with ethical issues. The dependence of the WMA on funding from American physicians and pharmaceutical industry representatives in the 1960s resulted in the adoption of a policy, the 1964 DoH, that might have been significantly different if the Association had been financially independent. Although, as Robert Carson et al. point out, the WMA currently has a much greater and more diverse membership and arguably a more democratic structure than in 1964, certain national medical associations still exercise greater influence than others and, inevitably, political considerations continue to play an important role in the approval process for new and revised policies, including the DoH.

IV. Commerce

Another major change in the context of medical research since the 1960s has been the increasing dominance of the pharmaceutical industry in the funding and conduct of research. The industry has long since surpassed governments as the primary source of such funding, and thanks to its highly successful lobbying of governments, it has consolidated its control over the benefits of research through the extension of legal protection of intellectual property and related laws and regulations.

Although it is widely recognized that the interests of business are not necessarily compatible with medical ethics, and therefore there is need for government regulation of commercial involvement in medical research, in fact governments have tended to give industry a significant role in the development of laws and regulations for such research. The pharmaceutical industry is a major, if not the dominant, partner in the ICH, whose headquarters is located in the office of the

International Federation of Pharmaceutical Manufacturers Associations in Geneva. As Dominique Sprumont et al. note, the ICH Good Clinical Practice Guidelines have been formally incorporated into the drug approval regulations of the EU, the U.S. FDA and the Ministry of Health, Labour and Welfare in Japan, and are used in other countries, including Canada and several in Asia. The principal ICH Guideline dates back to 1996 and is arguably in need of updating in the light of recent developments in research ethics, but ICH is an extremely secretive organization that has shown no sign of involving other interested groups in any revision process.

As noted above, the final content of the 1964 DoH was significantly influenced by commercial considerations. Although the WMA has become much less reliant on industry funding than in 1964, some of its member national medical associations retain close ties with the industry and may be reluctant to support WMA policies that are inimical to industry interests. However, as Robert Carlson et al. demonstrate, the 2000 version of the DoH contains provisions that did not please the industry and its supporters in the U.S. FDA and elsewhere. Subsequently, the WMA was accused of caving in to industry demands in its 2002 and 2004 notes of clarification to paragraphs 29 and 30 of the 2000 DoH, but a careful reading of these, admittedly somewhat ambiguous, notes shows that they do not diminish the fundamental rights of research subjects enunciated in the 2000 DoH.

V. Professionalism and Academic Freedom

Ulrich Tröhler describes the 1964 DoH somewhat disparagingly as "endors[ing] the paternalistic ethos of the health care professions that fosters patients' beneficence as defined by professionals." One may question his identification of paternalism and beneficence, but a more significant problem with this statement is its implicit denigration of professionalism. Physicians have a fiduciary responsibility to act in the best interests of their patients, whether or not they are research subjects. In the research context, this responsibility has traditionally taken the form of protection. In the 1960s, and subsequently, the physician's duty to protect potential or actual research subjects took precedence over an individual's right to participate in research insofar as individuals were not allowed to be research subjects if, in the physician's considered opinion, the potential harm to the individual would outweigh the potential benefits. Although there is some dispute as to whether the priority of protection over autonomy should be maintained in the 21st century, it would be wrong to criticize the 1964 DoH for incorporating it.

As noted above, much medical research in the 1960s was considered therapeutic in that the experimental intervention was intended, or at least hoped, to benefit the patient/research subject. In that context, there was no conflict between the role of the treating physician and the role of the researcher when the same person fulfilled both roles. With the introduction of double-blinded placebo-controlled clinical trials, the possibility of conflict between these roles presented a real challenge to physician-researchers. The various versions of the DoH have consistently reminded physicians that when such conflicts arise, their professional responsibility for the well-being of the patient takes precedence over their responsibility to advance knowledge. The lucrative inducements offered physicians to participate in clinical trials make this reminder more pertinent nowadays than ever before.

Another essential aspect of professionalism is self-regulation. The WMA initiated the process that led to the DoH because almost all medical researchers at that time were physicians. As the representative of the international medical community, the WMA was the appropriate organization for undertaking this task as part of its responsibility for setting ethical standards for physicians worldwide. This was in keeping with one of the original goals of the WMA, namely, to ensure that the atrocities committed by physicians during the Nazi era would never be repeated.

The role of the medical profession has undergone enormous change since the 1960s in response to the social and cultural forces described below. Medical professionalism is currently experiencing major challenges, both external and internal. Governments have severely limited the self-regulatory role of the profession, and managed care in its various forms has further eroded the clinical autonomy of physicians. Some physicians would rather consider themselves as businesspersons than as professionals and they try to influence professional organizations and governments to allow them to practise in accordance with conventional business models. Many physicians have close ties to industry and resist the efforts of their professional associations to regulate these relationships. Clearly, the concept of medical professionalism that shaped the 1964 DoH is no longer accepted by all physicians, but neither has it been replaced. The implications of this for research ethics are yet to be determined.

For many researchers, especially those who are not members of a regulated health profession, the concept of academic freedom plays a similar role to that of clinical autonomy for physicians. Granting researchers the freedom to generate new knowledge as they see fit has traditionally been considered to be in the best interests of both researchers and society in general. In the absence of licensing and disciplinary bodies for academic researchers, however, they have not been made as aware of their responsibilities as have their health professional counterparts. This was not especially problematic in the 1960s when almost all research on human subjects was conducted by physicians. However, with the rapid evolution of health research since then, many non-health professionals have become involved in research involving human subjects, including biochemists, biostatisticians, engineers and computer scientists.

In recent years numerous reports of scientific misconduct have resulted in calls for stricter regulation of scientists. Some measures have already been implemented, including U.S. requirements for training in the responsible conduct of research and international journal editors' rules designed to prevent the publication of research conducted unethically. The academic freedom of researchers is also increasingly constrained by the commercial control of research, as described above. Industry, and government granting agencies as well, tend to favour applied over fundamental research and companies often seek to control the dissemination of research results, especially if they are unfavourable to the sponsoring company's product. In reaction to recent scandals involving pharmaceutical products such as Vioxx that were marketed in spite of (suppressed) data on their toxicity, the industry has reluctantly agreed to participate in registries of clinical trials that will include negative as well as positive results for the products under investigation.[2] This is a sign that academic freedom can flourish in the 21st century if it is aligned with the public interest.

VI. Society and Culture

Societies and cultures differ markedly among themselves and it is risky to make general statements about the changes that have taken place around the world since the 1960s. However, it is safe to say that significant changes have taken place almost everywhere, even in the most traditional and conservative societies. Some of the social and cultural forces for change listed below are strongly opposed in certain quarters but even there, these forces have had major impacts. The list that follows is of necessity illustrative rather than exhaustive.

Human Rights: Although the U.N. Universal Declaration on Human Rights had been adopted in 1948, its acceptance and implementation in the 1960s was far from universal. The same can be said for its implications for medical research. Ulrich Tröhler correctly notes that the 1964 DoH is based on professional obligations rather than human rights, although the two are not incompatible. As human rights became more prominent in the decades after 1964, WMA policies began to incorporate a human rights perspective, most notably in its 1981 Declaration of Lisbon on the Rights of the Patient (amended in 1995 and 2005). The 2000 DoH clearly reflects this perspective, despite considerable differences of opinion both within and outside the WMA regarding the nature and extent of the human rights of research subjects during and following clinical trials.

Consumerism: Whereas the development and implementation of human rights protection was directed from "above", by the United Nations and national governments, consumerism represented a "bottom up" approach to the same issues. From the 1960s onwards, individuals in many countries have banded together to assert their "rights" to better treatment from businesses, governments, health care institutions and other providers of goods and services. Some of these consumer groups represent specific constituencies, such as senior citizens or automobile owners, while others, for example patients' rights associations, focus on particular sectors. Through such tactics as lobbying corporations and governments, well-publicized comparative evaluations of products and services, and public educational campaigns, these groups empower ordinary individuals to exercise greater autonomy in access to and choice of such goods. It must be acknowledged

2   See, for example, Mike Adams: Merck caught in scandal to bury Vioxx heart attack risks, intimidate scientists and keep pushing dangerous drugs; Vioxx lawsuits now forming (http://www.newstarget.com/002155.html).

that their influence on medical research, especially at the international level, has been somewhat limited to date, and the fledgling International Association of Patient Organizations will need to find considerable resources in order to become an active dialogue partner with organizations such as the WMA and WHO.

Communications Technology: At the time of the 1964 DoH, the only source of information about a medical research project for potential subjects was the physician researcher. This explains in part the heavy emphasis on the physician's responsibility for the protection of research subjects in that document. Since then, the rapid development of communications technology, especially home computers and the Internet, has provided many individuals with easy access to information about medical research, including research on conditions that affect them. Since much of this information is inaccurate, however, the duty of the researcher to provide potential research subjects with all the information needed to ensure fully informed consent remains paramount. The 2000 DoH is considerably more detailed on this point than its predecessors.

Culture: In 1964, medical research was confined to a very few countries, mainly in North America and Europe. As noted above, the first DoH had to deal with cultural differences regarding the appropriateness of using prisoners and institutionalized children as research subjects, but for the most part its developers could assume a common cultural basis for its recommendations. By 1997, however, when the most recent revision of the DoH began, medical research had expanded around the globe, generating considerable controversy about the application of Western research ethics in non-Western societies.

Like many other international organizations, the WMA tries to establish globally accepted standards while recognizing and respecting cultural differences. During the 1997-2000 revision process, two culturally related issues in particular demanded attention. ("Culture" as used here, includes economic factors.) The first was whether the Western requirement that competent adults give individual informed consent for their participation in medical research should prevail in countries where the husband or community elders normally make such decisions for others. This issue was decided somewhat perfunctorily in the affirmative. Much more contentious was the matter of "double standards" in research ethics, in particular whether interventions that are considered unacceptable in high income countries (e.g., placebos for trials of conditions where effective treatments exist) can be used in low and middle income countries. The 2000 DoH opposes such double standards, although in doing so it has incurred the displeasure of the pharmaceutical industry and the U.S. FDA, among others.

VII. Ethics

Of all the changes that have taken place in the context of medical research since the 1960s, perhaps the most far reaching have been in ethics. As is well known, the word "bioethics" did not exist before 1970. The ethics of medical research was medical ethics, i.e., the ethics of the medical profession. As Ulrich Tröhler and Dominique Sprumont et al. recount, the 1964 DoH was followed by numerous other documents on research ethics, emanating from governmental, intergovernmental and nongovernmental bodies. After its initial concentration on clinical ethical issues, the new field of bioethics turned its attention to research ethics and this has been one of its major foci ever since.

The shift from medical ethics to bioethics resulted in the displacement of physicians from the centre of research ethics in favour of research subjects. This can be seen already in the 1975 DoH where the physician's responsibility to protect subjects is no longer his or hers alone but is now shared with an ethics committee. In subsequent versions of the DoH and related documents, the autonomy of the research subject receives ever-greater prominence. The 2000 DoH marks a further development in this direction with its insistence that research subjects have a right to benefit from the results of the research in which they have participated.

The roles and activities of research ethics committees have greatly expanded since they first appeared in the 1970s. Whereas initially they only provided advice to researchers, who were free to accept or reject it, now they usually have the authority to approve or reject protocols. Many committees are expected to monitor research projects to ensure that they are being implemented properly. Since many proposed studies involve complex ethical issues related to consent, confidentiality, protection of vulnerable subjects, etc., education of committee members is a necessity. The exponential growth of medical research has resulted in a considerable workload for committee members, most of whom are volunteers with heavy employment responsibilities. In response to these considerations, research ethics governance and administration has become a major concern of medical research authorities and funders.

The final change in the context of research ethics to be mentioned here is its globalization. The WMA may have been the first international organization to deal with research ethics but it now shares the field with many other groups, including intergovernmental bodies such as WHO, UNAIDS and UNESCO, NGOs such as CIOMS, and the aforementioned ICH. Unfortunately, there are significant discrepancies among the documents produced by these organizations, although they all claim to support the "fundamental principles" of medical research ethics.

VIII. Have the Principles Changed?

Can the principles of research ethics remain unchanged in the face of such major changes in its context? And if they can, and do, might they become irrelevant? To answer these questions, it is first necessary to define the term "principle" and then to determine what it would mean for a principle to change. We can then attempt to identify "the fundamental and universal principles laid down in the [1964] Declaration [of Helsinki]" (Dominique Sprumont et al. (2007) in this volume) and compare it to the 2000 version to see if in fact the principles have changed.

The conventional meaning of "principle" has two aspects: it expresses a value, i.e., something that is considered very important, and it serves as a premise from which other assertions follow. Both values and premises are posited rather than deduced or proven. Therefore, the choice of principles cannot be defended or refuted by logic or science. Since principles are an essential element of ethical decision-making and behaviour, it is not surprising that ethics is pluralistic. Indeed, what is surprising is that there exists a considerable degree of consensus on the principles of research ethics.

Principles can change in two ways. First, they can be replaced by other principles, either absolutely or in a rank order. It is commonly held that autonomy has displaced beneficence in Western ethics. Second, they can change in how they are interpreted or applied. For example, the principle of respect for human life in traditional medical ethics has been interpreted in recent years not to exclude abortion.

Dominique Sprumont et al. have shown that there is a widespread belief, enunciated in such documents as the ICH GCP and the EU Clinical Trials Directive, in the existence of a set of ethical principles for medical research that have their origin in the DoH, presumably the 1964 version. It is noteworthy that the Nuremberg Code is not mentioned in this respect, although as Ulrich Tröhler and Susan Lederer show, both the 1954 WMA Principles for Those in Research and Experimentation and the 1964 DoH draw heavily from the Code.

A detailed comparison of the Nuremberg Code, the 1954 WMA Principles, and the 1964 and 2000 versions of the DoH is beyond the scope of this chapter. Instead, let us see whether the principles of the 1964 DoH are identical to those of the 2000 version.

The 1964 DoH is divided into four sections: Introduction, Basic Principles, Clinical Research Combined with Professional Care, and Non-Therapeutic Clinical Research. Although only the second section has the word "principles" in its title, it can safely be assumed that the contents of the third and fourth sections are also principles. The 2000 DoH has three sections: Introduction, Basic Principles for All Medical Research, and Additional Principles for Medical Research Combined with Medical Care. A comparison of the two sets of principles gives rise to the following observations:

- All of the principles in the 1964 DoH are incorporated in the 2000 version, although the wording has usually been modified. Whether such modifications constitute changes to the principles is a matter of interpretation. For example, it could be argued that the wording of paragraph 17 in the 2000 DoH, "Medical research involving human subjects should only be conducted if the importance of the objective outweighs the inherent risks and burdens to the subject" is significantly different from Basic Principle 3 in the 1964 DoH, "Clinical research cannot legitimately be carried out unless the importance of the objective is in proportion to the inherent risk to the subject."

- The "fundamental distinction [...] between clinical research in which the aim is essentially therapeutic for a patient, and the clinical research, the essential object of which is purely scientific and without therapeutic value to the person subjected to the research" in the 1964 DoH was all but discarded in the 2000 version. The principles for Clinical Research Combined With Professional Care have been retained but the 2000 version states that such treatment is not research unless the results are recorded, evaluated, and, where appropriate, published.

- The 2000 DoH is considerably more demanding than the 1964 version in its requirements for protection of vulnerable subjects and for the information that potential research subjects must be given.

- There are many additional principles in the 2000 DoH that do not appear in the 1964 version, including paragraph 12 on respect for the environment and for animals used in research, paragraph 13 on the requirement for ethics committee approval of every research project, paragraphs 19 and 30 on the right of research populations and individual research subjects to have access to the benefits of research, paragraph 25 on the need to obtain the assent of minor children to participate in research, paragraph 27 on the ethical obligations of authors and publishers, and paragraph 29 on the comparators to be used in clinical trials.

IX. Conclusion

No one would deny that the DoH has changed since 1964. As noted above, the major differences between this version and the latest one concern the structure of the documents, the wording of the principles, the requirements of some of the shared principles and the addition of several principles in the 2000 version. Dominique Sprumont et al. contend that, "Whether someone refers to the first, 1964 version of the Declaration or to the latest one, the underlying principles have not changed." However, according to the above-mentioned description of how principles can change, this statement is debatable at best. Although all of the 1964 principles have been retained in some form, they have been significantly reordered and reworded. More importantly, because the 2000 DoH contains additional principles, it would be inaccurate to say that the principles of the DoH have not changed. Indeed, if these changes had not been made, the DoH would no longer occupy centre stage in international research ethics but would be simply a historical curiosity.

The changes in the 2000 DoH were, for the most part, responses to the evolving context of medical research and research ethics. This context, in all its facets, will continue to evolve and consequently there will be need for future revisions of the DoH. Rather than bemoaning such change, even where principles are involved, those concerned about research ethics should recognize its necessity and strive for ever-greater improvements in the protection and empowerment of research subjects in the DoH and related documents.

Jonathan D. Moreno

Helsinki into the Future
An Epilogue

The remarkable scholarship on offer in this volume is testimony to the intense intellectual and organizational activity that has been devoted to a framework of protections for human research subjects. These efforts have intensified since the first Helsinki Declaration and are now codified in much the same spirit within the specific laws of many nations. In spite of the many shortcomings of the current experiment protections regime, including both the ambiguities in the current standards as well as what many agree are inadequate systems of enforcement, it is hard to deny that much has been clarified and much international consensus has been reached since the trials of the Nazi doctors in Nuremberg.

One notable exception to the fairly comprehensive and evolving conceptual scheme in place is medical research for national security purposes. With the notable exception of Ulf Schmidt's review of the 1953 sarin gas death of Ronald Maddison, the focus of these papers and of the research ethics literature generally is on human experiments in the civilian context. A continuing challenge for the regulation of human experiments lies in the area of military studies, a complex historic and policy problem that only promises to become more complex as the technological possibilities follow on increasingly sophisticated science.

These days when one mentions military medical research the topic that normally first comes to mind is biological and chemical weapons. But these agents have a long history, one that intensified in the Japanese and to a lesser extent German experiments during World War II (I say "lesser" because the Imperial Japanese research program was of a far greater scale and sophistication in the biochemical field than that of Nazi Germany). The sarin gas experiment involving Ronald Maddison was motivated partly by a desire to learn more about newer agents that were far more lethal than the old nitrogen mustard gases. In the same era as the ill-fated Porton Down testing here were attempts by the United States Central Intelligence Agency and the U.S. Army to learn about hallucinogens, with unwitting or poorly informed subjects that included psychiatric patients and soldiers. Chemical weapons were also sprayed over soldiers and naval vessels. Although international treaties supposedly outlawed offensive "BCW" research, the Soviets continued their secret program through the early 1990s, though whether systematic human experiments were conducted is not known.

In 1994-1995 the administration of President Bill Clinton authorized a massive and unprecedented investigation of rumoured federal sponsored experiments involving ionizing radiation.[1] The Advisory Committee on Human Radiation Experiments, for which I served as senior staff, requested and received the declassification of thousands of documents, constructing a narrative of research conducted from World War II to the mid-1970s. A small number of abuses were clearly documented, including observational studies of human effects, and remedies were recommended. One vivid lesson of the radiation experiments investigation was the moral hazard associated with a government's ability to categorize activities as other than human experiments, thus in effect avoiding regulation that would otherwise apply. Thus over 200,000 soldiers and marines deployed to witness Cold War atomic tests in close proximity to ground zero were considered to be participants in training exercises, not medical experiments.

Another important lesson of the human radiation experiments revelations, at least in the United States, was the fact that the national security establishment had taken seriously the question of human research policy long before the civilian medical world had. In particular, the Department of Defence adopted a policy of voluntary written consent for atomic, biological and chemical weapons in a top secret 1953 document signed by the Secretary of Defence. It is noteworthy that, by contrast, it took another decade for the World Medical Association to adopt its first version of Helsinki. Unfortunately, both the historical record and the Clinton Administration's response to the radiation advisory committee report demonstrate that the application of these enlightened policies was, at best, inconsistent. As is well known, various human radiation experiments took place during the Cold War in violation of the consent policy, a fact that was recognized as early as 1975 by the Army Inspector General when the LSD experiments controversy surfaced.

Today the U.S. armed forces are governed by the same regulations that are supposed to bind all other federal agencies that sponsor or conduct human experiments, including basic requirements for prior review and informed consent. Indeed, it is not too much to say that the bureaucratic obstacles to using soldiers in research are as great as for any population of potential research subjects.

However, a number of new issues confront the national security establishment, especially in the post-9/11 environment. For example, there has never been a satisfactory resolution of the question of whether human experiments can ethically be conducted in secret. Although no U.S. administration has ever stated that ethical conventions in human studies could be suspended without specific advance review by authorities, it is by no means clear what conditions would make secret experiments permissible. My own view is that "ethical secret human experiments" is an oxymoron, because ethics requires the oxygen of transparency and public accountability.

The "war on terrorism" also raises questions about epidemiological studies. During the Cold War, for example, there were numerous secret cases of environ-

---

1   Moreno (1999/2001).

mental releases of nerve gases and toxins in order to test the way these agents would behave under various conditions. These tests included the intentional venting of radioactive gases from nuclear production facilities and spraying of nerve gas on ships at sea and soldiers on manoeuvres. Today the regulatory obstacles against such activities would be far greater, but how far authorities could go in protecting the public health is not a settled question.

A different set of issues is created by the nature of the novel science potentially of interest to defence planners, particularly in the burgeoning field of neuroscience.[2] Some neuroscientific experiments raise multiple sorts of questions. For instance, neuropharmaceuticals, brain implants, or other techniques for altering mental function like deep brain stimulation (DBS), could be of considerable interest in improving soldiers' warfighting capacity. But what does informed consent mean when the experiment itself alters cognition at a basic level? At what point is the "person" who gave consent at an earlier time not precisely the same "person" whose personality has been altered? Although this issue is not unique to the national security context, defence planners have the resources and rationale to drive science in powerful new directions such as these.

Science is more, not less, likely to be a critical aspect of military endeavours in the 21st century. A critical question is whether a voluntary, professional standard such as the Helsinki Declaration is up to the task ahead. Recently we have seen the U.S. psychiatric and psychological organizations struggle with the problem of the appropriate professional role in the interrogation of detainees in the hands of intelligence agencies. A difficult question is whether international treaties may need to address more explicitly this sort of problem, with all the hazards and vagaries of such diplomatic processes.

But that is for the future. I conclude with a last word about the past. We should remind ourselves of the ultimate lesson of the sort of historical work so well described in this volume, a lesson to which we may become inured through all the important details of the particular studies. As Andreas Frewer notes, investigations of past ethical violations are not "mere history." Their implications for the present are frequently exemplified in the reaction to those investigations on the part of powerful forces that would prefer to forget. Thus it is all the more vital that this field continue to be ploughed.

References

Moreno, J. D. (1999/2001): Undue Risk: Secret State Experiments on Humans. New York: W. H. Freeman Publishers; New York: Routledge Publishers.
Moreno J. D. (2006): Mind Wars: Brain Research and National Defense. Washington, D.C.: Dana Press.

---

2   Moreno (2006).

IV.
Key Documents on the
History of Research Ethics

Circular of the Reich Minister of the Interior Concerning Guidelines for New Therapy and Human Experimentation, 28 February 1931[1]

The Reich Health-Council (Reichsgesundheitsrat) has set great store in ensuring that all physicians receive information with regard to the following Guidelines. The Council has agreed that all physicians in open and closed health care institutions should sign a commitment to these guidelines when entering their employment.

Final Draft of Guidelines for New Therapy and Human Experimentation

1. Medical science, if it is not to come to a standstill, cannot refrain from introducing in suitable cases New Therapy using as yet insufficiently tested agents and methods. Also, medical science cannot dispense completely with Human Experimentation. Otherwise, progress in diagnosis, therapy, and prevention of disease would be hindered or even rendered impossible.

    The special rights to be granted to the physician under these new guidelines must be balanced by the special duty of the physician to be aware of the grave responsibility which he bears for the life and health of each individual undergoing New Therapy or Human Experimentation.

2. The term *New Therapy* used in these Guidelines defines therapeutic experimentation and modes of treatment of humans which serve the process of healing, i.e. pursuing in specific individual cases the recognition, healing or prevention of an illness or suffering, or the removal of a bodily defect, even though the effects and consequences of the therapy can not yet be adequately determined on the basis of available knowledge.

3. The term *Human Experimentation*, as defined in the Guidelines, means operations and modes of treatment on humans carried out for research purposes which are non-therapeutic; it includes the side-effects and consequences which can not yet be adequately determined on the basis of available knowledge.

4. Any New Therapy must be in accord with the principles of medical ethics and the rules of the medical arts and sciences, both in its design and in its realization.

---

1   Reichsgesundheitsblatt 55 (1931), 6, pp. 174-175 [Veröffentlichungen des Reichsgesundheitsamtes]; see also Frewer, A./Schmidt, U. (2007): Standards der Forschung. Historische Entwicklung und ethische Grundlagen klinischer Studien. Frankfurt: Peter Lang, pp. 254-255 and Sass, H.-M. (1983): Reichsrundschreiben 1931: Pre-Nuremberg German Regulations Concerning New Therapy and Human Experimentation, The Journal of Medicine and Philosophy 8 (1983), 2, pp. 99-111, here pp. 104-106.

A consideration and calculation of possible harms must be undertaken to determine whether they stand in a suitable relationship to expected benefits.

New Therapy may only be initiated after first being tested in animal experimentation, where this is at all possible.

5. New Therapy may only be applied if consent or proxy consent has been given in a clear and undebatable manner following earlier appropriate information.

New Therapy may only be introduced without consent if it is urgently required, and cannot be postponed because of a need to save life or prevent severe damage to health, and if prior consent could not be obtained owing to special circumstances.

6. Introduction of New Therapy in the treatment of children and minors under eighteen requires especially careful examination.

7. Medical ethics rejects any exploitation of social and economic need in conducting New Therapy.

8. New Therapy using living micro-organisms requires heightened caution, especially in the case of live pathogens. Such therapy may only be considered permissible if a relative degree of harmlessness in the procedure can be assumed, and if the achievement of equal benefits by other means cannot be expected under any given circumstances.

9. In medical ethics, polyclinics, hospitals or other health care institutions, New Therapy may only be conducted by the chief physician himself or, at his specific request and with his full responsibility, by another physician.

10. A written report on any new therapy is required, containing information on therapy design, its justification and execution. Such a report shall state especially that the subject, or his or her legal representative, has been adequately informed and has given consent. If New Therapy is applied without consent, according to (5.2), the report must clearly outline these pre-conditions.

11. Publication of results of New Therapy must respect the patient's dignity and the commandments of humanity.

12. Numbers 1 through 11 of these Guidelines are equally applicable to Human Experimentation (Art. 3). In addition, the following requirements for such experimentation apply:

a) Without consent, non-therapeutic research is under no circumstances permissible.

b) Any human experimentation which could as well be carried out in animal experimentation is not permissible. Only after all basic information has been obtained should Human Experimentation begin. This information should first be obtained by means of scientific biological or laboratory research and animal experimentation for reasons of clarification and safety. Given these presuppositions, unfounded or random Human Experimentation is impermissible.

c) Experimentation with children or minors is impermissible if it endangers the child or minor in the slightest degree.

d) Experimentation with dying persons conflicts with the principles of medical ethics and therefore is impermissible.

13. Assuming that, in accordance with these Guidelines, physicians and, in parti-
    cular, responsible directors in charge of medical institutions will be guided by
    a strong sense of responsibility toward the patients entrusted to them, it also is
    to be hoped that they will maintain a readiness responsibly to seek relief,
    improvement, protection or cure for the patient along new paths, when the
    accepted and actual state of medical science, according to their medical
    knowledge, no longer seems adequate.
14. In academic teaching, already, every opportunity should be uses to stress the
    special duties of a physician undertaking New Therapy or Human
    Experimentation; these special responsibilities also apply to the publication of
    the results of New Therapy and Human Experimentation.

The Nuremberg Code (1947)[1]

1. The voluntary consent of the human subject is absolutely essential. This means that the person involved should have legal capacity to give consent; should be so situated as to be able to exercise free power of choice, without the intervention of any element of force, fraud, deceit, duress, over-reaching, or other ulterior form of constraint or coercion; and should have sufficient knowledge and comprehension of the elements of the subject matter involved as to enable him to make an understanding and enlightened decision. This latter element requires that before the acceptance of an affirmative decision by the experimental subject there should be made known to him the nature, duration, and purpose of the experiment; the method and means by which it is to be conducted; all inconveniences and hazards reasonably to be expected; and the effects upon his health or person which may possibly come from his participation in the experiment.
   The duty and responsibility for ascertaining the quality of the consent rests upon each individual who initiates, directs or engages in the experiment. It is a personal duty and responsibility which may not be delegated to another with impunity

2. The experiment should be such as to yield fruitful results for the good of society, unprocurable by other methods or means of study, and not random and unnecessary in nature.

3. The experiment should be so designed and based on the results of animal experimentation and a knowledge of the natural history of the disease or other problem under study that the anticipated results will justify the performance of the experiment.

4. The experiment should be so conducted as to avoid all unnecessary physical and mental suffering and injury.

5. No experiment should be conducted where there is an a priori reason to believe that death or disabling injury will occur; except, perhaps, in those experiments where the experimental physicians also serve as subjects.

6. The degree of risk to be taken should never exceed that determined by the humanitarian importance of the problem to be solved by the experiment.

7. Proper preparation should be made and adequate facilities provided to protect the experimental subject against even remote possibilities of injury, disability, or death.

8. The experiment should be conducted only by scientifically qualified persons. The highest degree of skill and care should be required through all stages of the experiment of those who conduct or engage in the experiment.

---

1   NDT-Records, frames 11568-11569.

9. During the course of the experiment the human subject should be at liberty to bring the experiment to an end if he has reached the physical or mental state where continuation of the experiment seems to him to be impossible.
10. During the course of the experiment the scientist in charge must be prepared to terminate the experiment at any stage, if he has probable cause to believe, in the exercise of the good faith, superior skill, and careful judgement required of him, that a continuation of the experiment is likely to result in injury, disability, or death to the experimental subject.

See also Oppitz, U.-D. (1999): Das Urteil gegen Karl Brandt und andere, in: Frewer, A. et al. (Hrsg.) (1999): Medizinverbrechen vor Gericht. Das Urteil im Nürnberger Ärzteprozeß gegen Karl Brandt und andere sowie aus dem Prozeß gegen Generalfeldmarschall Erhard Milch. Mit einem Vorwort von T. v. Uexküll. Erlanger Studien zur Ethik in der Medizin, Band 7, Erlangen, Jena: Palm & Enke, pp. 123-125, and Schmidt, U. (2004): Justice at Nuremberg. Leo Alexander and the Nazi Doctors' Trial. St Antony's Series, Houndsmill, New York.

World Medical Association, Declaration of Helsinki I, 18th World Medical Assembly, Helsinki, Finland, June 1964[1]

It is the mission of the doctor to safeguard the health of the people. His or her knowledge and conscience are dedicated to the fulfilment of this mission.

The Declaration of Geneva of the World Medical Association binds the physician with the words, "The health of my patient will be my first consideration"; and the International Code of Medical Ethics declares that "Any act or advice which could weaken physical or mental resistance of a human being may be used only in his interest."

Because it is essential that the results of laboratory experiments be applied to human beings to further scientific knowledge and to help suffering humanity, the World Medical Association has prepared the following recommendations as a guide to each doctor in clinical research. It must be stressed that the standards as drafted are only a guide to physicians all over the world. Doctors are not relieved from criminal, civil, and ethical responsibilities under the laws of their own countries.

In the field of clinical research a fundamental distinction must be recognized between clinical research in which the aim is essentially therapeutic for a patient, and clinical research the essential object of which is purely scientific and without therapeutic value to the person subjected to the research.

I.   BASIC PRINCIPLES

1. Clinical research must conform to the moral and scientific principles that justify medical research, and should be based on laboratory and animal experiments or other scientifically established facts.
2. Clinical research should be conducted only by scientifically qualified persons and under the supervision of a qualified medical man.
3. Clinical research cannot legitimately be carried out unless the importance of the objective is in proportion to the inherent risk to the subject.
4. Every clinical research project should be preceded by careful assessment of inherent risks in comparison to foreseeable benefits to the subject or to others.
5. Special caution should be exercised by the doctor in performing clinical research in which the personality of the subject is liable to be altered by drugs or experimental procedures.

---

1   Annas, G. J./Grodin, M. A. (eds.) (1992): The Nazi Doctors and the Nuremberg Code. Human Rights in Human Experimentation. New York, Oxford: Oxford University Press, pp. 331-333.

II. CLINICAL RESEARCH COMBINED WITH PROFESSIONAL CARE

1. In the treatment of the sick person the doctor must be free to use a new therapeutic measure if in his judgement it offers hope of saving life, re-establishing health, or alleviating suffering.

    If at all possible, consistent with patient psychology, the doctor should obtain the patient's freely given consent after the patient has been given a full explanation. In case of legal incapacity consent should also be procured from the legal guardian; in case of physical incapacity the permission of the legal guardian replaces that of the patient.

2. The doctor can combine clinical research with professional care, the objective being the acquisition of new medical knowledge, only to the extent that clinical research is justified by its therapeutic value for the patient.

III. NON-THEARPEUTIC CLINICAL RESEARCH

1. In the purely scientific application of clinical research carried out on a human being it is the duty of the doctor to remain the protector of the life and health of that person on whom clinical research is being carried out.

2. The nature, the purpose, and the risk of clinical research must be explained to the subject by the doctor.

3a. Clinical research on human beings cannot be undertaken without his free consent, after he had been fully informed; if he is legally incompetent the consent of the legal guardian should be procured.

3b. The subject of clinical research should be in such a mental, physical, and legal state as to be able to exercise fully his power of choice.

3c. Consent should as a rule be obtained in writing. However, the responsibility for clinical research always remains with the research worker; it never falls on the subject, even after consent is obtained.

4a. The investigator must respect the right of each individual to safeguard his personal integrity, especially if the subject is in a dependent relationship to the investigator.

4b. At any time during the course of clinical research the subject or his guardian should be free to withdraw permission for research to be continued. The investigator or the investigating team should discontinue the research if in his or their judgement it may, if continued, be harmful to the individual.

World Medical Association, Declaration of Helsinki II
29th World Medical Assembly, Tokyo, Japan, October 1975[1]

It is the mission of the medical doctor to safeguard the health of the people. His or her knowledge and conscience are dedicated to the fulfilment of this mission.

The Declaration of Geneva of the World Medical Association binds the doctor with the words, "The health of my patient will be my first consideration"; and the International Code of Medical Ethics declares that "Any act or advice which could weaken physical or mental resistance of a human being may be used only in his interest."

The purpose of biomedical research involving human subjects must be to improve diagnostic, therapeutic and prophylactic procedures and the understanding of the aetiology and pathogenesis of disease.

In current medical practice most diagnostic, therapeutic and prophylactic procedures involve hazards. This applies *a fortiori* to biomedical research.

Medical progress is based on research which ultimately must rest in part on experimentation involving human subjects.

In the field of biomedical research a fundamental distinction must be recognized between medical research in which the aim is essentially diagnostic or therapeutic for a patient, and medical research, the essential object of which is purely scientific and without therapeutic value to the person subjected to the research.

Special caution must be exercised in the conduct of research which may affect the environment, and the welfare of animals used for research must be respected.

Because it is essential that the results of laboratory experiments be applied to human beings to further scientific knowledge and to help suffering humanity, the World Medical Association has prepared the following recommendations as a guide to every doctor in biomedical research involving human subjects. They should be kept under review in the future. It must be stressed that the standards as drafted are only a guide to physicians all over the world. Doctors are not relieved from criminal, civil and ethical responsibilities under the laws of their own countries.

---

1   Annas, G. J./Grodin, M. A. (eds.) (1992): The Nazi Doctors and the Nuremberg Code. Human Rights in Human Experimentation. New York, Oxford: Oxford University Press, pp. 333-336.

I.   BASIC PRINCIPLES

1.   Biomedical research involving human subjects must conform to the generally accepted scientific principles and should be based on adequately performed laboratory and animal experimentation and on a thorough knowledge of the scientific literature.

2.   The design and performance of each experimental procedure involving human subjects should be clearly formulated in an experimental protocol which should be transmitted to a specially appointed independent committee for consideration, comment and guidance.

3.   Biomedical research involving human subjects should be conducted only by scientifically qualified persons and under the supervision of a clinically competent medical person. The responsibility for the human subject must always rest with a medically qualified person and never rest on the subject of the research, even though the subject has given his or her consent.

4.   Biomedical research involving human subjects cannot legitimately be carried out unless the importance of the objective is in proportion to the inherent risk to the subject.

5.   Every biomedical research project involving human subjects should be preceded by careful assessment of predictable risks in comparison with foreseeable benefits to the subject or to others. Concern for the interests of the subject must always prevail over the interests of science and society.

6.   The right of the research subject to safeguard his or her integrity must always be respected. Every precaution should be taken to respect the privacy of the subject and to minimize the impact of the study on the subject's physical and mental integrity and on the personality of the subject.

7.   Doctors should abstain from engaging in research projects involving human subjects unless they are satisfied that the hazards involved are believed to be predictable. Doctors should cease any investigation if the hazards are found to outweigh the potential benefits.

8.   In publication of the results of his or her research, the doctor is obliged to preserve the accuracy of the results. Reports of experimentation not in accordance with the principles laid down in this Declaration should not be accepted for publication.

9.   In any research on human beings, each potential subject must be adequately informed of the aims, methods, anticipated benefits and potential hazards of the study and the discomfort it may entail. He or she should be informed that he or she is at liberty to abstain from participation in the study and that he or she is free to withdraw visor her consent to participa-

tion at any time. The doctor should then obtain the subject's freely-given informed consent, preferably inheriting.

10. When obtaining informed consent for the research project the doctor should be particularly cautious if the subject is in a dependent relationship to him or her or may consent under duress. In that case the informed consent should be obtained by a doctor who is not engaged in the investigation and who is completely independent of this official relationship.

11. In case of legal incompetence, informed consent should be obtained from the legal guardian in accordance with national legislation. Where physical or mental incapacity makes it impossible to obtain informed consent, or when the subject is a minor, permission from the responsible relative replaces that of the subject in accordance with national legislation.

12. The research protocol should always contain a statement of the ethical considerations involved and should indicate that the principles enunciated in the present Declaration are complied with.

II. MEDICAL RESEARCH COMBINED WITH PROFESSIONAL CARE (Clinical Research)

1. In the treatment of the sick person, the doctor must be free to use a new diagnostic and therapeutic measure, if in his or her judgement it offers hope of saving life, re-establishing health or alleviating suffering.

2. The potential benefits, hazards and discomfort of a new method should be weighed against the advantages of the best current diagnostic and therapeutic methods.

3. In any medical study, every patient – including those of a control group, if any – should be assured of the best proven diagnostic and therapeutic method.

4. The refusal of the patient to participate in a study must never interfere with the doctor-patient relationship.

5. If the doctor considers it essential not to obtain informed consent, the specific reasons for this proposal should be stated in the experimental protocol for transmission to the independent committee (I, 2).

6. The doctor can combine medical research with professional care, the objective being the acquisition of new medical knowledge, only to the extent that medical research is justified by its potential diagnostic or therapeutic value for the patient.

III. NON-THEARPEUTIC BIOMEDICAL RESEARCH INVOLVING HU-
MAN SUBJECTS (Non-Clinical Biomedical Research)

1. In the purely scientific application of medical research carried out on a human being, it is the duty of the doctor to remain the protector of the life and health of that person on whom biomedical research is being carried out.

2. The subjects should be volunteers – either healthy persons or patients for whom the experimental design is not related to the patient's illness.

3. The investigator or the investigating team should discontinue the research if in his/her or their judgment it may, if continued, be harmful to the individual.

4. In research on man, the interest of science and society should never take precedence over considerations related to the well-being of the subject.

Convention for the Protection of Human Rights and Dignity of the Human Being with regard to the Application of Biology and Medicine: Convention on Human Rights and Biomedicine, Oviedo, 4 April 1997

Preamble

The member States of the Council of Europe, the other States and the European Community, signatories hereto,

Bearing in mind the Universal Declaration of Human Rights proclaimed by the General Assembly of the United Nations on 10 December 1948;

Bearing in mind the Convention for the Protection of Human Rights and Fundamental Freedoms of 4 November 1950;

Bearing in mind the European Social Charter of 18 October 1961;

Bearing in mind the International Covenant on Civil and Political Rights and the International Covenant on Economic, Social and Cultural Rights of 16 December 1966;

Bearing in mind the Convention for the Protection of Individuals with regard to Automatic Processing of Personal Data of 28 January 1981;

Bearing also in mind the Convention on the Rights of the Child of 20 November 1989;

Considering that the aim of the Council of Europe is the achievement of a greater unity between its members and that one of the methods by which that aim is to be pursued is the maintenance and further realisation of human rights and fundamental freedoms;

Conscious of the accelerating developments in biology and medicine;

Convinced of the need to respect the human being both as an individual and as a member of the human species and recognising the importance of ensuring the dignity of the human being;

Conscious that the misuse of biology and medicine may lead to acts endangering human dignity;

Affirming that progress in biology and medicine should be used for the benefit of present and future generations;

Stressing the need for international co-operation so that all humanity may enjoy the benefits of biology and medicine;

Recognising the importance of promoting a public debate on the questions posed by the application of biology and medicine and the responses to be given thereto;

Wishing to remind all members of society of their rights and responsibilities;

Taking account of the work of the Parliamentary Assembly in this field, including Recommendation 1160 (1991) on the preparation of a convention on bioethics;

Resolving to take such measures as are necessary to safeguard human dignity and the fundamental rights and freedoms of the individual with regard to the application of biology and medicine,

Have agreed as follows:

Chapter I – General provisions

Article 1 – Purpose and object

Parties to this Convention shall protect the dignity and identity of all human beings and guarantee everyone, without discrimination, respect for their integrity and other rights and fundamental freedoms with regard to the application of biology and medicine.

Each Party shall take in its internal law the necessary measures to give effect to the provisions of this Convention.

Article 2 – Primacy of the human being

The interests and welfare of the human being shall prevail over the sole interest of society or science.

Article 3 – Equitable access to health care

Parties, taking into account health needs and available resources, shall take appropriate measures with a view to providing, within their jurisdiction, equitable access to health care of appropriate quality.

Article 4 – Professional standards

Any intervention in the health field, including research, must be carried out in accordance with relevant professional obligations and standards.

Chapter II – Consent

Article 5 – General rule

An intervention in the health field may only be carried out after the person concerned has given free and informed consent to it.

This person shall beforehand be given appropriate information as to the purpose and nature of the intervention as well as on its consequences and risks.

The person concerned may freely withdraw consent at any time.

Article 6 – Protection of persons not able to consent

Subject to Articles 17 and 20 below, an intervention may only be carried out on a person who does not have the capacity to consent, for his or her direct benefit.

Where, according to law, a minor does not have the capacity to consent to an intervention, the intervention may only be carried out with the authorisation of his or her representative or an authority or a person or body provided for by law.

The opinion of the minor shall be taken into consideration as an increasingly determining factor in proportion to his or her age and degree of maturity.

Where, according to law, an adult does not have the capacity to consent to an intervention because of a mental disability, a disease or for similar reasons, the intervention may only be carried out with the authorisation of his or her representative or an authority or a person or body provided for by law.

The individual concerned shall as far as possible take part in the authorisation procedure.

The representative, the authority, the person or the body mentioned in paragraphs 2 and 3 above shall be given, under the same conditions, the information referred to in Article 5.

The authorisation referred to in paragraphs 2 and 3 above may be withdrawn at any time in the best interests of the person concerned.

Article 7 – Protection of persons who have a mental disorder

Subject to protective conditions prescribed by law, including supervisory, control and appeal procedures, a person who has a mental disorder of a serious nature may be subjected, without his or her consent, to an intervention aimed at treating his or her mental disorder only where, without such treatment, serious harm is likely to result to his or her health.

Article 8 – Emergency situation

When because of an emergency situation the appropriate consent cannot be obtained, any medically necessary intervention may be carried out immediately for the benefit of the health of the individual concerned.

Article 9 – Previously expressed wishes

The previously expressed wishes relating to a medical intervention by a patient who is not, at the time of the intervention, in a state to express his or her wishes shall be taken into account.

Chapter III – Private life and right to information

Article 10 – Private life and right to information

Everyone has the right to respect for private life in relation to information about his or her health.

Everyone is entitled to know any information collected about his or her health. However, the wishes of individuals not to be so informed shall be observed.

In exceptional cases, restrictions may be placed by law on the exercise of the rights contained in paragraph 2 in the interests of the patient.

Chapter IV – Human genome

Article 11 – Non-discrimination

Any form of discrimination against a person on grounds of his or her genetic heritage is prohibited.

Article 12 – Predictive genetic tests

Tests which are predictive of genetic diseases or which serve either to identify the subject as a carrier of a gene responsible for a disease or to detect a genetic predisposition or susceptibility to a disease may be performed only for health purposes or for scientific research linked to health purposes, and subject to appropriate genetic counselling.

Article 13 – Interventions on the human genome

An intervention seeking to modify the human genome may only be undertaken for preventive, diagnostic or therapeutic purposes and only if its aim is not to introduce any modification in the genome of any descendants.

Article 14 – Non-selection of sex

The use of techniques of medically assisted procreation shall not be allowed for the purpose of choosing a future child's sex, except where serious hereditary sex-related disease is to be avoided.

Chapter V – Scientific research

Article 15 – General rule

Scientific research in the field of biology and medicine shall be carried out freely, subject to the provisions of this Convention and the other legal provisions ensuring the protection of the human being.

Article 16 – Protection of persons undergoing research

Research on a person may only be undertaken if all the following conditions are met:

there is no alternative of comparable effectiveness to research on humans;
the risks which may be incurred by that person are not disproportionate to the potential benefits of the research;

the research project has been approved by the competent body after independent examination of its scientific merit, including assessment of the importance of the aim of the research, and multidisciplinary review of its ethical acceptability;

the persons undergoing research have been informed of their rights and the safeguards prescribed by law for their protection;

the necessary consent as provided for under Article 5 has been given expressly, specifically and is documented. Such consent may be freely withdrawn at any time.

Article 17 – Protection of persons not able to consent to research

Research on a person without the capacity to consent as stipulated in Article 5 may be undertaken only if all the following conditions are met:

the conditions laid down in Article 16, sub-paragraphs i to iv, are fulfilled;

the results of the research have the potential to produce real and direct benefit to his or her health;

research of comparable effectiveness cannot be carried out on individuals capable of giving consent;

the necessary authorisation provided for under Article 6 has been given specifically and in writing; and

the person concerned does not object.

Exceptionally and under the protective conditions prescribed by law, where the research has not the potential to produce results of direct benefit to the health of the person concerned, such research may be authorised subject to the conditions laid down in paragraph 1, sub-paragraphs i, iii, iv and v above, and to the following additional conditions:

the research has the aim of contributing, through significant improvement in the scientific understanding of the individual's condition, disease or disorder, to the ultimate attainment of results capable of conferring benefit to the person concerned or to other persons in the same age category or afflicted with the same disease or disorder or having the same condition;

the research entails only minimal risk and minimal burden for the individual concerned.

Article 18 – Research on embryos in vitro

Where the law allows research on embryos in vitro, it shall ensure adequate protection of the embryo.

The creation of human embryos for research purposes is prohibited.

Chapter VI – Organ and tissue removal from living donors for transplantation purposes

Article 19 – General rule

Removal of organs or tissue from a living person for transplantation purposes may be carried out solely for the therapeutic benefit of the recipient and where there is no suitable organ or tissue available from a deceased person and no other alternative therapeutic method of comparable effectiveness.

The necessary consent as provided for under Article 5 must have been given expressly and specifically either in written form or before an official body.

Article 20 – Protection of persons not able to consent to organ removal

No organ or tissue removal may be carried out on a person who does not have the capacity to consent under Article 5.

Exceptionally and under the protective conditions prescribed by law, the removal of regenerative tissue from a person who does not have the capacity to consent may be authorised provided the following conditions are met:

there is no compatible donor available who has the capacity to consent;

the recipient is a brother or sister of the donor;

the donation must have the potential to be life-saving for the recipient;

the authorisation provided for under paragraphs 2 and 3 of Article 6 has been given specifically and in writing, in accordance with the law and with the approval of the competent body;

the potential donor concerned does not object.

Chapter VII – Prohibition of financial gain and disposal of a part of the human body

Article 21 – Prohibition of financial gain

The human body and its parts shall not, as such, give rise to financial gain.

Article 22 – Disposal of a removed part of the human body

When in the course of an intervention any part of a human body is removed, it may be stored and used for a purpose other than that for which it was removed, only if this is done in conformity with appropriate information and consent procedures.

Chapter VIII – Infringements of the provisions of the Convention

Article 23 – Infringement of the rights or principles

The Parties shall provide appropriate judicial protection to prevent or to put a stop to an unlawful infringement of the rights and principles set forth in this Convention at short notice.

Article 24 – Compensation for undue damage

The person who has suffered undue damage resulting from an intervention is entitled to fair compensation according to the conditions and procedures prescribed by law.

Article 25 – Sanctions

Parties shall provide for appropriate sanctions to be applied in the event of infringement of the provisions contained in this Convention.

Chapter IX – Relation between this Convention and other provisions

Article 26 – Restrictions on the exercise of the rights

No restrictions shall be placed on the exercise of the rights and protective provisions contained in this Convention other than such as are prescribed by law and are necessary in a democratic society in the interest of public safety, for the prevention of crime, for the protection of public health or for the protection of the rights and freedoms of others.

The restrictions contemplated in the preceding paragraph may not be placed on Articles 11, 13, 14, 16, 17, 19, 20 and 21.

Article 27 – Wider protection

None of the provisions of this Convention shall be interpreted as limiting or otherwise affecting the possibility for a Party to grant a wider measure of protection with regard to the application of biology and medicine than is stipulated in this Convention.

Chapter X – Public debate

Article 28 – Public debate

Parties to this Convention shall see to it that the fundamental questions raised by the developments of biology and medicine are the subject of appropriate public discussion in the light, in particular, of relevant medical, social, economic, ethical and legal implications, and that their possible application is made the subject of appropriate consultation.

Chapter XI – Interpretation and follow-up of the Convention

Article 29 – Interpretation of the Convention

The European Court of Human Rights may give, without direct reference to any specific proceedings pending in a court, advisory opinions on legal questions concerning the interpretation of the present Convention at the request of:

the Government of a Party, after having informed the other Parties;
the Committee set up by Article 32, with membership restricted to the Representatives of the Parties to this Convention, by a decision adopted by a two-thirds majority of votes cast.

Article 30 – Reports on the application of the Convention

On receipt of a request from the Secretary General of the Council of Europe any Party shall furnish an explanation of the manner in which its internal law ensures the effective implementation of any of the provisions of the Convention.

Chapter XII – Protocols

Article 31 – Protocols

Protocols may be concluded in pursuance of Article 32, with a view to developing, in specific fields, the principles contained in this Convention.
The Protocols shall be open for signature by Signatories of the Convention. They shall be subject to ratification, acceptance or approval. A Signatory may not ratify, accept or approve Protocols without previously or simultaneously ratifying accepting or approving the Convention.

Chapter XIII – Amendments to the Convention

Article 32 – Amendments to the Convention

The tasks assigned to "the Committee" in the present article and in Article 29 shall be carried out by the Steering Committee on Bioethics (CDBI), or by any other committee designated to do so by the Committee of Ministers.
Without prejudice to the specific provisions of Article 29, each member State of the Council of Europe, as well as each Party to the present Convention which is not a member of the Council of Europe, may be represented and have one vote in the Committee when the Committee carries out the tasks assigned to it by the present Convention.
Any State referred to in Article 33 or invited to accede to the Convention in accordance with the provisions of Article 34 which is not Party to this Convention may be represented on the Committee by an observer. If the European Community is not a Party it may be represented on the Committee by an observer.

In order to monitor scientific developments, the present Convention shall be examined within the Committee no later than five years from its entry into force and thereafter at such intervals as the Committee may determine.

Any proposal for an amendment to this Convention, and any proposal for a Protocol or for an amendment to a Protocol, presented by a Party, the Committee or the Committee of Ministers shall be communicated to the Secretary General of the Council of Europe and forwarded by him to the member States of the Council of Europe, to the European Community, to any Signatory, to any Party, to any State invited to sign this Convention in accordance with the provisions of Article 33 and to any State invited to accede to it in accordance with the provisions of Article 34.

The Committee shall examine the proposal not earlier than two months after it has been forwarded by the Secretary General in accordance with paragraph 5. The Committee shall submit the text adopted by a two-thirds majority of the votes cast to the Committee of Ministers for approval. After its approval, this text shall be forwarded to the Parties for ratification, acceptance or approval.

Any amendment shall enter into force, in respect of those Parties which have accepted it, on the first day of the month following the expiration of a period of one month after the date on which five Parties, including at least four member States of the Council of Europe, have informed the Secretary General that they have accepted it.

In respect of any Party which subsequently accepts it, the amendment shall enter into force on the first day of the month following the expiration of a period of one month after the date on which that Party has informed the Secretary General of its acceptance.

Chapter XIV – Final clauses

Article 33 – Signature, ratification and entry into force

This Convention shall be open for signature by the member States of the Council of Europe, the non-member States which have participated in its elaboration and by the European Community.

This Convention is subject to ratification, acceptance or approval. Instruments of ratification, acceptance or approval shall be deposited with the Secretary General of the Council of Europe.

This Convention shall enter into force on the first day of the month following the expiration of a period of three months after the date on which five States, including at least four member States of the Council of Europe, have expressed their consent to be bound by the Convention in accordance with the provisions of paragraph 2 of the present article.

In respect of any Signatory which subsequently expresses its consent to be bound by it, the Convention shall enter into force on the first day of the month following the expiration of a period of three months after the date of the deposit of its instrument of ratification, acceptance or approval.

Article 34 – Non-member States

After the entry into force of this Convention, the Committee of Ministers of the Council of Europe may, after consultation of the Parties, invite any non-member State of the Council of Europe to accede to this Convention by a decision taken by the majority provided for in Article 20, paragraph d, of the Statute of the Council of Europe, and by the unanimous vote of the representatives of the Contracting States entitled to sit on the Committee of Ministers.

In respect of any acceding State, the Convention shall enter into force on the first day of the month following the expiration of a period of three months after the date of deposit of the instrument of accession with the Secretary General of the Council of Europe.

Article 35 – Territories

Any Signatory may, at the time of signature or when depositing its instrument of ratification, acceptance or approval, specify the territory or territories to which this Convention shall apply. Any other State may formulate the same declaration when depositing its instrument of accession.

Any Party may, at any later date, by a declaration addressed to the Secretary General of the Council of Europe, extend the application of this Convention to any other territory specified in the declaration and for whose international relations it is responsible or on whose behalf it is authorised to give undertakings. In respect of such territory the Convention shall enter into force on the first day of the month following the expiration of a period of three months after the date of receipt of such declaration by the Secretary General.

Any declaration made under the two preceding paragraphs may, in respect of any territory specified in such declaration, be withdrawn by a notification addressed to the Secretary General. The withdrawal shall become effective on the first day of the month following the expiration of a period of three months after the date of receipt of such notification by the Secretary General.

Article 36 – Reservations

Any State and the European Community may, when signing this Convention or when depositing the instrument of ratification, acceptance, approval or accession, make a reservation in respect of any particular provision of the Convention to the extent that any law then in force in its territory is not in conformity with the provision. Reservations of a general character shall not be permitted under this article.

Any reservation made under this article shall contain a brief statement of the relevant law.

Any Party which extends the application of this Convention to a territory mentioned in the declaration referred to in Article 35, paragraph 2, may, in respect of the territory concerned, make a reservation in accordance with the provisions of the preceding paragraphs.

Any Party which has made the reservation mentioned in this article may withdraw it by means of a declaration addressed to the Secretary General of the Council of Europe. The withdrawal shall become effective on the first day of the month following the expiration of a period of one month after the date of its receipt by the Secretary General.

Article 37 – Denunciation

Any Party may at any time denounce this Convention by means of a notification addressed to the Secretary General of the Council of Europe.

Such denunciation shall become effective on the first day of the month following the expiration of a period of three months after the date of receipt of the notification by the Secretary General.

Article 38 – Notifications

The Secretary General of the Council of Europe shall notify the member States of the Council, the European Community, any Signatory, any Party and any other State which has been invited to accede to this Convention of:

any signature;

the deposit of any instrument of ratification, acceptance, approval or accession;

any date of entry into force of this Convention in accordance with Articles 33 or 34;

any amendment or Protocol adopted in accordance with Article 32, and the date on which such an amendment or Protocol enters into force;

any declaration made under the provisions of Article 35;

any reservation and withdrawal of reservation made in pursuance of the provisions of Article 36;

any other act, notification or communication relating to this Convention.

In witness whereof the undersigned, being duly authorised thereto, have signed this Convention.

Done at Oviedo (Asturias), this 4th day of April 1997, in English and French, both texts being equally authentic, in a single copy which shall be deposited in the archives of the Council of Europe. The Secretary General of the Council of Europe shall transmit certified copies to each member State of the Council of Europe, to the European Community, to the non-member States which have parti-cipated in the elaboration of this Convention, and to any State invited to accede to this Convention.

World Medical Association, Declaration of Helsinki (2004)
Ethical Principles for Medical Research Involving Human Subjects

Adopted by the 18th WMA General Assembly, Helsinki, Finland, June 1964,
and amended by the
29th WMA General Assembly, Tokyo, Japan, October 1975
35th WMA General Assembly, Venice, Italy, October 1983
41st WMA General Assembly, Hong Kong, September 1989
48th WMA General Assembly, Somerset West, Republic of South Africa,
October 1996
and the 52nd WMA General Assembly, Edinburgh, Scotland, October 2000
Note of Clarification on Paragraph 29 added by the WMA General Assembly,
Washington 2002
Note of Clarification on Paragraph 30 added by the WMA General Assembly,
Tokyo 2004

A. INTRODUCTION

1. The World Medical Association has developed the Declaration of Helsinki as a statement of ethical principles to provide guidance to physicians and other participants in medical research involving human subjects. Medical research involving human subjects includes research on identifiable human material or identifiable data.

2. It is the duty of the physician to promote and safeguard the health of the people. The physician's knowledge and conscience are dedicated to the fulfillment of this duty.

3. The Declaration of Geneva of the World Medical Association binds the physician with the words, "The health of my patient will be my first consideration," and the International Code of Medical Ethics declares that, "A physician shall act only in the patient's interest when providing medical care which might have the effect of weakening the physical and mental condition of the patient."

4. Medical progress is based on research which ultimately must rest in part on experimentation involving human subjects.

5. In medical research on human subjects, considerations related to the well-being of the human subject should take precedence over the interests of science and society.

6. The primary purpose of medical research involving human subjects is to improve prophylactic, diagnostic and therapeutic procedures and the understanding of the aetiology and pathogenesis of disease. Even the best proven prophylactic, diagnostic, and therapeutic methods must continuously be challenged through research for their effectiveness, efficiency, accessibility and quality.

7. In current medical practice and in medical research, most prophylactic, diagnostic and therapeutic procedures involve risks and burdens.

8. Medical research is subject to ethical standards that promote respect for all human beings and protect their health and rights. Some research populations are vulnerable and need special protection. The particular needs of the economically and medically disadvantaged must be recognized. Special attention is also required for those who cannot give or refuse consent for themselves, for those who may be subject to giving consent under duress, for those who will not benefit personally from the research and for those for whom the research is combined with care.

9. Research Investigators should be aware of the ethical, legal and regulatory requirements for research on human subjects in their own countries as well as applicable international requirements. No national ethical, legal or regulatory requirement should be allowed to reduce or eliminate any of the protections for human subjects set forth in this Declaration.

B. BASIC PRINCIPLES FOR ALL MEDICAL RESEARCH

10. It is the duty of the physician in medical research to protect the life, health, privacy, and dignity of the human subject.

11. Medical research involving human subjects must conform to generally accepted scientific principles, be based on a thorough knowledge of the scientific literature, other relevant sources of information, and on adequate laboratory and, where appropriate, animal experimentation.

12. Appropriate caution must be exercised in the conduct of research which may affect the environment, and the welfare of animals used for research must be respected.

13. The design and performance of each experimental procedure involving human subjects should be clearly formulated in an experimental protocol. This protocol should be submitted for consideration, comment, guidance, and where appropriate, approval to a specially appointed ethical review committee, which must be independent of the investigator, the sponsor or any other kind of undue influence. This independent committee should be in conformity with the laws and regulations of the country in which the research experiment is performed. The committee has the right to monitor ongoing trials. The researcher has the obligation to provide monitoring information to the committee, especially any serious adverse events. The researcher should also submit to the committee, for review, information regarding funding, sponsors, institutional affiliations, other potential conflicts of interest and incentives for subjects.

14. The research protocol should always contain a statement of the ethical considerations involved and should indicate that there is compliance with the principles enunciated in this Declaration.

15. Medical research involving human subjects should be conducted only by scientifically qualified persons and under the supervision of a clinically competent medical person. The responsibility for the human subject must always rest with a medically qualified person and never rest on the subject of the research, even though the subject has given consent.

16. Every medical research project involving human subjects should be preceded by careful assessment of predictable risks and burdens in comparison with foreseeable benefits to the subject or to others. This does not preclude the participation of healthy volunteers in medical research. The design of all studies should be publicly available.

17. Physicians should abstain from engaging in research projects involving human subjects unless they are confident that the risks involved have been adequately assessed and can be satisfactorily managed. Physicians should cease any investigation if the risks are found to outweigh the potential benefits or if there is conclusive proof of positive and beneficial results.

18. Medical research involving human subjects should only be conducted if the importance of the objective outweighs the inherent risks and burdens to the subject. This is especially important when the human subjects are healthy volunteers.

19. Medical research is only justified if there is a reasonable likelihood that the populations in which the research is carried out stand to benefit from the results of the research.

20. The subjects must be volunteers and informed participants in the research project.

21. The right of research subjects to safeguard their integrity must always be respected. Every precaution should be taken to respect the privacy of the subject, the confidentiality of the patient's information and to minimize the impact of the study on the subject's physical and mental integrity and on the personality of the subject.

22. In any research on human beings, each potential subject must be adequately informed of the aims, methods, sources of funding, any possible conflicts of interest, institutional affiliations of the researcher, the anticipated benefits and potential risks of the study and the discomfort it may entail. The subject should be informed of the right to abstain from participation in the study or to withdraw consent to participate at any time without reprisal. After ensuring that the subject has understood the information, the physician should then obtain the subject's freely-given informed consent, preferably in writing. If the consent cannot be obtained in writing, the non-written consent must be formally documented and witnessed.

23. When obtaining informed consent for the research project the physician should be particularly cautious if the subject is in a dependent relationship with the physician or may consent under duress. In that case the informed consent should be obtained by a well-informed physician who is not engaged in the investigation and who is completely independent of this relationship.

24. For a research subject who is legally incompetent, physically or mentally incapable of giving consent or is a legally incompetent minor, the investigator must obtain informed consent from the legally authorized representative in accordance with applicable law. These groups should not be included in research unless the research is necessary to promote the health of the population represented and this research cannot instead be performed on legally competent persons.

25. When a subject deemed legally incompetent, such as a minor child, is able to give assent to decisions about participation in research, the investigator must obtain that assent in addition to the consent of the legally authorized representative.

26. Research on individuals from whom it is not possible to obtain consent, including proxy or advance consent, should be done only if the physical/mental condition that prevents obtaining informed consent is a necessary characteristic of the research population. The specific reasons for involving research subjects with a condition that renders them unable to give

informed consent should be stated in the experimental protocol for consideration and approval of the review committee. The protocol should state that consent to remain in the research should be obtained as soon as possible from the individual or a legally authorized surrogate.

27. Both authors and publishers have ethical obligations. In publication of the results of research, the investigators are obliged to preserve the accuracy of the results. Negative as well as positive results should be published or otherwise publicly available. Sources of funding, institutional affiliations and any possible conflicts of interest should be declared in the publication. Reports of experimentation not in accordance with the principles laid down in this Declaration should not be accepted for publication.

C. ADDITIONAL PRINCIPLES FOR MEDICAL RESEARCH COMBINED WITH MEDICAL CARE

28. The physician may combine medical research with medical care, only to the extent that the research is justified by its potential prophylactic, diagnostic or therapeutic value. When medical research is combined with medical care, additional standards apply to protect the patients who are research subjects.

29. The benefits, risks, burdens and effectiveness of a new method should be tested against those of the best current prophylactic, diagnostic, and therapeutic methods. This does not exclude the use of placebo, or no treatment, in studies where no proven prophylactic, diagnostic or therapeutic method exists.

30. At the conclusion of the study, every patient entered into the study should be assured of access to the best proven prophylactic, diagnostic and therapeutic methods identified by the study.

31. The physician should fully inform the patient which aspects of the care are related to the research. The refusal of a patient to participate in a study must never interfere with the patient-physician relationship.

32. In the treatment of a patient, where proven prophylactic, diagnostic and therapeutic methods do not exist or have been ineffective, the physician, with informed consent from the patient, must be free to use unproven or new prophylactic, diagnostic and therapeutic measures, if in the physician's judgement it offers hope of saving life, re-establishing health or alleviating suffering. Where possible, these measures should be made the object of research, designed to evaluate their safety and efficacy. In all cases, new information should be recorded and, where appropriate, published. The other relevant guidelines of this Declaration should be followed.

Note:

Note of clarification on paragraph 29 of the WMA Declaration of Helsinki

The WMA hereby reaffirms its position that extreme care must be taken in making use of a placebo-controlled trial and that in general this methodology should only be used in the absence of existing proven therapy. However, a placebo-controlled trial may be ethically acceptable, even if proven therapy is available, under the following circumstances:

- Where for compelling and scientifically sound methodological reasons its use is necessary to determine the efficacy or safety of a prophylactic, diagnostic or therapeutic method; or

- Where a prophylactic, diagnostic or therapeutic method is being investigated for a minor condition and the patients who receive placebo will not be subject to any additional risk of serious or irreversible harm.

All other provisions of the Declaration of Helsinki must be adhered to, especially the need for appropriate ethical and scientific review.

Note:

Note of clarification on paragraph 30 of the WMA Declaration of Helsinki

The WMA hereby reaffirms its position that it is necessary during the study planning process to identify post-trial access by study participants to prophylactic, diagnostic and therapeutic procedures identified as beneficial in the study or access to other appropriate care. Post-trial access arrangements or other care must be described in the study protocol so the ethical review committee may consider such arrangements during its review.

The Declaration of Helsinki (Document 17.C) is an official policy document of the World Medical Association, the global representative body for physicians. It was first adopted in 1964 (Helsinki, Finland) and revised in 1975 (Tokyo, Japan), 1983 (Venice, Italy), 1989 (Hong Kong), 1996 (Somerset-West, South Africa) and 2000 (Edinburgh, Scotland). Note of clarification on Paragraph 29 added by the WMA General Assembly, Washington 2002.

9.10.2004

Source: See www.wma.net/e/policy/b3.htm

List of Contributors

Till Bärnighausen
Dr. med., Boston, Dept. Population & International Health, Harvard School of Public Health, current address: Mtubabtuba, South Africa.

Kenneth Boyd
Prof., M.D., The University of Edinburgh, Old College, South Bridge, Edinburgh EH8 9YL, United Kingdom.

Robert Carlson
Ph.D., The University of Edinburgh, Old College, South Bridge, Edinburgh EH8 9YL, United Kingdom.

Dietrich von Engelhardt
Prof. Dr. phil., Institute for the History of Medicine and Science, University of Lübeck, Königstrasse 42, 23552 Lübeck, Germany.

Andreas Frewer
Prof. Dr. med., M.A. History, Ethics and Philosophy of Medicine, Medizinische Hochschule Hannover, Carl-Neuberg-Strasse 1, D-30625 Hannover; History of Medicine and Medical Ethics, University Erlangen-Nuremberg, Germany.

Sara Girardin
Dr. phil., Institute of Health Law, Av. 1er-Mars 26, 2000 Neuchâtel, Switzerland.

Susan Lederer
Prof., Ph.D., Section of the History of Medicine, Yale University School of Medicine, 333 Cedar St., New Haven, CT 06520-8015, USA.

Trudo Lemmens
Prof., Ph.D., Faculty of Law, University of Toronto, 78 Queen's Park, Toronto, Ontario, M5S 2C5, Canada.

Kati Myllymäki
M.D., Sosiaali-ja terveysministeriö, PL 33, 00023 Valtioneuvosto, Finnland.

Jonathan Moreno
Prof., M.D., Center for Bioethics, University of Pennsylvania, 3401 Market Street, Philadelphia, PA 19104, USA.

Povl Riis
Prof., M.D., Nerievej 7, DK-2900 Hellerup, Denmark.

Ulf Schmidt
Prof., Ph.D., Professor of Modern History, School of History, Rutherford College, University of Kent, Canterbury, CT2 7NX, United Kingdom.

Dominique Sprumont
Prof. Dr., Institute of Health Law, Av. 1er-Mars 26, 2000 Neuchâtel, Switzerland.

Ulrich Tröhler
Prof. Dr. med. PhD (London), FRCP (Edinburgh), Emeritus Professor for the History and Epistemology of Medicine at the Institut für Sozial-und Präventiv-medizin University of Berne, Switzerland.

David Webb
Ph.D., The University of Edinburgh, Old College, South Bridge, Edinburgh EH8 9YL, United Kingdom.

David Willcox
Ph.D., School of History, Rutherford College, University of Kent, Canterbury, CT2 7NX, United Kingdom.

John Williams
Prof., Ph.D., World Medical Association, 13, ch. Du Levant, CIB - Bâtiment A, 01210 Ferney-Voltaire, France.

Acknowledgements

This collection of essays is the result of a joint effort of scholars from Canada, Denmark, Finland, France, Germany, Great Britain, Switzerland and the United States to study and better understand the history of research ethics, and commemorate the 40th anniversary of the Declaration of Helsinki in 2004.

The book would not exist without the unflinching support, commitment as well patience from all the authors who contributed to this volume. We are truly grateful to them for having embarked on what turned out be a journey on largely uncharted territory in the history of modern medical research ethics. Our special thanks also goes to the organizations which generously supported this work from the very beginning, in particular the German Fritz Thyssen Stiftung, the Medical University, Hanover, and the University of Kent. We are particularly indebted to all the hard work which Irene Hirschberg, Florian Bruns and our colleagues from the Institute for the History, Ethics and Philosophy in Medicine at the Medical University, Hanover, spent on this project. We are also really grateful to the staff of the Leibniz-Haus in Hanover where we held the conference on the subject of this book. Their hospitality and professionalism ensured a successful conference outcome and made the subsequent collaboration among the authors of this volume all the more enjoyable.

A book of this nature could not have been written without the contribution and feedback from colleagues and experts around the world. They all deserve our deepest gratitude and thanks. We are particularly grateful to the staff of the archive of the World Medical Association for their support, and to Irene Hulst from Holland for having provided us with previously unpublished images of key personalities and events that led to the formulation of the Declaration of Helsinki. We would also like to thank Thomas Schaber, Angela Hoeld and Harald Schmitt from Steiner Publishers for all their support and commitment to this project, and to David Willcox and Geetha Naren for having proof-read and edited the manuscript.

Finally, we would like to thank our respective families for having supported this book project since its inception. They, more than anyone else, know of the many difficulties this project had to overcome. I, Andreas Frewer, am particularly grateful to Andrea Jost, our children and friends for their enormous patience. And I, Ulf Schmidt, would like to thank Katia Mai and our lovely dog Bella for having ensured that life goes on and is perhaps also sometimes less serious than some of the issues discussed in the present book. I am deeply grateful to them for having 'disturbed' me time and again for their share of affection which they both so well-deserve.

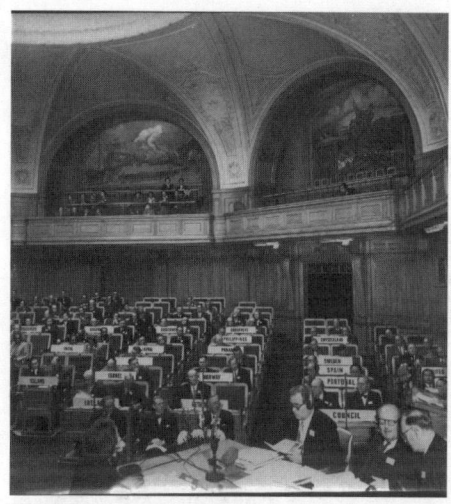

Figure 1
World Medical Association, 5th General
Assembly in Stockholm/Sweden (1951)
Source: Irene Hulst, Private Archive.

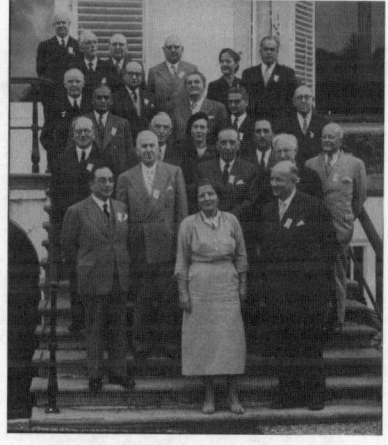

Figure 2
World Medical Association, 7th General Assembly
in Soestdijk/Netherlands (1953).
Source: Irene Hulst, Private Archive.

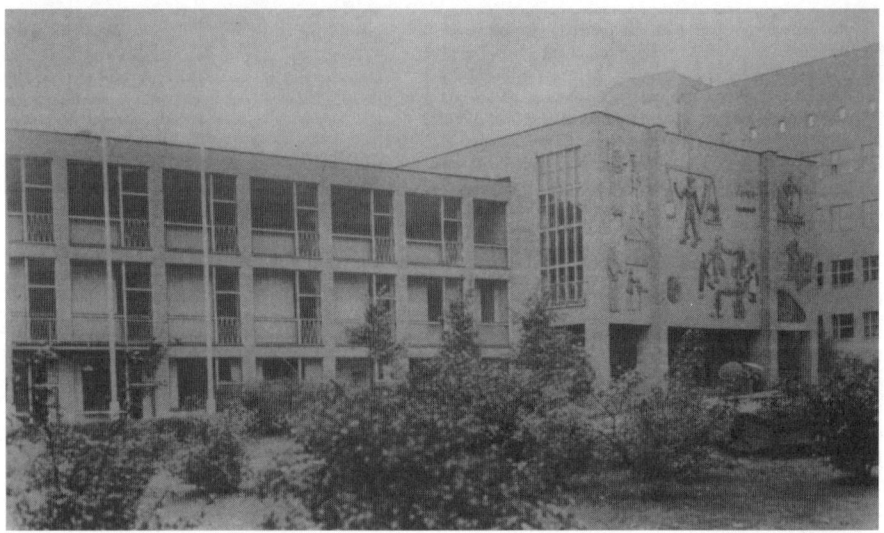

Figure 3
Helsinki School of Economics, Helsinki/Finland (1964).
Source: World Medical Journal (1964).

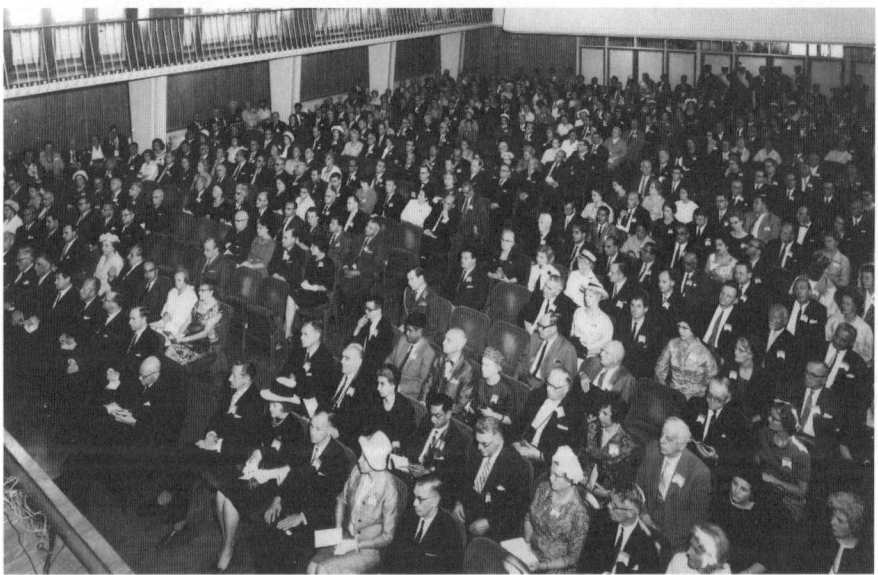

Figure 4
World Medical Association, 18th General Assembly in Helsinki (1964).
The meeting took place at the Helsinki School of Economics.
Source: Photo Archive of the Finnish Medical Association.

Declaration of Helsinki

RECOMMENDATIONS GUIDING DOCTORS IN CLINICAL RESEARCH

Introduction

IT IS THE MISSION OF THE DOCTOR TO SAFEGUARD THE health of the people. His knowledge and conscience are dedicated to the fulfillment of this mission.

The Declaration of Geneva of the World Medical Association binds the doctor with the words: "The health of my patient will be my first consideration" and the International Code of Medical Ethics which declares that "Any act or advice which could weaken physical or mental resistance of a human being may be used only in his interest."

Because it is essential that the results of laboratory experiments be applied to human beings to further scientific knowledge and to help suffering humanity, The World Medical Association has prepared the following recommendations as a guide to each doctor in clinical research. It must be stressed that the standards as drafted are only a guide to physicians all over the world. Doctors are not relieved from criminal, civil and ethical responsibilities under the laws of their own countries.

In the field of clinical research a fundamental distinction must be recognized between clinical research in which the aim is essentially therapeutic for a patient, and the clinical research, the essential object of which is purely scientific and without therapeutic value to the person subjected to the research.

I. Basic Principles

1. Clinical research must conform to the moral and scientific principles that justify medical research and should be based on laboratory and animal experiments or other scientifically established facts.

2. Clinical research should be conducted only by scientifically qualified persons and under the supervision of a qualified medical man.

3. Clinical research cannot legitimately be carried out unless the importance of the objective is in proportion to the inherent risk to the subject.

4. Every clinical research project should be preceded by careful assessment of inherent risks in comparison to foreseeable benefits to the subject or to others.

5. Special caution should be exercised by the doctor in performing clinical research in which the personality of the subject is liable to be altered by drugs or experimental procedure.

II. Clinical Research Combined with Professional Care

1. In the treatment of the sick person, the doctor must be free to use a new therapeutic measure, if in his judgment it offers hope of saving life, reestablishing health, or alleviating suffering.

If at all possible, consistent with patient psychology, the doctor should obtain the patient's freely given consent after the patient has been given a full explanation. In case of legal incapacity, consent should also be procured from the legal guardian; in case of physical incapacity the permission of the legal guardian replaces that of the patient.

2. The doctor can combine clinical research with professional care, the objective being the acquisition of new medical knowledge, only to the extent that clinical research is justified by its therapeutic value for the patient.

III. Non-Therapeutic Clinical Research

1. In the purely scientific application of clinical research carried out on a human being, it is the duty of the doctor to remain the protector of the life and health of that person on whom clinical research is being carried out.

2. The nature, the purpose and the risk of clinical research must be explained to the subject by the doctor.

3a. Clinical research on a human being cannot be undertaken without his free consent after he has been informed; if he is legally incompetent, the consent of the legal guardian should be procured.

3b. The subject of clinical research should be in such a mental, physical and legal state as to be able to exercise fully his power of choice.

3c. Consent should, as a rule, be obtained in writing. However, the responsibility for clinical research always remains with the research worker; it never falls on the subject even after consent is obtained.

4a. The investigator must respect the right of each individual to safeguard his personal integrity, especially if the subject is in a dependent relationship to the investigator.

4b. At any time during the course of clinical research the subject or his guardian should be free to withdraw permission for research to be continued.

The investigator or the investigating team should discontinue the research if in his or their judgment, it may, if continued, be harmful to the individual.

Figure 5
Declaration of Helsinki (English version).
Source: World Medical Journal (1964).

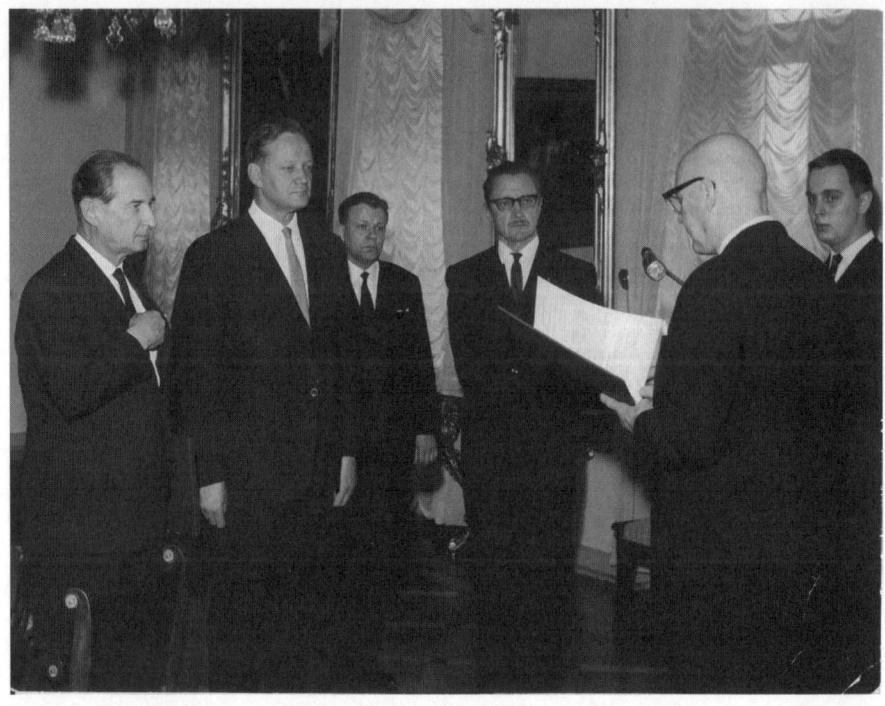

Figure 6
The representatives of the Finnish Medical Association present the Declaration of Helsinki (1964)
to the President of the Republic of Finland, Urho Kekkonen.

Note:

We are grateful for the support of Marit Henriksson (Finnish Medical Association).

For a complete chronology of General Assemblies and Council Sessions of the World Medical Association see http://www.wma.net/e/history/assemblies.htm.

GESCHICHTE UND PHILOSOPHIE DER MEDIZIN /
HISTORY AND PHILOSOPHY OF MEDICINE

Herausgegeben von Andreas Frewer

1. **Frank Stahnisch / Florian Steger**, Hrsg: **Medizin, Geschichte und Geschlecht**. Körperhistorische Rekonstruktionen von Identitäten und Differenzen. 2005. 318 S. m. 35 Abb. auf 18 Tafeln, kt.   8564-9

2. **Ulf Schmidt / Andreas Frewer**, Eds.: **History and Theory of Human Experimentation**. The Declaration of Helsinki and modern Medical Ethics. 2007. 370 S. m. 6 Abb., geb.   8862-6

3. **Martin Mattulat: Medizinethik in historischer Perspektive**. Zum Wandel ärztlicher Moralkonzepte im Werk von Georg Benno Gruber (1884–1977). 2007. 187 S. m. 23 Abb., geb.   8863-3

4. **Hinderk Conrads / Brigitte Lohff: Carl Neuberg – Biochemie, Politik und Geschichte**. Lebenswege und Werk eines fast verdrängten Forschers. 2006. 221 S. u. 28 Abb. auf 16 Taf., geb.   8894-7

5. **Brigitte Lohff / Hinderk Conrads: From Berlin to New York**. Life and work of the almost forgotten German-Jewish biochemist Carl Neuberg (1877–1956). With a bibliography of Carl Neuberg's publications by Michael Engel and Brigitte Lohff. Transl. from the German by Anthony Mellor-Stapelberg. 2007. 294 S. sowie 28 Abb. auf 16 Taf., geb.   9062-9

FRANZ STEINER VERLAG STUTTGART

ISSN 1860-6199